Human Eye Imaging and Modeling

T0289907

Human Eye Imaging and Modeling

Edited by
E.Y.K. Ng
Jen Hong Tan
U. Rajendra Acharya
Jasjit S. Suri

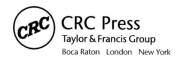

CRC Press
Taylor & Francis Group
Boca Raton   London   New York

CRC Press is an imprint of the
Taylor & Francis Group, an **informa** business

CRC Press
Taylor & Francis Group
6000 Broken Sound Parkway NW, Suite 300
Boca Raton, FL 33487-2742

First issued in paperback 2017

ISBN 13: 978-1-138-07165-0 (pbk)
ISBN 13: 978-1-4398-6993-2 (hbk)

Library of Congress Cataloging-in-Publication Data

Human eye imaging and modeling / editors, E. Y. K. Ng ... [et al.].
    p. ; cm.
   Includes bibliographical references and index.
   Summary: "This comprehensive, multi-contributed reference work details the latest state-of-the art techniques relating to all aspects of eye imaging, textural imaging, and modeling of the human eye in 2D and 3D. Drawing on the expertise of well-known professors and lecturers in the field, it covers theory, principles, and the results of human eye imaging. It focuses on the latest techniques in computer-based imaging and detection methods as well as eye imaging under diabetes retinopathy stages and glaucoma processes. Extensive references at the end of each chapter facilitate further learning"--Provided by publisher.
   ISBN 978-1-4398-6993-2 (hardback : alk. paper)
   I. Ng, Y. K. Eddie.
   [DNLM: 1. Eye Diseases--diagnosis. 2. Diagnostic Imaging. 3. Models, Biological. 4. Ocular Physiological Phenomena. WW 141]

617.7'15--dc23

2012009445

Visit the Taylor & Francis Web site at
http://www.taylorandfrancis.com

and the CRC Press Web site at
http://www.crcpress.com

Contents

SECTION II

Preface

The human eye is one of the most important organs of the human body. Many advanced image processing and mathematical modeling techniques have been used recently to diagnose various eye diseases at the early stages. Fundus optical images can help to extract important salient features which may aid the ophthalmologists in their diagnosis. Application of numerical simulations to develop a human eye model using principles of fluid dynamics and heat transfer can help to predict inner temperatures of the eye from its surface temperature. Correlating variations in the ocular surface temperature of the thermogram predict monitoring the health of the eye.

This book has two major sections. Section I is dedicated to imaging of the fundus and infrared imaging, while Section II is dedicated to mathematical modeling of the human eye. Section I covers topics such as imaging of fundus and infrared images, diagnosis of diabetes retinopathy and glaucoma, estimation of tear evaporation of dry eye, and discussion on the various instruments and formal modeling related to the design of a physical solution for the glaucoma detection. Section II covers computer simulation of the human eye based on principles of heat transfer and various bioheat equations to predict interior temperatures based on the surface temperature. A brief description of the layout of these chapters in these sections is presented.

SECTION I

Prolonged diabetes slowly affects the circulatory system, including the retina. As diabetes progresses, a patient's vision may begin to deteriorate; this deterioration may lead to diabetic retinopathy (DR). In DR, the retinal microvasculature is subjected to progressive pathological alterations leading to complications like retinal nonperfusion, increase in vascular permeability, and pathologic proliferation of retinal blood vessels. Chapter 1 discusses the classification of normal and abnormal nonproliferative diabetic retinopathy (NPDR) and proliferative diabetic retinopathy (PDR) classes. The cluster center features are extracted from the digital fundus images using fuzzy c-means clustering (FCM) and fed to the support vector machine (SVM) classifier to discriminate normal and abnormal classes.

VAMPIRE is a software tool for efficient semiautomatic assessment of the retinal vasculature with large collections of fundus camera images. It is also an international collaborative project of (currently) four image processing groups and five clinical centers. The tool aims to minimize the amount of time spent by a user with no image processing background to quantify features of the retinal vasculature, currently optic disc location, vessel width, branching angles and coefficients, vessel tortuosity, and fractal dimension. Chapter 2 discusses the VAMPIRE modules, reporting purpose, algorithms, and current validation. Example images are shown throughout.

Optical Coherence Tomography (OCT) and Heidelberg Retinal Tomography (HRT) are used to diagnose glaucoma. These methods are rather expensive and difficult to integrate into an electronic workflow. In contrast, glaucoma detection based on digital fundus images is cost effective, because inexpensive general-purpose electronic components can be used to build the detection system. Furthermore, fundus images are digital to begin with, so there is no break in the processing chain. This digital setup makes it very easy to integrate the glaucoma detection system into a clinical workflow. Chapter 3 explains how a formal and model-driven design approach helps to address these issues and therefore allows us to build reliable and safe biomedical processing systems, such as the glaucoma detector. The main body of this chapter describes the systems engineering design methodology, extended with formal modeling, to design a physical solution for the glaucoma detection problem.

Computer-aided software forms an important part of most medical imaging systems in the diagnosis of diseases. They could be constructed using several basic image processing techniques and be applied in the retinal image analysis to segment and quantify regions of interest. Chapter 4 discusses the assessment of the optic nerve and explains the problems and the level of complexity linked with each retinal imaging task.

Glaucoma is the worst form of ophthalmic disease due to its irreversible and progressive nature. In glaucoma, the optic nerve encounters gradual damage as a result of the elevated intraocular pressure (IOP) due to the blockade in the flow of aqueous humor. Due to its irreversibility, timely diagnosis is crucial in proper management of the glaucomatous condition. Chapter 5 surveys the various instruments, including their patents, used in the diagnosis and management of glaucoma. The instruments surveyed herein are grouped under the categories of tonometers, goniolens, imaging techniques, and corneal pachymetry. The key contribution of this chapter is to bring all these instruments under one roof and describe them in detail.

A number of modalities are currently used for imaging of ocular surface diseases and many more will be used in the future. The front surface of the eye is more accessible to noninvasive imaging techniques than other parts of the eye or human body. Although clinical management of many ocular surface diseases requires proper imaging for diagnosis and monitoring, there are many limitations associated with the use of such imaging. Chapter 6 evaluates a range of imaging modalities based on how frequently they are used.

Ocular surface temperature is an important feature that can be used to understand the physiology and pathology of the eye. Numerous examinations on ocular surface temperature are made today using infrared thermography, to reveal its relationship with ocular diseases such as dry eye, glaucoma, cataract, and so on. The studies in this field can be further advanced by the introduction of better localization technique and analytical methodology. Recent examples of such advancement—such as the application of snake algorithm in the localization, image warping and cross co-occurrence matrix in the analysis of surface temperature, and the derivation of the rate of tear evaporation—are discussed in detail in Chapter 7.

Infrared thermography efficiently and intuitively captures the distribution of temperature across the surface and is now widely applied to investigate the physiology and pathology at the ocular surface. However, there is no investigation on the estimation of the rate of tear evaporation based on ocular thermography. Earlier studies on the measurement of evaporation rate largely based on the change in relative humidity returned only a single value and did not permit observation of the variation in the rate over time. Also, researchers could not observe left-right difference in the evaporation rate and were prone to error since they had no efficient way to exclude evaporation from the facial area and moments when an eye blinks. Chapter 8 attempts to derive and develop a measuring methodology on tear evaporation rate with none of the above constraints and disadvantages.

Dry eye syndrome is one of the most common eye diseases in developed countries. However, clinical diagnostic methods for dry eye syndrome are invasive methods that are uncomfortable for patients. Chapter 9 presents the use of infrared thermal imaging to examine the quality of the normal and abnormal tear films, as well as the temporal and spatial characteristics. The results may lead to the implementation of infrared thermal imaging systems to facilitate noncontact diagnosis of dry eye syndrome.

SECTION II

Chapter 10 reviews the state of knowledge regarding biomechanical modeling of the eye, with a particular focus on corneal biomechanics. First, the relevant anatomical, morphological, and physiological aspects of normal corneal function are summarized. Pathophysiology is addressed using the example of keratoconus—a disease of the cornea involving the changes to the corneal microstructure as well as to its macrostructure, which gradually causes a conic-like corneal shape that distorts vision. Biomechanical modeling is described as a tool to study the normal corneal performances as well as the function of the cornea in pathological conditions, both in the context of basic research and towards clinical applications.

Experimental measurements of temperature during laser surgery in a functioning human eye are also currently not available. To overcome these difficulties, numerical analysis is performed and solution methods proposed to limit thermal damage during surgery. Chapter 11 deals with the modeling of the human eye during retinal laser surgery using both finite element and finite volume methods.

Chapter 12 presents a framework for computational modeling and simulation of the human eye system. Making use of geometric modeling and computer graphics techniques, the proposed approach is able to handle both synthetic and in vivo corneal topography data from which it is possible to visualize and analyze retinal images of a specific eye.

Chapter 13 proposes the weighted extended-basis splines (web-splines) approach in the finite element method (FEM) for bioheat problems for two-dimensional (2D) and three-dimensional (3D) structures. This newly developed computational approach is employed to calculate the steady-state temperature distribution in a normal human eye. As a first step, the human eye is evaluated in two dimensions. The simulation results are verified using the values reported in the literature, and show better efficiency in terms of the accuracy level.

The most important issue in surgical application of lasers is the assessment of the temperature variation of tissues when subjected to the high-intensity laser radiation before the operation. Therefore, to minimize any damage of intraocular tissues due to heating, a mathematical model based on the space-time dependent Pennes' bioheat transfer equation, having taken into account different types of heat transfer processes, is presented in Chapter 14. The detailed geometry of the human eye has been developed to give a realistic representation of the actual eye.

Computer simulation of the thermal states of biological bodies, usually governed by the Pennes bioheat equation involving blood perfusion and metabolic heat generation, has received increasing attention and can be used for noninvasive diagnosis with simple surface temperature measurement. Chapter 15 deals with the simulation of transient bioheat transfer in the human eye by considering the thermal effect of blood perfusion rates in the sclera, the choroid, retina layers, and the optic nerve. The role of blood supply to the sclera in moderating temperature is studied via comparison between results from a model considering the presence of blood perfusion rate and those from a model in the absence of blood perfusion rate.

Computational modeling is an effective tool for the detection of eye abnormalities and a valuable assistant to hyperthermia treatments. In all these diagnoses and treatments, predicting the temperature distribution accurately is very important. However, the standard FEM currently used for such purposes has strong reliance on element meshes and the discretized system exhibits "overly stiff" behavior. To overcome this shortcoming, Chapter 16 formulates an edge-based smoothed finite element method (ES-FEM) in 2D and a face-based smoothed finite element method (FS-FEM) in 3D to compute bioheat transfer in the human eyes. The ES-FEM and FS-FEM use triangular (2D) and tetrahedron (3D) elements that can be generated automatically for complicated domains and hence are particularly suited for modeling human eyes.

Chapter 17 presents a mathematical model for the calculation of the bioheat transfer in the human eye, taking into account convective mass transport in the anterior chamber. The developed model contains all the necessary anatomical detail for predicting temperature distributions and convective flow velocities of the aqueous humor, providing useful information for biomedical and clinical applications.

In summary, this book aims to enrich the lives of people suffering from eye abnormalities with various novel image imaging and modeling algorithms.

E. Y. K. Ng
Jen Hong Tan
U. Rajendra Acharya
Jasjit S. Suri

Contributors

U. Rajendra Acharya
Department of Electronics and
   Computer Engineering
Ngee Ann Polytechnic
Singapore

Roy Asher
Department of Biomedical
   Engineering
Faculty of Engineering
Tel Aviv University
Tel Aviv, Israel

Leandro Paganotti Brazil
Institute of Computer Science and
   Mathematics
University of São Paulo
São Carlos, Brazil
Wernher von Braun Center for
   Advanced Research
Campinas, Brazil

Odemir Martinez Bruno
Physics Institute of San Carlos
University of São Paulo
São Carlos, Brazil

David O. Chang
United Integrated Services Co. Ltd.
Taiwan

Joe Chang
United Integrated Services Co. Ltd.
Taiwan

Shu Wen Chang
Department of Ophthalmology
Far Eastern Memorial Hospital
Taiwan

Subhagata Chattopadhyay
School of Computer Studies
National Institute of Science and
   Technology
Orissa, India

Huihua Kenny Chiang
Institute of Biomedical Engineering
National Yang-Ming University
Taiwan

Khai Sing Chin
VAMPIRE Project
School of Computing
University of Dundee
Dundee, United Kingdom

Mario Cvetkovic
Faculty of Electrical Engineering
Mechanical Engineering and Naval
   Architecture
University of Split
Split, Croatia

Baljean Dhillon
Princess Alexandra Eye Pavilion
National Health Service Lothian
Edinburgh, United Kingdom

Alexander Doney
VAMPIRE Project
Diabetes Genetics Group
Ninewells Hospital
Dundee, United Kingdom

Oliver Faust
Department of Electronics and
   Computer Engineering
Ngee Ann Polytechnic
Singapore

Amit Gefen
Department of Biomedical
  Engineering
Faculty of Engineering
Tel Aviv University
Tel Aviv, Israel

Andrea Giachetti
VAMPIRE Project
Department of Computer Science
University of Verona
Verona, Italy

Lingam Gopal
Medical Research Foundation
Sankara Nethralaya
Nungambakkam, Chennai, India

ZC He
State Key Laboratory of Advanced
  Technology for Vehicle Body
  Design & Manufacture
Hunan University
Changsha, Peoples' Republic of China

Andreas Karampatzakis
Department of Physics
Aristotle University of Thessaloniki
Thessaloniki, Greece

M. Muthu Rama Krishnan
Department of Electronics and
  Computer Engineering
Ngee Ann Polytechnic
Singapore

Fulya Callialp Kunter
Department of Electrical and Electronic
  Engineering
Bogazici University
Bebek, Istanbul, Turkey

W. Lan
Singapore Eye Research Institute
Singapore

Augustinus Laude
National Healthcare Group Eye Institute
Tan Tock Seng Hospital
Singapore

S.Y. Lee
Singapore Eye Research Institute
Singapore

Eric Li
Center for Advance Computations in
  Engineering Science
Department of Mechanical Engineering
National University of Singapore
Singapore

Teik-Cheng Lim
School of Science and Technology
SIM University
Singapore

GR Liu
Center for Advance Computations in
  Engineering Science
Department of Mechanical Engineering
National University of Singapore
Singapore

Cheng-Kai Lu
School of Engineering
Edinburgh University
Edinburgh, United Kingdom

Carmen A. Lupascu
VAMPIRE Project
Department of Mathematics and
  Informatics
University of Palermo
Palermo, Italy

Thomas J. MacGillivray
VAMPIRE Project
Clinical Research Imaging Center
University of Edinburgh
Edinburgh, United Kingdom

Alan F. Murray
School of Engineering
Edinburgh University
Edinburgh, United Kingdom

Arunn Narasimhan
Heat Transfer and Thermal Power
    Laboratory
Department of Mechanical
    Engineering
Indian Institute of Technology Madras
Chennai, India

E.Y.K. Ng
School of Mechanical and Aerospace
    Engineering
College of Engineering
Nanyang Technological University
Singapore

Andres Peratta
Ashurst Lodge
Wessex Institute of Technology
Ashurst, Southampton
United Kingdom

Adria Perez-Rovira
VAMPIRE Project
School of Computing
University of Dundee
Dundee, United Kingdom

Andrea Petznick
Singapore Eye Research Institute
Singapore

Dragan Poljak
Faculty of Electrical Engineering
Mechanical Engineering and Naval
    Architecture
University of Split
Split, Croatia

Qing-Hua Qin
School of Engineering
Australian National University
Canberra, ACT, Australia

Theodoros Samaras
Department of Physics
Aristotle University of Thessaloniki
Thessaloniki, Greece

S. Selim Seker
Department of Electrical and Electronic
    Engineering
Bogazici University
Bebek, Istanbul, Turkey

Tai Yuan Su
Institute of Biomedical Engineering
National Yang-Ming University
Taiwan

Jasjit S. Suri
Global Biomedical Technologies, Inc.
Roseville, California
(Affiliated) Research Professor
Biomedical Engineering Department
Idaho State University
Pocatello, Idaho

G. Swapna
Department of Applied Electronics &
    Instrumentation
Government Engineering College
Kozhikode, Kerala, India

Toshiyo Tamura
Department of Medical System
    Engineering
Chiba University
Chiba, Japan

Jen Hong Tan
Department of Electronics and
    Computer Engineering
Ngee Ann Polytechnic
Singapore

Vincent Tan
Center for Advance Computations in
    Engineering Science
Department of Mechanical Engineering
National University of Singapore
Singapore

Tong Boon Tang
Department of Electrical and
    Electronics Engineering
Universiti Teknologi Petronas
Tronoh, Perak, Malaysia

Domenico Tegolo
VAMPIRE Project
Department of Mathematics and
    Informatics
University of Palermo
Palermo, Italy

Louis Tong
Singapore Eye Research Institute
Singapore

Emanuele Trucco
VAMPIRE Project
School of Computing
University of Dundee
Dundee, United Kingdom

David Varssano
Cornea and External Disease Service
Department of Ophthalmology
Tel Aviv Sourasky Medical Center
Sackler Faculty of Medicine
Tel Aviv University
Tel Aviv, Israel

Hui Wang
Institute of Scientific and Engineering
    Computation
Henan University of Technology
Zhengzhou, China

Peter J. Wilson
VAMPIRE Project
Department of Ophthalmology
Ninewells Hospital
Dundee, United Kingdom

Wong Li Yun
Department of Electronics and
    Computer Engineering
Ngee Ann Polytechnic
Singapore

Section I

1 Automated Identification of Diabetes Retinopathy Using Artificial Intelligence Techniques

M. Muthu Rama Krishnan, Wong Li Yun,
U. Rajendra Acharya, G. Swapna, and Jasjit S. Suri

CONTENTS

1.1   INTRODUCTION

Diabetes mellitus is a metabolic disorder of multiple etiologies characterized by hyperglycemia with disturbances of carbohydrate and lipid metabolisms result-ing from defects in insulin secretion or insulin action or both. Insulin level may be decreased due to the decrease in the beta cell mass and there may also be functional/relative disturbances of beta cells as a result of stress [1]. Diabetes mellitus was recognized and distinguished as two types as early as 700–200 BC. Earlier than 1980 it was believed to be a genetically based disorder or resulting due to dietary indiscretions. In 1980, the World Health Organization (WHO) classified diabetes into clinical classes and statistical risk groups. Impaired glucose tolerance (IGT), diabetes mellitus, and gestational diabetes are included in clinical classes. Potential abnormality of glucose tolerance is included in statistical risk groups. Degree of insulin deficiency and the etiology were used in combination to classify diabetes. Diabetes may be associated with symptoms or without symptoms depending on the severity of the metabolic abnormality. Some common symptoms are thirst, polyuria (frequent urination) and weight loss. It may also progress to ketoacidosis and coma. Broadly diabetes has been divided into two main types: insulin-dependent, or type 1, diabetes and non-insulin-dependent, or type 2, diabetes [2,3].

1.1.1   Types of Diabetes

1.1.1.1   Type 1 Diabetes or Insulin-Dependent Diabetes Mellitus (IDDM)

IDDM occurs due to autoimmune destruction of insulin-producing beta cells of the pancreas, rendering the pancreas unable to synthesize and secrete insulin. The symptoms of type 1 diabetes are polyuria, polydipsia (increased thirst), polyphagia (increased hunger), and loss of body weight. Type 1 diabetes affects 5 to 10% of people [4]. In type 1 diabetes, insulin is required for survival and to prevent the development of ketoacidosis and coma. Type 1 diabetes can occur at any age though common in young individuals [5].

1.1.1.2   Type 2 Diabetes or Non-Insulin-Dependent Diabetes Mellitus (NIDDM)

NIDDM is most common and is characterized by combination of insulin resistance (a physiological condition in which insulin becomes less effective in lowering the blood sugar level) and inadequate insulin secretion. Type 2 diabetes affects 90 to 95% of people. The major symptoms of type 2 diabetes are polydipsia, polyuria, polyphagia, blurry vision, fatigue, and irritability [6]. Type 2 diabetes occurs mainly due to nurture and nature. The external factors are sedentary habits, inappropriate diet, and obesity. In addition, mutation of pancreatic cells may occur in type 2 diabetes [7,8].

1.1.1.3 Gestational Diabetes

Gestational diabetes is a form of diabetes that affects pregnant women. It is believed that the hormones produced during pregnancy reduce the woman's receptivity to insulin, leading to high blood sugar level. Gestational diabetes affects 4% of pregnant women. The symptoms of gestational diabetes are fatigue, nausea, vomiting, increased urination, bladder infections, and blurred vision. Gestational diabetes may be a temporary phase; it may disappear after pregnancy [9].

1.1.2 Prevalence of Diabetes

In the last few years the status of diabetes has been changed from being considered as a mild disorder to one of the major causes of morbidity and mortality. The prevalence of diabetes is swiftly mounting all over the world. High prevalence of diabetes was found among urban Asian Indians (7.3%) when compared with rural prevalence rate (3.1%). Diabetes is the fifth deadliest disease in the United States. The total annual economic cost of diabetes in 2002 was estimated to be US $132 billion [10]. The global prevalence of diabetes is expected to rise from 2.8% in 2000 to 4.4% of the global population by 2030 [11].

1.1.3 Diabetic Retinopathy (DR)

Diabetes affects the circulatory system including that of the retina. Twenty years after the onset of diabetes, almost all patients with type 1 diabetes and over 60% of patients with type 2 diabetes will have some degree of retinopathy [11]. The tiny blood vessels that nourish the retina are damaged by the increased glucose level, which leads to blindness. This tiny blood vessel will leak blood and fluid on the retina, forming features such as microaneurysms, hemorrhages, hard exudates, cotton wool spots, or venous loops [12,13]. Laser treatment can now prevent blindness in the majority of these cases. Hence, early screening and identification of patients with retinopathy will help to prevent loss of vision. DR can be broadly classified as nonproliferative diabetic retinopathy (NPDR) and proliferative diabetic retinopathy (PDR). Depending on the presence of features on the retina, the stages of DR can be identified [13].

1.1.4 Anatomy of an Eye

The eyes are an important sense organ of our body. Four-fifths of all of the information the brain receives comes from the eye. The eye is a hollow, spherical organ about 2.5 cm in diameter. It has a wall composed of three layers. The outermost layer is composed of the cornea and sclera. The middle layer consists of the choroid, ciliary body, and iris. The innermost is the retina. Its interior spaces are filled with fluids that support the walls and maintain the shape of the eye [11]. Figure 1.1 shows the

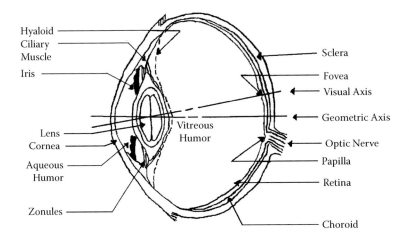

FIGURE 1.1   Simple diagram of the parts of the eye.

cross-sectional structure of the eye. The important parts of the eye are discussed in the following sections.

1.1.4.1   The Cornea

The cornea is a transparent medium situated in the front of the eye covering the iris, pupil, and anterior chamber that helps to focus incoming light with a water content of 78%. The cornea is elliptical in shape with a vertical and horizontal diameter of 11 and 12 mm, respectively. The cornea is supplied with oxygen and nutrients through tear-fluid and does not have blood vessels in it. The function of the cornea is to refract and transmit light [14].

1.1.4.2   The Aqueous Humor

The eye contains aqueous fluid in the front part between the lens and the cornea. Aqueous fluid supplies the cornea and lens with nutrients and oxygen [14].

1.1.4.3   The Iris

The iris is a thin, pigmented, circular structure in the eye that regulates the amount of light that enters the eye. The function of the iris is to control the size of the pupil by adjusting it to the intensity of the lighting conditions. By expanding the size of the pupil, the iris allows more light to enter. This reflex known as the accommodation reflex expands the pupil to allow more light to enter when focusing on distant objects or in the darkness [14].

1.1.4.4   The Pupil

The pupil is the opening in the center of the iris. The size of the pupil determines the amount of light that enters the eye. The pupil size is controlled by the dilator and sphincter muscles of the iris. It appears black because most of the light entering the pupil is absorbed by the tissues inside the eye [14].

1.1.4.5 The Lens

The lens is a transparent, biconvex structure in the eye that, along with the cornea, helps to refract light to be focused on the retina [14]. Changing the shape of the lens results in the change of the focal distance of the eye and hence helps to have sharp images on the retina.

1.1.4.6 The Vitreous Humor

The vitreous is a clear fluid that fills the eyeball (between the lens and the retina). It is the largest domain of the human eye. The fluid contains more than 95% water [14].

1.1.4.7 The Sclera

The sclera is the white opaque tissue that acts as the eye's protective outer coat. Six tiny muscles connect to it around the eye and control the eye's movements. The optic nerve is attached to the sclera at the very back of the eye [14].

1.1.4.8 The Optic Disc

The optic disc (optic nerve head or the blind spot) is the place where the optic nerve attaches to the eye. There are no light-sensitive rods or cones to respond to a light stimulus at this point. This causes a break in the visual field called the blind spot or the physiological blind spot [14].

1.1.4.9 The Retina

The retina is a thin layer of neural cells that lines the inner back of the eye. It is light sensitive and absorbs light. The image signals are received and sent to the brain. The retina contains two kinds of light receptors: rods and cones. The rods absorb light in black and white. The rods are responsible for night vision. The cones are color sensitive and absorb stronger light. The cones are responsible for color vision [14].

1.1.4.10 The Macula

The macula is the area around the fovea. It is an oval-shaped, highly pigmented yellow spot near the center of the retina as shown in Figure 1.2. It is a small and highly sensitive part of the retina responsible for detailed central vision [14].

1.1.4.11 The Fovea

The fovea is the most central part of the macula. The visual cells located in the fovea are packed tightest, resulting in optimal sharpness of vision. Unlike the retina, it has no blood vessels to interfere with the passage of light striking the foveal cone mosaic [14].

There are four progressive stages of diabetic retinopathy:

1. Mild nonproliferative retinopathy (Mild NPDR): In this earliest stage, small areas of balloon-like swelling called microaneurysms develop in the tiny blood vessels of the retina. Approximately 40% of people with diabetes have at least mild signs of DR [16].

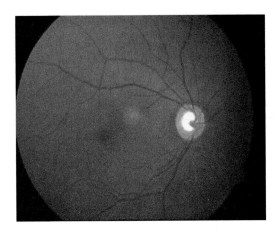

FIGURE 1.2   Location of macula, fovea, and optic disc. (Please see color insert.)

2. Moderate nonproliferative retinopathy (Moderate NPDR): In this second stage, the blood vessels nourishing the retina are blocked. Numerous microaneurysms and retinal hemorrhages are present. Cotton wool spots and a limited amount of venous beading can also be seen. Sixteen percent of the patients with moderate NPDR develop PDR within a year [15].

3. Severe nonproliferative retinopathy (Severe NPDR): This is the third stage in the progression of DR. In this stage, several areas of the retina are deprived of their blood supply due to the blockage of more blood vessels. This is characterized by any one of the following characteristics:
   • Numerous hemorrhages and microaneurysms in all four quadrants of the retina;
   • Venous beading in two or more quadrants;
   • Intraretinal microvascular abnormalities in at least one quadrant;
   • Fifty percent chance of progression to PDR in 1 year.
   Patients with two or more of these features are graded as very severe NPDR [15].

4. Proliferative retinopathy (PDR): This is the advanced stage in which the retina is deprived of sufficient blood supply and hence gives signals that will lead to the growth of new blood vessels. These new blood vessels are thin and fragile. They grow along the retina and also along the surface of the clear vitreous gel that fills the inside of the eye. The leakage of the blood vessels may lead to blindness. About 3% of people in this condition may suffer severe visual loss [15].

Figure 1.3 shows the typical fundus images of normal, NPDR, and PDR class.

Early detection of retinopathy is very important. If undetected and untreated, prolonged diabetic retinopathy may lead to blindness. Traditionally, ophthalmologists detect different stages of diabetic retinopathy by retinal examination using indirect biomicroscopy [15]. There is an alternative method of detecting diabetic retinopathy

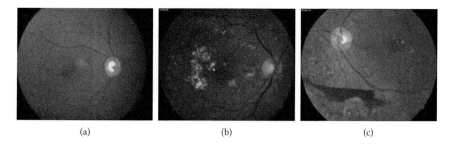

(a)   (b)   (c)

FIGURE 1.3 Typical images of (a) normal, (b) NPDR, and (c) PDR. (Please see color insert.)

by extracting salient features from retinopathy images and processing them. All works used the retinal fundus photographs as an input for their work to extract useful features like exudates, microaneurysms, hemorrhages, lesions, and cotton wool spots, which can be further analyzed to detect the presence of diabetic retinopathy.

Several authors have investigated a number of classification methods for the segmentation of the vessels [16]. Chaudhuri et al. [17] proposed a two-dimensional linear kernel with a Gaussian profile for segmentation of the vasculature. The profile of the filter is designed to match that of a blood vessel, which typically has a Gaussian or a Gaussian derivative profile. Morphological operators have been applied to vasculature segmentation (Zana and Klein [18,19]) and also to microaneurysm extraction. Morphological processing for identifying specific shapes has the advantage of speed and noise resistance. Artificial neural networks have been extensively investigated for segmenting retinal features such as the vasculature (Akita and Kuga [20]) making classifications based on statistical probabilities rather than objective reasoning.

Many authors have investigated neural networks for the detection of microaneurysms and/or hemorrhages. An early approach by Gardner et al. [21] used a back propagation neural network to detect microaneurysms and/or hemorrhages. The green channel images are used for the analysis. The images were divided into 20×20 pixel or 30×30 pixel windows, which were individually graded manually by a trained observer. The sub-images were classified as normal without vessel, normal vessel, exudate, and hemorrhage/microaneurysm. The authors reported detection rates for hemorrhages of 73.8% for both sensitivity and specificity. Spencer et al. [22] proposed a morphological transformation to segment microaneurysms within fluorescein angiograms. The authors reported a sensitivity of 82% and specificity of 86% in comparison to a clinician, with 100 false positive pixels per image reported. Cree et al. [23] refined this technique using alternative region growing and classification algorithms. This approach automatically determined the macular region and included an automated process for image registration to allow sequential comparisons of microaneurysm turnover, based on a registration of longitudinal images. The automated detection algorithm achieved a sensitivity of 82% and specificity of 84% in previously unseen image data. Hipwell et al. [24] proposed a method for the detection of microaneurysms in red-free images. The images were initially processed by shade correction of the image, followed by removal of vessels and other distractors by the top-hat transformation. A Gaussian

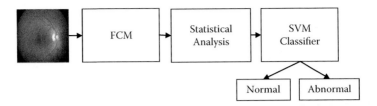

FIGURE 1.4   Block diagram of automated DR detection system. (Please see color insert.)

matched filter was applied to retain candidate microaneurysms for subsequent classification. The system produced a sensitivity of 81%, with 93% specificity. However, this was achieved only when images with questionable HMA present were excluded.

Sinthanayothin et al. [25] identified exudates in color images based on the same recursive region-growing technique described above to define an "exudate" and "non-exudate" image. After thresholding to produce a binary image, the regions containing the exudates were overlaid onto the original image. Ege et al. [26] reported the detection of exudates and cotton wool spots with sensitivity of 99% and 80%, respectively. In comparison with a general clinical ophthalmologist, Lee et al. [27] reported sensitivities of 96% and 80% and specificities of 93% and 93% for hard exudates and cotton wool spots.

In the study described in this chapter, three salient features, namely the red, green, and blue centroids, were extracted using fuzzy c-means clustering (FCM) and classified as Normal and Abnormal (NPDR and PDR) using the SVM classifier. Figure 1.4 shows the proposed system for identification of these two classes.

1.2   MATERIALS AND METHODS

1.2.1   IMAGE ACQUISITION

In this work, 181 normal and 317 abnormal (158 NPDR and 159 PDR) retinal photographs were studied. These patient data were provided by the Kasturba Medical Hospital, Manipal, India. Images taken with Ziess Visucamlite fundus camera interfaced to the computer were stored in 24 bit JPEG format with an image size of 256 × 256 pixels.

1.2.2   FEATURE EXTRACTION

In this work fuzzy c-means clustering algorithm was used to extract features, which were fed to the SVM classifier to discriminate normal and abnormal classes. The steps involved in automated detection are shown in Figure 1.2. First the Red (R), Green (G), and Blue (B) centroids were extracted from the digital fundus images. These three features were subjected to statistical analysis (Student's t-test) to find the clinically significant features and then fed to the SVM classifier for automated detection. These steps are explained below in detail.

1.2.2.1   Fuzzy c-Means Clustering (FCM)

FCM is a clustering method where one input data piece is allowed to belong to two or more clusters [28]. The FCM, with the help of a membership function, allows the data to belong to more than one class or group. This approach develops classes that are, in general, softly overlapping with the degree of overlap being controlled by a user-specified parameter. The partitions are determined by the learning procedure of the clustering. FCM clustering is used to group regions within each image using the RGB vector as an input. The FCM clustering technique is as follows:

$$\text{Let } z_j(k) = \begin{pmatrix} R_j^k \\ G_j^k \\ B_j^k \end{pmatrix}, \text{ where } j = 1,2,...,6, \text{ and let } x = \begin{pmatrix} R^{nn} \\ G^{nn} \\ B^{nn} \end{pmatrix} \tag{1.1}$$

where
R, G, B is the red, blue, and green layers of the image, respectively; nn = any pixel in image.

The following paragraphs describe the steps of the clustering technique.

We choose six initial cluster centers, namely $z_1(1), z_2(1), z_3(1), z_4(1), z_5(1), z_6(1)$. Six clusters were used because they best visually distinguish the various parts on the captured fundus image of the eye. The parts correspond to the background of the image, optic disc, blood vessels, exudates, and microaneurysms.

The fuzzy c-means clustering algorithm optimizes [28] the following objective function

$$J = \sum_{i=1}^{N}\sum_{j=1}^{c} u_{ji}^m \|x_i - V_j\|^2 \tag{1.2}$$

where u_{ji} is the fuzzy membership having m as the weighting exponent and with pattern x_i such that it can associate with the cluster j having centroid V_j. The fuzzy membership has the property such that

$$\sum_{j=1}^{c} u_{ji} = 1 \ \forall i \tag{1.3}$$

The algorithm works similarly to k-means algorithm. The update equations for the cluster center and the fuzzy membership are as follows:

$$V_j^{(new)} = \frac{\sum_{i=1}^{N}(u_{ji})^m x_i}{\sum_{i=1}^{N}(u_{ji})^m} \tag{1.4}$$

$$u_{ji}^{(new)} = \frac{\left(\dfrac{1}{\left\|x_i - V_j^{(new)}\right\|}\right)^{\frac{2}{(m-1)}}}{\displaystyle\sum_{l=1}^{c}\left(\dfrac{1}{\left\|x_i - V_l^{(new)}\right\|}\right)^{\frac{2}{(m-1)}}} \qquad (1.5)$$

The iterations are stopped when $\left\|U^{(new)} - U\right\|_F < \varepsilon$, a predefined small real number and $U = \{u_{ji}, 1 \leq j \leq c, 1 \leq i \leq N\}$.

After all images are processed using FCM, the brightest and darkest cluster centroids of each are removed as they represent the optic disc region and background, respectively. These regions do not contain important features that aid automatic detection of normal and diabetic retinopathy. The remaining cluster centroids are fed into an SVM classifier to distinguish the normal and abnormal classes.

1.2.2.2 Self-Organizing Map (SOM)

SOM is trained to classify normal and diabetic retinopathy classes based on three centroids. Self-organizing feature maps (SOFM) learn to classify input vectors according to how they are grouped in the input space [29]. Thus, self-organizing maps learn both the distribution (as do competitive layers) and topology of the input vectors they are trained on.

The principal goal of SOM is to transform the input feature pattern of arbitrary dimension into a one- or two-dimensional discrete map, and to perform this transformation adaptively in a topologically ordered fashion. The neurons in the layer of an SOFM are arranged originally in physical positions according to a topology function. The function hextop arranges the neurons in a hexagonal topology. Distances between neurons are calculated from their positions with a distance function [29].

The stages of the SOM algorithm can be summarised [29] as follows:

1. *Initialization*—Choose random values for the initial weight vectors W_j.
2. *Sampling*—Draw a sample training input vector x from the input space.
3. *Matching*—Find the winning neuron $I(x)$ with weight vector closest to input vector.
4. *Updating*—Apply the weight update equation $\Delta W_{ji} = \eta(t) T_{j,I(x)}(t)(x_i - W_{ji})$.
5. *Continuation*—Keep returning to step 2 until the feature map stops changing.

In this work we have used SOM in order to visualize the weight vectors of normal and abnormal groups.

1.3 STATISTICAL ANALYSIS

When the number of extracted features is high, it is often found that some of these features are redundant. Using a larger number of redundant features, or in other words, a high-dimensional feature vector, to train the classifier will result in increased computational complexity and also will lead to poor training and non-convergence of the classifiers. Therefore during the feature selection phase, only highly significant, discriminating, and unique features are retained. To select such features, we used the Student's t-test [30]. For every feature, a null hypothesis that the averages of the feature for the two classes are equal is assumed. Then, a t-statistic, which is the ratio of difference between the means of the feature for the two classes to the standard error between class means, and the corresponding p-value are calculated. The p-value is the probability of rejecting the null hypothesis given that the null hypothesis is true. If the p-value is less than 0.01 or 0.05, the null hypothesis can be confidently rejected implying that the means are not equal in both classes, and hence the feature has clearly different values for both the classes, and therefore is highly discriminating.

1.4   CLASSIFICATION

In this work, support vector machine (SVM) classifiers with linear, polynomial kernel with order 1, order 2, order 3, and radial basis function (RBF) kernels were used to select the best kernel function based on highest classification accuracy. It is briefly described here.

1.4.1   SUPPORT VECTOR MACHINE (SVM)

The cluster center features after test of significance are fed to support vector machine (SVM) [31–33] to classify normal and abnormal fundus images. It is a set of related supervised learning methods used for classification and regression. Let us denote a feature vector by $\underline{x} = (x_1, x_2 \ldots x_n)$ and its class label by y such that $y = \{+1, -1\}$. Therefore, consider the problem of separating n training patterns belonging to two classes as $(\underline{x}_i, y_i)$, $\underline{x}_i \in R^n$, $y_i = \{+1, -1\}$, $i = 1, 2, \ldots n$. The SVM is based on the idea of margin maximization and it can be found by solving the following optimization problem

$$\min \frac{1}{2} w^T w + C \sum_{i=1}^{l} \xi_i^2 \tag{1.6}$$

$$s.t. y_i(w^T x_i + b) \geq 1 - \xi_i, i=1, l, \xi_i \geq 0$$

The decision function for linear SVMs is given as $g(x) = w^T x + b$. In this formulation, we have the training data set $\{x_i, y_i\}$ $i = 1, \ldots, l$, where $x_i \in R^n$ are the training data points or the tissue sample vectors, y_i are the class labels, l is the number of samples, and n is the number of features in each sample. By solving the optimization problem (1.6), i.e., by finding the parameters w and b for a given training set, we are effectively designing a decision hyperplane over an n-dimensional input space that produces the maximal margin in the space. Generally, the optimization problem (1.6) is solved by changing it into the dual problem below:

$$\max L_d(\alpha) = \sum_{i=1}^{l} \alpha_i - \frac{1}{2} \sum_{i,j=1}^{l} y_i y_j \alpha_i \alpha_j x_i^T x_j \tag{1.7}$$

$$\text{Subject to } 0 \leq \alpha_i \leq C, i = 1, \ldots, l$$

$$\sum_{i=1}^{l} \alpha_i y_i = 0 \tag{1.8}$$

In this setting, one needs to maximize the dual objective function $L_d(\alpha)$ with respect to the dual variables α_i and the constraint $0 \leq \alpha_i \leq C$, where C is the penalty parameter, which is determined by the user. The optimization problem can be solved by various established techniques for solving general quadratic programming problems with inequality constraints. In this experiment, we used Binary SVM algorithm to discriminate normal and abnormal classes.

1.5 DIAGNOSTIC MEASURES

The performance of the classifier needs to be evaluated. In this study, performance of the classifier was evaluated using three parameters: accuracy, sensitivity, and specificity. They are briefly explained in the following sections.

1.5.1 OVERALL CLASSIFICATION ACCURACY

In this study, the overall classification accuracy (or the overall performance) for the datasets are measured using the equation [34]

$$\text{Accuracy } (T) = \sum_{i=1}^{T} \frac{Assess(t_i)}{|T|}, t_i \in T \ldots \tag{1.9}$$

$$\text{Assess } (t) = \begin{cases} 1, if \ classify(t) \equiv correct \ classification, \\ 0, otherwise \end{cases} \tag{1.10}$$

where T is the set of data items to be classified (the test set), $t \in T$, t_i is the class of item t, and classify (t) returns the classification of t by the classifier.

1.5.2 CONFUSION MATRIX

The actual and predicted classifications of a classification system are shown in the confusion matrix [34]. Performance of such a system is commonly evaluated using the data in the matrix. Table 1.1 shows the typical confusion matrix for a two-class classifier.

1.5.3 SENSITIVITY AND SPECIFICITY

We define sensitivity and specificity of the classifier as follows:

$$\text{Sensitivity} = \frac{TP}{TP + FN} \% \tag{1.11}$$

$$\text{Specificity} = \frac{TN}{FP + TN} \%$$ (1.12)

Sensitivity is thus a measure of accuracy of diagnosis of DR (true) cases. Specificity is a measure of accuracy of diagnosis of normal (false) cases.

1.6 RESULTS

Figure 1.5 shows the images before and after FCM clustering. The grayscale image output after clustering has six different distinct gray values. Each of the gray values represents one cluster. Observations of these images show that the FCM cluster the features of the DR images well. The optic disc and background are well grouped and clearly defined. Hence the optic disc and background of the image do not contribute as features that determine the diabetes retinopathy stages.

In this study, features having p-value of less than 0.05 were considered significant. Among the extracted six cluster centers, three features were found to be significant. These significant features and their ranges for both the normal and abnormal classes are presented in Table 1.2. It can be seen from Table 1.2 that these values are higher for normal and lower for abnormal cases. It indicates the abnormal fundus

TABLE 1.1
Representation of Confusion Matrix

	Predicted	
Actual	**Negative**	**Positive**
Negative	TN	FP
Positive	FN	TP

TP: True Positive: A patient predicted with DR when he/she actually has DR.
TN: True Negative: A patient predicted healthy when he/she actually is healthy.
FP: False Positive: A patient predicted with DR when he/she actually is healthy.
FN: False Negative: A patient predicted healthy when he/she actually has DR.

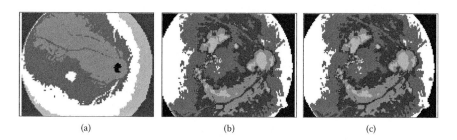

(a)   (b)   (c)

FIGURE 1.5 Results of K-means clustering algorithm with six clusters for (a) normal, (b) NPDR, and (c) PDR of Figure 1.3.

images having defects, namely microaneurysms, hard exudates, cotton wool spots, and hemorrhages. Moreover, Figure 1.6 shows the weight vectors derived from SOM for normal and abnormal (NPDR and PDR) classes, which helps to visualize the discrimination between the two classes. In Figure 1.6, we can see that NPDR and PDR classes are clearly separated from the normal class.

In this study, a three-fold stratified cross validation method was used to test the SVM classifier with various kernel functions. The entire data set was split into three equal parts (roughly), each part containing a similar proportion of samples belonging to both classes. Two parts of the data (training set) were used for classifier development and the built classifier was evaluated using the remaining one part (test set) (i.e., 360 images were used for training and 138 images for testing each time). This procedure was repeated three times using a different part as the test set in each case.

TABLE 1.2

Summary Statistics of the Features of Normal and Abnormal Groups

Features	Normal	Abnormal	p-Value
Red centroid	132.49 ± 76.83	114.37 ± 70.89	<0.0001
Green centroid	86.49 ± 69.27	75.36 ± 60.03	<0.0001
Blue centroid	52.41 ± 61.02	33.99 ± 42.17	<0.0001

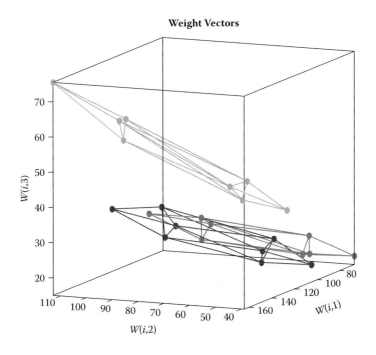

Weight Vectors

FIGURE 1.6 Weight vectors of SOM: Green indicates normal; red and blue indicate NPDR and PDR classes, respectively. (Please see color insert.)

TABLE 1.3

Classification Results of Normal and Abnormal Groups Using SVM Classifier with Different Kernel Functions

SVM Kernels	TN	FN	TP	FP	Accuracy (%)	PPV (%)	Sensitivity (%)	Specificity (%)
Linear kernel	21	9	75	33	69.08	69.08	88.89	38.27
Polynomial kernel with order 1	21	9	75	33	69.08	69.08	88.89	38.27
Polynomia kernel with order 2	28	10	74	26	73.67	73.79	87.69	51.85
Polynomial kernel with order 3	29	9	75	25	75.60	75.04	89.68	53.70
RBF kernel	41	6	78	13	86.23	86.16	92.46	76.54

Average of the accuracy, sensitivity, specificity, and positive predictive accuracy was calculated for all three trials to obtain the overall performance measures.

Table 1.3 presents the classification results of the eye fundus image data using the extracted cluster center features. The first column indicates the kernel functions used for SVM classifier. The next four columns present the number of True Negatives (TN), False Negatives (FN), True Positives (TP), and False Positives (FP). The classification accuracy is shown in column 6. Columns 7, 8, and 9 show the positive predictive accuracy, sensitivity, and specificity, respectively. It is also evident from the results that the RBF kernel performed better than other kernel functions with an accuracy of 86.23% with sensitivity and specificity of 92.46% and 76.54%, respectively.

1.7 DISCUSSION

The exudates, hemorrhages, and microaneurysms were used for computer-based screening of the DR subjects [25]. The sensitivity and specificity for exudates detection were 88.5% and 99.7%, respectively. The algorithm achieved a sensitivity of 77.5% and specificity of 88.7% for detection of hemorrhages and microaneurysms.

Singalavanija et al. [35] differentiated DR from a normal retina using image-processing algorithms. In their method, retinal images were preprocessed using adaptive local contrast enhancement. Their system, based on a multilayer perceptron neural network, yielded a sensitivity of 74.8% and a specificity of 82.7%.

A decision support system for the early detection of the DR (presence of the microaneurysms) was proposed by Kahai et al. [36]. The detection rule was based on a binary-hypothesis testing problem with yes-no decisions. The Bayesian classifier was used to discriminate the fundus images for the early detection of the DR. This system was able to identify accurately the presence of microaneurysms with a sensitivity of 100% and specificity of 67%.

Wong et al. [37] classified normal, mild DR, moderate DR, severe DR, and PDR stages using morphological features and feed-forward neural network. In their work, the area and perimeter of the RGB components of the blood vessels are chosen as the features for the classifier. The average classification accuracy of their system was 84%, the sensitivity was 90%, and the specificity was 100%.

Using the area of the exudates, blood vessels, and texture parameters, the fundus images were classified into normal, NPDR, and PDR [38]. They demonstrated a classification accuracy of 93%, a sensitivity of 90%, and a specificity of 100%.

Classification of nonproliferative diabetic retinopathy (NPDR) based on the three types of lesions, namely hemorrhages and microaneurysms, hard exudates, and a cotton wool spot was proposed [27]. This method was accurate in detecting the different key features in the fundus images. The accuracy of detection of hemorrhages was 85.3%, microaneurysms 87.5%, hard exudates and cotton wool spots 93.1%.

A computer-aided system was developed using image processing and pattern recognition techniques to detect early lesions of diabetic retinopathy, namely hemorrhages and microaneurysms, hard exudates, and cotton wool spots [39]. This system was able to diagnose diabetes retinopathy with an accuracy of more than 90% of the cases.

The vessel tracker algorithm was developed to determine the retinal vascular network captured using fundus camera [40]. These algorithms were developed to detect the optic disc, bright lesions such as cotton wools spots, and dark lesions such as hemorrhages. This algorithm identifies arteries and veins with an accuracy of 78.4% and 66.5%, respectively.

The fundus images were subjected to the segmentation to extract the lesions and later fed to the neural network for classification [41]. The system showed a sensitivity of 95.1% and a specificity of 46.3%.

Larsen et al. have used image processing algorithm for the detection of hemorrhages and microaneurysms to diagnose diabetic retinopathy [42]. Their algorithm yielded a specificity of 71.4% and a resulting sensitivity of 96.7% in detecting diabetic retinopathy when applied at a tentative threshold setting for use in diabetic retinopathy screening.

Recently, Acharya et al. [43] automatically identified normal, mild DR, moderate DR, severe DR, and PDR stages using the higher-order spectra features and SVM classifier [43]. They obtained an average accuracy of 82% in identifying the unknown class, with a sensitivity of 82% and a specificity of 88%. They also extracted four salient features, namely blood vessels, microaneurysms, exudates, and hemorrhages from normal and DR images using morphological image processing and then classified using SVM classifier with an accuracy of 85.9%, sensitivity of 82.3%, and specificity of 86.4% [44]. Table 1.4 shows the summary of these works.

In this work, we classify normal and abnormal (NPDR and PDR) classes using FCM and SVM classifier. We used SOM to visualize the discrimination between the two classes. Our proposed system is able to identify the unknown class accurately with an efficiency of more than 86% using RBF kernel and the sensitivity and specificity of the systems are 92.46% and 76.54%, respectively. However, the accuracy of the system can be further increased by adding more features such as blood vessels, exudates, microaneurysms, hemorrhages, and texture. Also, when more diverse DR images are taken under identical lighting conditions and orientations, this may improve the results in diagnosing the correct class of the unknown input image.

TABLE 1.4

Summary of Automated Diabetic Retinopathy Detection System Studies

Author	Objective of the Work	Method Used	Result
Singalavanija et al. (2002) [25]	Detection of exudates, microaneurysms, and hemorrhages	Recursive region growing algorithm and moat operator	Exudates detection Sensitivity—88.5% Specificity—99.7% Hemorrhages and microaneurysms detection Sensitivity—77.5% Specificity—88.7%
Singalavanija et al. (2006) [35]	Classification of normal and abnormal	Multi-layer perceptron neural network	Sensitivity—74.8% Specificity—82.7%
Kahai et al. (2006) [36]	Detection of DR	Bayesian classifier	Sensitivity—100% Specificity—67%
Wong et al. (2008) [37]	Classification of normal, moderate DR, severe DR, and prolific DR stages	Area and perimeters of RGB components of blood vessels, neural network	Accuracy—84% Sensitivity—90% Specificity—100%
Nayak et al. (2008) [38]	Classification of normal, NPDR and PDR classes	Artificial neural network	Accuracy—93% Sensitivity—90%, Specificity—100%
Lee et al. (2001) [39]	Detection of early lesions of DR	Image processing and pattern recognition	Accuracy more than 90%
Englmeier et al. (2004) [40]	Detection of retinal vasculature	Multiresolution method	Accuracy to detect arteries—78.4% Accuracy to detect veins—66.5%
Usher et al. (2004) [41]	Detection of DR using fundus lesions	Artificial neural network	Sensitivity—95.1% Specificity—46.3%
Larsen et al. (2003) [42]	Detection of hemorrhages and microaneurysms to diagnose DR	Tentative threshold setting	Sensitivity—96.7% Specificity—71.4%
Acharya et al. (2008) [43]	Classification of normal, mild DR, moderate DR, severe DR, and prolific DR classes	HOS features and SVM classifier	Accuracy—82%
Acharya et al. (2009) [44]	Classification of moderate DR, mild DR, severe DR, and prolific DR stages	Image processing and SVM techniques	Sensitivity—82% Specificity—86% PPV—95%
This study	Classification of normal and abnormal	Cluster center features and SVM	Accuracy—86.23% Sensitivity—92.46% Specificity—76.54%

1.8   CONCLUSION

Diabetic retinopathy is a complication of diabetes and a leading cause of blindness. Hence it is very important to diagnose DR at an early stage efficiently. In the present work, an automated technique was proposed to identify the DR class using image-processing and data-mining techniques. The cluster center features were extracted from the raw images using FCM and fed to the SVM for classification. The system can identify normal and abnormal classes with an average accuracy of more than 86%, a sensitivity of 92.46%, and a specificity of 76.54%. The performance can be further increased with more diverse data and better features.

REFERENCES

1. Dineshkumar, B., Mitra, A., and Manjunatha, M. (2010) Studies on the anti-diabetic and hypolipidemic potentials of mangiferin (Xanthone Glucoside) in streptozotocin-induced Type 1 and Type 2 diabetic model rats, *International Journal of Advances in Pharmaceutical Science* 1, 75–85.
2. Chandra, A., Mahdhi, A. A., Ahmad, S., and Singh, R. K. (2007) Indian herbs result in hypoglycemic responses in streptozotocin-induced diabetic rats, *Nutrition Research* 27, 161–168.
3. Kuzuya, T., Nakagawa, S., Satoh, J., Kanazawa, Y., Iwamoto, Y., Kobayashi, M., Nanjo, K., Sasaki, A., Seino, Y., Ito, C., Shima, K., Nonaka, K., and Kodowaki, T. (2002) Report of the committee on the classification and diagnostic criteria of diabetes mellitus, *Diabetes Research and Clinical Practice* 55, 65–85.
4. American Diabetes Association. (2008) Diagnosis and classification of diabetes mellitus, *Diabetes Care* 31, S55–S60.
5. Kyvik, K. O., Nystrom, L., Gorus, F., Songini, M., Oestman, J., Castell, C., Green, A., Guyrus, G., Ionescu-Trigoviste, C., McKinney, P. A., Michalkova, D., Ostrauskas, R., and Raymond, N. T. (2004) The epidemiology of type 1 diabetes mellitus is not the same in young adults as in children, *Diabetologia* 47, 377–384.
6. Sharma, A., Rastogi, T., Bhartiya, M., Shasany, A. K., and Khanuja, S. P. S. (2007) Type 2 diabetes mellitus: phylogenetic motifs for predicting protein functional site, *Journal of Biosciences* 32, 999–1004.
7. Ramachandran, A., Snehalatha, C., and Viswanathan, V. (2002) Burden of type 2 diabetes and its complications—the Indian Scenario, *Current Science* 83, 1471–1476.
8. Scheen, A. J. (2003) Pathophysiology of type 2 diabetes, *Acta Clinica Belgica* 58, 335–341.
9. American Diabetes Association. (2004) Gestational diabetes mellitus, *Diabetes Care* 27, S88–S90.
10. World Health Organization. Diabetes fact sheet. http://www.who.int/mediacenter/factsheets/fs312/en/index.html, last accessed 14th April 2011.
11. Wild, S., Roglic, G., Green, A., Sicree, R., and King, H. (2004) Global prevalence of diabetes: estimates for the year 2000 and projections for 2030, *Diabetes Care* 27, 1047–1053.
12. World Health Organization. Estimated number of adults with diabetes. http://www.who.int/diabetes/actionnow/en/diabprev.pdf, last accessed 30th July 2011.
13. Sarah Wild, et al. (2004) Global prevalence of diabetes, estimates for the year 2000 and projections for 2030, *Diabetes Care*, 27(5).
14. Rajendra Acharya, U., Ng, E. Y. K., Jasjit S. Suri. *Image Modeling of the Human Eye*, London: Artech House, 2008.

15. The Expert Committee on the Diagnosis and Classification of Diabetes Mellitus. (2011) Report of the Expert Committee on the Diagnosis and Classification of Diabetes Mellitus, *Diabetes Care* 34, S66–S68.
16. Winder, R. J., Morrow, P. J., McRitchie, I. N., Bailie, J. R., and Hart, P. M. (2009) Algorithms for digital image processing in diabetic retinopathy, *Comput Med Imaging Graph* 33(8), 608–622.
17. Chaudhuri, S., Chatterjee, S., Katz, N., Nelson, M., and Goldbaum, M. (1989) Detection of blood vessels in retinal images using two-dimensional matched filters, *IEEE Trans Med Imaging* 8, 263–269.
18. Zana, F. and Klein, J. C. (1997) Robust segmentation of vessels from retinal angiography. In *Proceedings of International Conference on Digital Signal Processing, IEEE*, 1087–1090.
19. Zana, F. and Klein, J. (1999) A multimodal registration algorithm of eye fundus images using vessels detection and Hough transform. *IEEE Trans Med Imaging* 18, 419–428.
20. Akita, K. and Kuga, H. (1982) A computer method of understanding ocular fundus images, *Pattern Recognit* 15, 431–443.
21. Gardner, G., Keating, D., Williamson, T. H., and Ell, A. T. (1996) Automatic detection of diabetic retinopathy using an artificial neural network: a screening tool, *Br J Ophthalmol* 80, 940–944.
22. Spencer, T., Olson, J. A., McHardy, K. C., Sharp, P. F., and Forrester, J. V. (1996) An image-processing strategy for the segmentation and quantification of microaneurysms in fluorescein angiograms of the ocular fundus, *Comp Biomed Res* 29, 284–302.
23. Cree, M. J., Olson, J. A., McHardy, K. C., Sharp, P. F., and Forrester, J. V. (1997) A fully automated comparative microaneurysm digital detection system, *Eye* 11, 622–628.
24. Hipwell, J. H., Strachan, F., Olson, J. A., McHardy, K. C., Sharp, P. F., and Forrester, J. V. (2000) Automated detection of microaneurysms in digital red-free photographs: a diabetic retinopathy screening tool. *Diab Med*, 17, 588–594.
25. Sinthanayothin, C., Boyce, J. F., Williamson, T. H., Cook, H. L., Mensah, E., Lal, S., et al. (2002) Automated detection of diabetic retinopathy on digital fundus images. *Diabet Med* 19, 105–112.
26. Ege, B. M., Hejlesen, O. K., Larsen, O. V., Moller, K., Jennings, B., Kerr, D., et al. (2000) Screening for diabetic retinopathy using computer based image analysis and statistical classification, *Comput Methods Programs Biomed* 62, 165–175.
27. Lee, S. C., Lee, E. T., Kingsley, R. M., Wang, Y., Russell, D., Klein, R., et al. (2001) Comparison of diagnosis of early retinal lesions of diabetic retinopathy between a computer system and human experts. *Arch Ophthalmol* 119, 509–515.
28. Bezdek, J. C. (1981) *Pattern Recognition with Fuzzy Objective Function Algorithms*, New York, Plenum Press.
29. Kohonen, T. and Somervuo, P. (1998) Self-organizing maps of symbol strings, *Neurocomputing* 21(1–3), 19–30
30. Gun, A. M., Gupta, M. K., and Dasgupta, B. (2008) Fundamentals of statistics (Vols I & II), 4th ed. World Press Private Ltd.
31. Burges, C. J. C. (1998) A tutorial on Support Vector Machines for pattern recognition, *Data Mining and Knowledge Discovery* 2, 121–167.
32. Vapnik, V. (1998) *Statistical Learning Theory*, 2nd ed., New York, Wiley, 760.
33. El-Naqa, I., Yang, Y., Wernick, M. N., Galatians, N. P., and Nishikawa, M. R. (2002) A Support Vector Machine approach for detection of microcalcifications, *IEEE Trans Med Imaging* 21, 1552–1563.
34. Kohavi, R. and Provost, F. (1998) Glossary of terms. Editorial for the Special Issue of *Applications of Machine Learning and the Knowledge Discovery Process* 30, 2–3.
35. Singalavanija, A., Supokavej, J., Bamroongsuk, P., Sinthanayothin, C., Phoojaruenchanachai, S., and Kongbunkiat, V. (2006) Feasibility study on computer-aided screening for diabetic retinopathy. *Jap. J. Ophthalmology* 50(4), 361–366.

36. Kahai, P., Namuduri, K. R., and Thompson, H. (2006) A decision support framework for automated screening of diabetic retinopathy. *Int J Biomed Imaging*, 2006: 1–8.

37. Wong, L. Y., Acharya, U. R., Venkatesh, Y. V., Chee, C., Lim, C. M., and Ng, E. Y. K. (2008) Identification of different stages of diabetic retinopathy using retinal optical images. *Inf Sci* 178(1), 106–121.

38. Nayak, J., Bhat, P. S., Acharya, U. R., Lim, C. M., and Kagathi, M. (2008) Automated identification of different stages of diabetic retinopathy using digital fundus images. *J. Med. Systems* 32(2), 107– 115.

39. Lee, S. C., Lee, E. T., Wang, Y., Klein, R., Kingsley, R. M., and Warn, A. (2005) Computer classification of nonproliferative diabetic retinopathy, *Archives of Ophthalmology* 123(6), 759–764.

40. Englmeier, K. H., Schmid, K., Hildebrand, C., Bichler, S., Porta, M., Maurino, M., and Bek, T. (2004) Early detection of diabetes retinopathy by new algorithms for automatic recognition of vascular changes, *European Journal of Medical Research* 9(10), 473–488.

41. Usher, D., Dumskyj, M., Himaga, M., Williamson, T. H., Nussey, S., Boyce, J. (2004) Automated detection of diabetic retinopathy in digital retinal images: a tool for diabetic retinopathy screening, *Diabetic Medicine* 21(1), 84–90.

42. Larsen, M., Godt, J., Larsen, N., Lund-Andersen, H., Sjolie, A. K., Agardh, E., Kalm, H., Grunkin, M., and Owens, D. R. (2003) Automated detection of fundus photographic red lesions in diabetic retinopathy, *Investigative Ophthalmology & Visual Science* 44(2), 761–66.

43. Acharya, U. R., Chua, K. C., Ng, E. Y. K., Wei, W., and Chee, C. (2008) Application of higher order spectra for the identification of diabetes retinopathy stages. *J Med Systems* 32(6), 481–488.

44. Acharya, U. R., Lim, C. M., Ng, E. Y. K., Chee, C., and Tamura, T. (2009) Computer-based detection of diabetes retinopathy stages using digital fundus images, *Proceedings of the Institution of Mechanical Engineers, Part H: Journal of Engineering in Medicine, Professional Engineering Publishing*, 223, 545–553.

2 VAMPIRE: Vessel Assessment and Measurement Platform for Images of the Retina

Thomas J. MacGillivray, Adria Perez-Rovira, Emanuele Trucco, Khai Sing Chin, Andrea Giachetti, Carmen A. Lupascu, Domenico Tegolo, Peter J. Wilson, Alexander Doney, Augustinus Laude, and Baljean Dhillon

CONTENTS

2.1   INTRODUCTION

We describe VAMPIRE, a software application for efficient, semi-automatic quantification of retinal vessel properties with large collections of fundus camera images. VAMPIRE is also an international collaborative project of four image processing groups and five clinical centers. VAMPIRE is an easy-to-use tool for clinical researchers allowing efficient quantification of features of the retinal vasculature with large sets of images (hundreds or thousands). Most of the processing is performed automatically before user intervention, which is kept at a minimum. The VAMPIRE interface provides easy-to-understand visual feedback of the features extracted and a set of tools that allows the user to easily identify, locate, and correct wrong measurements. No prior usage experience of image processing algorithms is assumed or required and the software is straightforward to use by those who are not computer literate.

Retinal microvascular abnormalities seen on fundal photography are associated with diabetes, hypertension, stroke, and cognitive impairment [1,2,3]. Often, diagnostic focus is placed on particular structural features of the vasculature such as the width of retinal vessels, branching angles, vessel tortuosity, and signs of retinopathy [4,5,6,7]. The retinal blood vessels are of similar size and physiology to the cerebral small vessels and may act as a surrogate marker for these cerebral small vessels. Abnormalities are often subtle and may be missed by visual observation or conventional retinal image inspection as performed by a human observer. Manual assessment of retinal fundus images is a time-consuming and laborious activity that effectively precludes the assessment of large numbers of patients thus hindering the detection of small differences. Hence the requirement for software tools that can process large numbers of images in an objective, effective, and efficient manner.

Some systems have been reported in recent years for semi-automatic assessment of retinal vessels. They include RISA, ROPtool, and ROPnet, designed within the context of retinopathy of prematurity, and AIAR, SiVA, and AVRnet in wider contexts. With the exception of AVRnet, which is under construction, no systems appear to be accessible publicly. In VAMPIRE, accurate segmentation of the retinal blood vessels and optic disc location is performed first, followed by the determination of the geometry at vessel bifurcations, the tortuosity of major vessels, and the branching complexity (through fractal dimension) of the vasculature. Most of the processing performed by VAMPIRE is hidden from the user, who is expected to provide only a minimal level of intervention after all measures have been calculated. The current, beta version of VAMPIRE includes modules for vessel detection, branching angle measurements, vessel width estimation, optic disc location, tortuosity estimation, and fractal analysis. VAMPIRE has already been used in several clinical and cognitive studies. The ultimate vision is to make VAMPIRE available as a public tool to support quantification and analysis of large collections of fundus camera images.

In this chapter we discuss related work and explain the VAMPIRE modules, reporting purpose, algorithms, and current validation. Example images are shown throughout. A discussion of current and future work concludes this chapter.

2.2   VAMPIRE OVERVIEW

2.2.1   USER INTERFACE

VAMPIRE allows the user to load a set of images of arbitrary size, limited only by memory constraints. Landmarks are detected automatically and efficient revision tools are provided so that the user can correct erroneous optic disk (OD) locations or discard images altogether. At the moment, no automatic quality assessment [8] is included. VAMPIRE then locates the full vasculature network and estimates branching coefficients, vessel widths, tortuosity, and fractal dimensions. Again, the user can revise results efficiently, making corrections or discarding images. All measures, together with metadata about the images, are saved by VAMPIRE in Excel files, ready for analysis. To date, VAMPIRE has been run on images of resolution ranging from approximately 400 × 400 to 3000 × 3000 pixels, acquired by various commercial instruments. These include fundus cameras (e.g., Canon CR-DGi non-mydriatic at 45° FOV (field of view), Canon EOS 20D, Canon EOS 10D, and Topcon TRC NW6 nonmydriatic retinograph with a 45° FOV), and a scanning laser ophthalmoscope (henceforth SLO), the OPTOS P200 ultra-wide field of view. VAMPIRE was run also on the main public datasets or retinal images, DRIVE [9], STARE [10], DIARETDB1 [11], and MESSIDOR [12].

2.2.2   LANDMARK LOCATION

2.2.2.1   Purpose

The purpose is to locate key retinal landmarks, namely the OD and the approximate path of the main arcade vessels. This in turn enables location of the fovea and the establishment of a retinal coordinates system.

2.2.2.2   Algorithm

The location of the OD contour is divided into two steps. First, the algorithm tries to find the fovea, the OD, and the main vessel arcades using independent weak detectors and choose the best triplet (formed by OD, fovea, and main vessel arcades) using anatomical information [13]. Second, after the algorithm has located a point inside the OD with high confidence, an elliptical shape model including an intensity model is fitted within a region centered on the located point to find the OD contour.

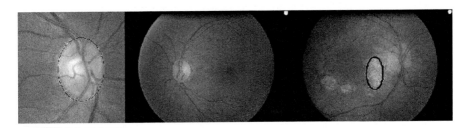

FIGURE 2.1 Examples of OD location. From left: ORIGA-light image, correct; Dundee images, correct and wrong. The latter is due to the false target created by the bright, circular lesions present.

2.2.2.3 Validation

The detection of the internal point has been validated with 230 images, including all the images in STARE, DRIVE, and DIARETDB1 public datasets, plus 20 cropped ultra-wide-field-of-view (200°) SLO images obtained with an OPTOS P200C SLO. Of these, 15 showed various lesions and 5 no lesion. Resolution was 3900 × 3092 pixels, cropped to 700 × 605 including macula and OD. OD location has been currently validated with two image sets: (a) the ORIGA-light set, courtesy of A-STAR Singapore, formed by 325 800 × 800 images cropped around the OD, which covers about 40% of the image area. Normal patients and glaucoma sufferers are included. On this set we achieve 100% correct location (defined as 90% or more of the estimated OD area overlapping the manually annotated one). (b) 286 2336 × 3504 images from the diabetes screening programme at Ninewells Hospital, Dundee, including healthy and diseased retinas. On this set we achieve, currently, 80% correct location (i.e., 240 correct results as defined above). Many errors are due to poor image quality (poor illumination or focus, OD absent or obscured by lesions). Figure 2.1 shows examples from the datasets.

2.2.3 VASCULATURE DETECTION

2.2.3.1 Purpose

The purpose is to locate the retinal vessel network and to generate a representation of its structure as vascular tree. This step is crucial to enable further measurements.

2.2.3.2 Algorithm

We conducted trials with various vessel detection algorithms, including Soares et al. [14] and Lupescu et al. [15]. Currently, VAMPIRE implements a version of Soares's algorithm. In essence, the algorithm applies a multiscale, two-dimensional (2D) Gabor wavelet transform to emphasize the appearance of vessels, followed by supervised pixel classification with a Bayesian classifier. Manually segmented images provide a labeled training set with two pixel classes, *vessel* and *nonvessel*. The authors of the technique report high accuracy values (0.9466 and 0.9480 from tests on DRIVE and STARE, respectively). VAMPIRE implements the high-performance supervised classification Gabor wavelet algorithm as a preprocessing tool to segment the retinal vasculature in fundus images and enable further measurements.

The notations and definitions in this section follow Soares et al. [14] in which the segmentation procedure is described in greater detail. The pixels of a fundus image are considered to be objects represented by feature vectors which allow the application of statistical classifiers to segment the image into two classes, *vessel* and *non-vessel*. Training sets for the classifier are constructed from manual segmentations of the images. Processing is performed on the green channel of the color images as this typically exhibits the greatest contrast between vessel and background. The green channel is first inverted so that vessels appear brighter than the background. See Figure 2.2. Before filtering with 2D Gabor wavelets, a preprocessing step extends the border around the edge of the FOV through an iterative approach of region growing the fundus image. The aim of this step is to remove the strong contrast difference between the retinal fundus and the region outside the aperture, thus preventing false detection of the FOV border as vessel. Following filtering, the image and filtered versions are shrunk back to the original FOV.

The Gabor wavelet is a complex exponentially modulated Gaussian. The 2D-Gabor wavelet is given by

$$\psi_G(x) = \exp(jk_0 x)\exp\left(-\frac{1}{2}|Ax|^2\right) \tag{2.1}$$

where $A = \text{diag}[\varepsilon -1/2, 1]$, and $\varepsilon \geq 1$ is a 2×2 diagonal matrix that defines the anisotropy of the filter, i.e., its elongation along the two coordinate axes. The parameter k_0 is a vector that defines the frequency of the complex exponential. Setting the parameter ε to 4 elongates the filter $k_0 = [0,3]$ gives a low frequency complex exponential with few significant oscillations. The combined effect on the filter of setting these parameters is a stronger response to vessel pixels in the fundus image while limiting noise and the emphasis of spurious areas in the FOV.

The Gabor wavelet transform is calculated for each fundus pixel at a selected scale value and from 0 to 170° in steps of 10°, and then the maximum is taken. Figure 2.2(b) shows the filter response for the image in Figure 2.2(a) and for a scale value of 2 pixels. Pixel features are the maximum modulus of the wavelet transform over multiple angles for multiple scales. As a result of the acquisition

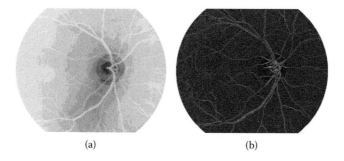

(a)   (b)

FIGURE 2.2   (a) Inverted green channel of a color fundus image. (b) Maximum modulus of Gabor wavelet transform over multiple angles and for a scale value of 2 pixels. Remaining parameters fixed at $\varepsilon = 4$ and $k_0 = [0,3]$.

process for fundus images, illumination is often non-uniform, with consequent variation of luminosity and contrast across the image [16]. As this may have an adverse affect on vessel segmentation, the image's feature space is normalized by its own means and standard deviations. Normalization is not attempted on the images themselves, as this may interfere negatively with the filtering stage of the segmentation process.

The final segmentation is achieved by supervised classification. Manually segmented images enable the creation of a labeled training set (used as gold standard for vessel detection) where pixels classes are defined as *vessel* and *nonvessel*. Only a subset of available vessel pixels is used for training in order to reduce computational processing time, and the probability distributions are estimated based on this selection. The segmentation is generated by a Bayesian classifier in which the class-conditional probability density functions are modeled with Gaussian mixtures formed by k_1 and k_2 Gaussians for *vessel* and *nonvessel*, respectively.

The pixel features used for classification were the pixel intensities of the inverted green channel and maximum Gabor transform response over angles $0°$ to $170°$ (in steps of $10°$) for filter scale sizes of 2, 3, 4, and 5 pixels. These scales were chosen so as to span the possible range of vessel widths throughout the images and increase the amount of vessels that could be automatically detected. One million random pixel samples were used to train the classifier and $k_1 = k_2 = 20$, as suggested by the authors of the technique in [14].

2.2.3.3 Validation

Classification of vessel labels by computerized approach was compared against manual segmentations by human observers to quantify performance and accuracy. Several of the computational segmentations warranted minor manual correction to remove prominent artifacts. Two authors, TMcG and APR, segmented manually a set of 20 fundus images. The segmentations of observer TMcG were taken as ground truth for the image database. The tracings of the second observer acted as a human reference for computerized segmentation performance assessment and had an accuracy of 0.9591. The accuracy of segmentation by computerized classification was 0.9570, computed as the total number of correctly classified vessel and nonvessel pixels divided by the sum of total number of pixels in FOV. Figure 2.3 shows three images, one from each public data set, and the respective segmentations.

2.2.4 Vessel Width

2.2.4.1 Purpose

The purpose is to determine accurately the width of retinal vessels at specific locations.

2.2.4.2 Algorithm

Determining vessel width is a deceptively simple task, as manual annotations by doctors used as gold standard vary. VAMPIRE adopts currently the length of the cross-section of the vessel mask found by the vasculature detection (Section 2.3) as its estimate of vessel width. The length is taken perpendicularly to the vessel's estimated axis.

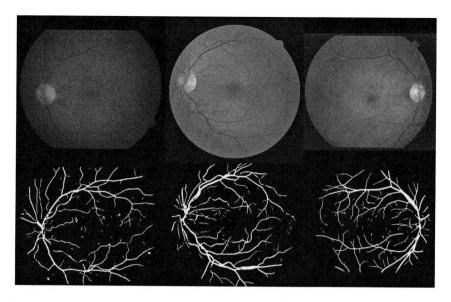

FIGURE 2.3   Images and vascular segmentation from data set (left to right) DIARETDB1 (1500 × 1152), DRIVE (565 × 584), STARE (700 × 605).

2.2.4.3   Validation

We compared manual (two observers) and automatic width estimates for 305 cross-sections of main and secondary vessels, both veins and arteries, from the 40-image set described in Section 2.3. The set includes healthy and diseased (diabetic retinopathy) images. 176 cross-sections were taken within the first two retinal zones around the OD. For vessels within 2 OD diameters of the OD (zone 1 and 2), considered normally in AVR studies, the mean of the *absolute* differences between observers (4.9 pixels) was higher than the mean of the differences between VAMPIRE and each observer (3.1 and 4.0 pixels). Similarly, the 95% confidence interval (CI) of the mean absolute differences between VAMPIRE and each observer (0.8 in both cases) was smaller than the 95% CI for the mean difference between the observers (0.98).

2.2.5   Vessel Tortuosity

2.2.5.1   Purpose

The purpose is to define and assess the degree of tortuosity of selected retinal vessels.

2.2.5.2   Algorithm

The tortuosity of retinal blood vessels is a diagnostic parameter assessed by ophthalmologists on the basis of examples and experience; no quantitative model is specified in clinical practice. All quantitative measures proposed to date for automatic image analysis purposes are functions of the curvature of the vessel skeleton. VAMPIRE implements a novel measure of tortuosity depending on both curvature and thickness [17], which was validated in 200 vessels selected by our clinical author from the public DRIVE database. Results are in good accordance with clinical judgment, similar to or better than that of four measures reported in the literature [17].

2.2.5.3 Validation

We carried out K-fold cross-validation tests [17] with a set of 200 vessels selected manually from 20 images, 10 vessels per image, from the public DRIVE set [9]. The vessels were chosen by a practicing ophthalmologist with 20 years' clinical experience, balancing the number of vessels in each class. We used larger-caliber and mainly first-order arterioles and venules to obtain a complete spectrum of tortuosity. Our choice was based on the assumption that the larger vessels inform the subjective assessment by the clinician on a first-pass scan. The images were acquired with a Canon CR5 nonmydriatic 3-CCD camera with 45° FOV. Each image was 768 × 584 pixels. Clinicians use a discrete scale of tortuosity; we adopted a common three-level scale (high, medium, absent). To assign each numeric value to one of the three classes, we used a logistic regression classifier [18].

2.2.6 BRANCHING COEFFICIENTS

2.2.6.1 Purpose

The purpose is to quantify bifurcation geometry, i.e., branching coefficient, which characterizes branching angles and cross-section area across a bifurcation.

2.2.6.2 Algorithm

Vessel centerlines are created from the binary vessel map (Section 2.3), and all intersecting junction points of three vessels are found. For each bifurcation junction point, an exclusion zone is defined based on the width of the parent vessel. A set number of points are extracted from each branch and a straight line fitted. For each junction, the three straight lines are used to find an improved junction point by a least-squares approach. The improved junction points, in conjunction with the previously extracted vessel branch points, are fitted with another straight line, this time anchored at the new bifurcation point. These fits are finally used to calculate junction angles. The bifurcation coefficient, b, is determined from the widths of parent, W, and that of the two child vessels, w_1, w_2, as [19]

$$b = \frac{w_1^2 + w_2^2}{W^2} \tag{2.2}$$

2.2.6.3 Validation

The agreement between human and computer measurements was assessed using 20 retinal images. On each, approximately five venule and five arteriole branching points were measured. Images were analyzed manually by two different raters using the angle measurement tool in *ImageJ* (http://rsbweb.nih.gov/ij/). Human measurements were then compared to the results obtained from VAMPIRE. The mean difference between the two human raters was 4.3° with 95% confidence interval (CI) of −13.9° to 22.4°; the mean difference between human and computer was 5.8° with 95% CI of −17.5° to 29°, showing good agreement.

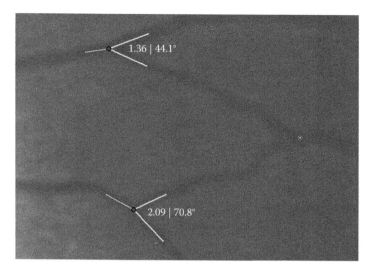

FIGURE 2.4 Two bifurcations detected by VAMPIRE with visualization of branching coefficients and angle values.

2.2.6.4 Examples

Figure 2.4 shows two bifurcations with the respective branching coefficient (1.36 and 2.09) and angles (44.1° and 70.8°). An unselected branching point can also be seen (right, marked by white circle and dot).

2.2.7 FRACTAL ANALYSIS

2.2.7.1 Purpose

The purpose is to compute monofractal and multifractal measures of the human retinal vasculature.

2.2.7.2 Algorithm

Fractal analysis characterizes complex, repeating geometrical patterns at various spatial scales. Fractal analysis has been tested, among others, with nonproliferative diabetic retinopathy [20], which has been found to yield a lower fractal dimension for the retinal vasculature than in control images. The cause for this discrepancy is not yet clear. Decreased fractal dimension has also been associated with aging and the presence of hypertension and retinopathy in type 1 diabetic patients aged 12–20 [21]. Monofractal analysis yields the fractal dimension, a dimensionless quantity which, in our case, measures the degree of branching complexity of the vasculature tree. However, a single fractal dimension is insufficient to describe the complexity of the retinal vasculature; multifractal analysis (MFA) is a better approach as it can resolve local density variations [22].

In the monofractal approach we measure a single fractal dimension using box-counting: the binary vessel map or skeleton is overlaid with a series of boxes of increasing size l, and the number of boxes N containing at least one object pixel is

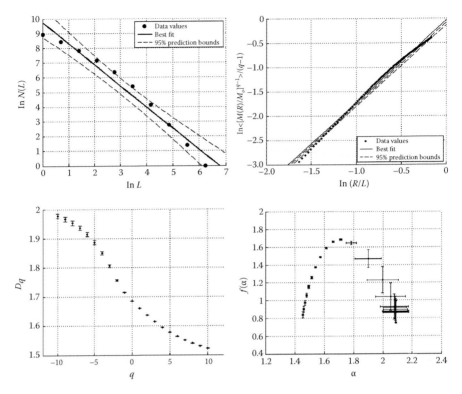

FIGURE 2.5 (a) Plot of ln $N(l)$ versus ln(l) where D_{box} is the slope of the best-fit straight line. Also shown are 95% prediction bounds for the fitted line, which determine the confidence interval for the calculated slope. (b) Plot of ln $\langle(M_i(R)/M0)^{q-1}\rangle / (q-1)$ versus ln (R/L) to estimate D_q, which is the slope of the best-fit straight line. Also shown are 95% prediction bounds for fitted line, which determine the confidence interval. (c) Generalized dimension spectrum D_q versus q. Error bars are calculated from standard error in the means and indicate 95% confidence interval. As the error bars do not overlap on the full range of q and D_q is a decreasing function, the segmented retinal vasculature is multifractal. (d) The corresponding $f(\alpha)$ spectrum. Error bars are calculated from the standard deviations of the means of α and $f(\alpha)$ and indicate 95% confidence interval. Peak position may be shifted by the onset of changes to the retinal vasculature.

counted [20]. The slope of ln $N(l)$ plotted against ln(l) obtained by least-squares fitting of a best-fit straight line yields the estimate of fractal dimension D_{box} and associated 95% CI. See Figure 2.5(a).

A geometrical multifractal is a pattern that is assumed to be composed of many fractals with different fractal dimensions depending on the scale; rather than evaluating a single fractal dimension, the complexity is instead described by deriving a spectrum of fractal dimensions [22]. Consider a structure with mass (i.e., number of object pixels) M_0 and linear size L, covered with a grid of boxes of linear size l. The generalized dimension D_q for the mass distribution is

$$\sum_i \left(\frac{M_i}{M_0}\right)^q \sim \left(\frac{l}{L}\right)^{(q-1)D_q} \tag{2.3}$$

where M_i is the mass or number of object pixels within the ith box, and q is a continuous and adjustable variable that makes it possible to examine fractal properties of the pattern at different scales [23]. Application of (3) to calculate D_q for $q < 0$ is hindered by the fact that boxes containing a small number of retinal vasculature pixels give anomalously large contribution to the sum on the left-hand side of (3), and so it is not possible to get reliable results. This problem is solved using the generalized sandbox method. This involves randomly selecting N of the M_0 points belonging to the structure, and for each point counting the number of object pixels $M_i(R)$ inside boxes of increasing linear dimension R, centered at the selected pixels. The sum on the left-hand side of equation (3) corresponds to taking an average of $(M_i(R)/M_0)^{q-1}$ according to the spatial probability distribution $M_i(R)/M_0$. When the box centers are chosen randomly the averaging is made over this distribution and therefore

$$\left\langle \left(\frac{M(R)}{M_0} \right)^{q-1} \right\rangle \sim \left(\frac{R}{L} \right)^{(q-1)D_q} \tag{2.4}$$

where $\langle ... \rangle$ denotes the average over the centers. Since in this method the boxes are centered on the structure there are no boxes containing too few non-object pixels.

For a segmented retinal image from the data sets used in our experiments, M_0 is approximately 30,000 pixels and the linear size L is approximately 600 pixels. To calculate the generalized dimension spectrum D_q plotted against q, 1,000 random points on the structure are selected, and the numbers of object pixels M_i inside boxes of linear size R and centered at the selected pixels counted. The counts are then used to calculate and plot $\ln \left\langle \left(M_i(R)/M_0 \right)^{q-1} \right\rangle$ against $\ln (R/L)$ for a range q values (-10 to 10), where the slope of the straight lines, obtained by least-squares fitting, corresponds to D_q (Figure 2.5(b)). Adjusting q allows fractal properties of the object at different scales to be extracted. For high q, D_q gives detail about high-density regions while for $q < 0$ it is geared toward low density regions. The procedure is repeated 100 times with different random choices of 1000 points for each structure. The final values of D_q are calculated as means over these repetitions. A 95% CI for each D_q was derived from $\pm 1.96 \times$ standard error (SE) of the mean estimate, where SE $= $ SD/$\sqrt{n}$ and SD is the standard deviation of D_q for $n = 100$ runs. See Figure 2.5(c).

Evaluating the spectrum $f(\alpha)$ provides a means of further quantifying a multifractal pattern [24]. Importantly, small changes to the retinal vasculature or abnormalities can change the spectrum in a quantifiable way [22]. Let $N(\alpha) = L - f(\alpha)$ represent the number of boxes such that the probability P_i of finding an object pixel within a given region i scales as $P_i = L^{\alpha i}$ where α_i is the exponent of singularity strength, and $f(\alpha)$ may be understood as the fractal dimension of the union of regions with singularity strengths between α and $\alpha + d\alpha$. The relationship between the $D(q)$ spectrum and the $f(\alpha)$ spectrum is expressed by the Legendre transform:

$$f(\alpha(q), \tau(q)) = q\alpha(q) - \tau(q) \tag{2.5}$$

where $\alpha(q) = d\tau(q)/dq$ and $\tau(q) \equiv (q-1)D_q$ is the mass correlation exponent of the q-th order. For a simple fractal, the fractal dimension is independent of q and is therefore represented by a single point $f(\alpha) = \alpha = D$ on the $f(\alpha)$ spectrum. Multifractal patterns produce a non-trivial spectrum. The derivatives are calculated as $d\tau(q)/dq \approx (\tau(q + \varepsilon) - \tau(q))/\varepsilon$ where $\varepsilon = 0.001$, except at $q = 1$ where $d\tau(q)/dq \approx (\tau(1 + \varepsilon) - \tau(1 - \varepsilon))/2\varepsilon$ is used. Over $n = 100$ runs, α and $f(\alpha)$ are evaluated at each q. Error values are calculated from $\pm 1.96 \times$ SD of the means of α and $f(\alpha)$ to give 95% CI. See Figure 2.5(d).

2.2.7.3 Validation

We tested MFA on the DRIVE and STARE datasets, and on our own image set. For each image database, monofractal and multifractal analysis was conducted on computer and ground truth manual segmentations as well as on skeletonized versions of these binary objects. Statistical methods [25] were employed to assess the agreement between results. The mean of the differences between pairs of fractal dimension measurements, the standard deviation of the differences, and the 95% limits of agreement were determined. The coefficient of repeatability (CR) was also calculated as the interval between upper and lower 95% levels of agreement and indicates the maximum difference that is likely to occur between two measurements.

Manual delineation of vessel pixels is a subjective process and so statistical methods were also employed to assess repeatability of fractal analysis when different observers performed segmentation. Pairs of fractal dimension measurements were again compared by determining the mean of the differences between each pair, the standard deviation of the differences, the limits of agreement, and CR.

In summary, our results showed that the 95% CI in fractal dimension was considerably smaller for multifractal analysis compared to the monofractal approach, i.e., less than ± 0.1% compared to approximately ± 7%. With reasonable image quality, the repeatability of fractal analysis performed on automatic vessel segmentations is close to that found when processing vessels traced manually by two human observers.

2.3 EXAMPLE OF VAMPIRE APPLICATIONS

We describe three studies on which VAMPIRE has been used to date.

2.3.1 LBC1936

This longitudinal study [1] investigated the determinants of differences in cognitive aging. Intelligence test data were collected on almost everyone born in Scotland in 1936 at age 11 in the Scottish Mental Survey of 1947. 1091 of these individuals were traced and retested. Study participants completed cognitive tests, gave details of their medical history and social background, completed psychosocial questionnaires, and underwent physical examination at age 70 and 73 years. Blood samples were collected for genetic analysis. Retinal photographs were taken with analysis and the participants underwent MR brain imaging.

2.3.2 ORCADES

This is a large genetic epidemiology study [26] that recruited 2000 volunteers to take advantage of the characteristics of the isolated Orkney population. Over 500 quantitatively varying risk factors for disease were considered, such as arterial stiffness, bone mineral density, and many lipid species. High-density genome-wide scan data will allow a variety of genetic analyses to be performed. Better knowledge of the genetic factors influencing disease should suggest new directions for treatment, for example, by identifying novel drug targets. Understanding the genetic basis of retinal vessel traits as a window to microvascular systems elsewhere in the body may provide insight into the pathogenesis of complex cardiovascular diseases.

2.3.3 LACUNAR STROKE

Lacunar stroke accounts for 25% of ischemic strokes, but the causes of cerebral small vessel abnormalities remain unknown. The retinal blood vessels have similar size and physiology as the cerebral small vessels and may act as a surrogate marker for these cerebral small vessels. 253 patients (129 lacunar stroke, 124 cortical stroke), mean age 68 years, were recruited. The results of this study [4] suggest that venular disease, a hitherto under-researched area, may play a role in the pathophysiology of lacunar stroke, and that retinal microvascular abnormalities can act as biomarkers for cerebral small vessel disease.

2.4 CONCLUSIONS

VAMPIRE is a software tool for efficient semi-automatic assessment of the retinal vasculature with large collections of fundus camera images. VAMPIRE is also an international collaborative project of (currently) four image processing groups and five clinical centers. The tool aims to minimize the amount of time spent by a user with no image processing background to quantify features of the retinal vasculature, current OD location, vessel width, branching angles and coefficients, vessel tortuosity, and fractal dimension. To guarantee the quality of data to be analyzed, the tool provides visual feedback and functions to correct wrong measurements manually.

VAMPIRE has already been used in several studies, which have also served as pilots to improve functionalities and interfaces. The ultimate vision is to make VAMPIRE available as a public tool to support quantification and analysis of large collections of fundus camera images. This vision brings several challenges of different types.

Current and future work focuses on the following areas. First, extending the validation of existing VAMPIRE modules. This requires gathering increasingly extensive collections of images, catalogued by different attributes (e.g., patient condition, imaging device) and, critically, annotated by multiple experts. Validation is an ongoing sub-project in VAMPIRE, in collaboration with (currently) five clinical centers internationally. Second, using VAMPIRE in further clinical, cognitive, and genetics studies. Third, developing further modules as required by requirements and feedback from researchers using VAMPIRE. Fourth, we are developing a novel parametric model of the intensity profile across vessels in fundus camera images, which is expected to improve the accuracy of width estimates significantly. Finally, deploying a substantial software engineering effort to maintain and grow a complex software application to which four different international groups are contributing.

REFERENCES

1. N. Patton, T. Aslam, T. J. MacGillivray, A. Pattie, I. J. Deary, and B. Dhillon, "Retinal vascular image analysis as a potential screening tool for cerebrovascular disease," *Journal of Anatomy*, vol. 206, pp. 318–348, 2005.
2. F. Doubal, P. Hokke, and J. Wardlaw, "Retinal microvascular abnormalities and stroke— a systematic review," *J. Neurol. Neurosurg. Psychiatry*, vol. 80, no. 2, pp. 158–165, 2009.
3. J. Ding, N. Patton, I. J. Deary, M. W. Strachan, F. G. Fowkes, R. J. Mitchell, and J. F. Price, "Retinal microvascular abnormalities and cognitive dysfunction: a systematic review," *Brit. J. Ophth*, vol. 92, no. 8, pp. 1017–1025, 2008.
4. F. N. Doubal, T. J. MacGillivray, P. E. Hokke, B. Dhillon, M. S. Dennis, and J. M. Wardlaw, "Differences in retinal vessels support a distinct vasculopathy causing lacunar stroke," *Neurology*, vol. 72, pp. 1773–1778, 2009.
5. N. Patton, T. M. Aslam, T. J. MacGillivray, I. J. Deary, B. Dhillon, R. H. Eikelboom, K. Yogesan, and I. J. Constable, "Retinal image analysis: concepts, applications and potential," *Prog. Retin. Eye Res.*, vol. 25, no. 1, pp. 99–127, 2006.
6. J. S. Wolffsohn, G. A. Napper, S-M. Ho, A. Jaworski, and T. L. Pollard, "Improving the description of the retinal vasculature and patient history taking for monitoring systemic hypertension," *Ophthalmic and Physiological Optics*, vol. 21, no. 6, pp. 441–449, 2002.
7. F. Doubal, B. Dhillon, M. S. Dennis, and J. M. Wardlaw, "Retinopathy in ischemic stroke subtypes," *Stroke*, vol. 40, no. 2, pp. 389–393, 2009.
8. A. D. Fleming, S. Philip, K. A. Goatman, J. A. Olson, and P. F. Sharp, "Automated assessment of diabetic retinal image quality based on clarity and field definition," *Investigative Ophthalmology and Visual Science*, vol. 47, no. 3, 2006.
9. J. Staal, M. D. Abramoff, M. Niemeijer, M. A. Viergever, and B. van Ginneken, "Ridge-based vessel segmentation in color images of the retina," *IEEE Transactions on Medical Imaging*, vol. 23, no. 4, pp. 501–509, 2004.
10. A. Hoover and M. Goldbaum, "Locating the optic nerve in a retinal image using the fuzzy convergence of the blood vessels," *IEEE Transactions on Medical Imaging*, vol. 22, no. 8, pp. 951–958, 2003.
11. T. Kauppi, V. Kalesnykiene, J. K. Kamarainen, L. Lensu, I. Sorri, A. Raninen, R. Voutilainen, J. Pietila, H. Kalviainen, and H. Uusitalo, "The DIARETDB1 diabetic retinopathy database and evaluation protocol," *Proc. Medical Image Understanding and Analysis (MIUA)*, pp. 61–65, 2007.
12. MESSIDOR: Digital Retinal Images (http://messidor.crihan.fr).
13. A. Perez-Rovira and E. Trucco, "Robust optic disk location via combination of weak detectors," *Journ. of Modern Optics*, vol. 57, no. 2, pp. 136–144, 2010.
14. J. V. B. Soares, J. J. G. Leandro, R. M. Cesar, H. F. Jelinek, and M. J. Cree, "Retinal vessel segmentation using the 2-D gabor wavelet and supervised classification," *IEEE Trans on Medical Imaging*, vol. 25, no. 9, pp. 1214–1222, 2006.
15. D. Tegolo C. Lupescu, and E. Trucco, "FABC: Retinal vessel segmentation using AdaBoost," *IEEE Trans. on Inf. Tech. in Biomedicine*, vol. 14, no. 5, pp. 1267–1274, 2010.
16. E. Grisan, A. Gianni, E. Ceseracciu, and A. Ruggeri, "Model-based illumination correction in retinal images," *Conf. Proc. IEEE ISBI*, pp. 6984–987, 2006.
17. E. Trucco, H. Azegrouz, and B. Dhillon, "Modeling the tortuosity of retinal vessels: does calibre play a role?," *IEEE Trans. on Biom. Engin.*, vol. 57, no. 9, pp. 2239–2247, 2010.
18. C. M. Bishop, *Pattern Recognition and Machine Learning*. New York: 599 Springer-Verlag, 2006.

19. N. Patton, A. Pattie, T. MacGillivray, T. Aslam, B. Dhillon, A. Gow, J. M. Starr, L. J. Whalley, and I. J. Deary, "The association between retinal vascular network geometry and cognitive ability in an elderly population," *Invest Ophthalmol Vis. Sci.*, vol. 48, no. 5, pp. 1995–2000, 2007.
20. A. Avakian, R. E. Kalina, E. H. Sage, A. H. Rambhia, K. E. Elliott, E. L. Chuang, J. I. Clark, J. Hwang, and P. Pasons-Wingerter, "Fractal analysis of region-based vascular changes in the normal and non-proliferative diabetic retina," *Curr. Eye Res.*, vol. 24, no. 4, pp. 274–280, 2002.
21. N. Cheung, K. C. Donaghue, G. Liew, S. L. Rogers, J. J. Wang, S. Lim, A. J. Jenkins, W. Hsu, M. L. Lee, and T. Y. Wong, "Quantitative assessment of early diabetic retinopathy using fractal analysis," *Diabetes Care*, vol. 32, pp. 106–110, 2009.
22. T. Stosic and B. D. Stosic, "Multifractal analysis of human retinal vessels," *IEEE Trans. Med. Imaging*, vol. 25, no. 8, pp. 1101–1107, 2006.
23. T. Vicsek, "Mass multifractals," *Physica A*, vol. 168, pp. 490–497, 1990.
24. A. Chabra and R. V. Jensen, "Direct determination of the f(α) singularity spectrum," Physical *Review Letters*, vol. 63, pp. 1327–1330, 1989.
25. J. M. Bland and D. G. Altman, "Statistical methods for assessing agreement between two methods of clinical measurement," *Lancet*, vol. 1, pp. 307–310, 1986.
26. R. McQuillan, A. L. Leutenegger, R. Abdel-Rahman, C. S. Franklin, M. Pericic, L. Barac-Lauc, N. Smolej Narancic, B. Janicijevic, O. Polasek, A. Tenesa, A. K. Macleod, S. M. Farrington, P. Rudan, C. Hayward, V. Vitart, I. Rudan, S. H. Wild, M. G. Dunlop, A. F. Wright, H. Campbell, and J. F. Wilson, "Runs of homozygosity in European populations," *American Journal of Human Genetics*, vol. 83, no. 3, pp. 359–372, 2008.

3 Formal Design and Development of a Glaucoma Classification System

Oliver Faust, U. Rajendra Acharya,
Jen Hong Tan, and Toshiyo Tamura

CONTENTS

3.1 INTRODUCTION

Glaucoma is a progressive optic neuropathy with characteristic structural changes in the optic nerve head which has a negative impact on the visual field [1]. Worldwide, it is the second leading cause of blindness [2]. It affects one in two hundred people aged fifty and younger, and one in ten over the age of eighty. In most cases, it is detected only after loss in vision. Vision loss is caused by damage to the optic nerve, which interrupts the image information transfer from the retina to the brain. Currently there is no cure for glaucoma. Hence, early detection and prevention is the only way to postpone, soften, or even avoid negative symptoms of this disease. There are two main types of glaucoma: primary open-angle glaucoma and angle-closure glaucoma. These occur due to increasing intraocular pressure (IOP). These two different types of glaucoma are briefly explained here.

1. Primary Open-Angle Glaucoma—This is the most common form of glaucoma. It describes a gradual process wherein the eye's drainage canals become clogged. Over time the IOP rises, because clogged canals cannot drain enough fluid out of the eye. In open-angle glaucoma, the entrances to the drainage canals are clear and work properly and the clogging problem occurs further inside the drainage canals (http://www.glaucoma.org). If open-angle glaucoma is not diagnosed and treated, it can cause a gradual loss of vision. This type of glaucoma develops slowly and sometimes without noticeable sight loss for many years. It usually responds well to medication, especially if diagnosed early and treated (http://www.glaucoma.org).

2. Angle-Closure Glaucoma (acute glaucoma or narrow-angle glaucoma)— This type of glaucoma is less common and is different from open-angle glaucoma. It happens when the drainage canals get blocked or covered over. The outer edge of the iris covers up drainage canal inlets, when the pupil enlarges too much or too quickly. One symptom of angle-closure glaucoma is that the iris is not as wide and open as it should be. Treatment of angle-closure glaucoma usually involves surgery to remove a small portion of the outer edge of the iris.

In current medical practice, glaucoma is detected using one of three tests: ophthalmoscopy, tonometry, and perimetry (http://www.clevelandsightcenter.org). Regular glaucoma checkups include two routine eye tests: tonometry and ophthalmoscopy.

Most glaucoma tests are time consuming and need special skills as well as equipment. There is an urgent need for new techniques to diagnose glaucoma at an early stage faster and more accurately, even with less skilled technicians. In recent years computer-based systems have made glaucoma screening easier [3]. Imaging systems, such as fundus camera, optical coherence tomography (OCT), Heidelberg retinal tomography (HRT), and scanning laser polarimetry have been extensively used for eye diagnosis [4]. HRT [5], confocal laser scanning tomography [6], and OCT [7] can show retinal nerve fiber damage even before the disease causes damage to the visual fields. However, the equipment cost is high and many hospitals cannot afford such systems. Fundus cameras can be used as a cost-effective alternative by many ophthalmologists to diagnose glaucoma. Digital signal processors extract features, such as the optic disk and blood vessels [8,9,10]. These features can provide us with useful information to diagnose glaucoma.

The application of artificial intelligence (AI) methods has been demonstrated to be an effective diagnostic procedure in the prediction of diseases. Several techniques have been used to automate the glaucoma detection process. A neuro-fuzzy method was proposed to diagnose glaucoma subjects with high sensitivity and specificity [11]. Fuzzy sets can be used to handle the uncertainty inherently present in the medical diagnosis process [12]. The results of 61 different tests were combined into one diagnosis to identify the presence or absence of the glaucoma. This method showed a classification efficiency of 75.8%. Nayak et al. have used preprocessing, morphological operations, and thresholding for the automatic detection of optic disc, blood vessels, and computation of the features. Their system was able to classify the glaucoma automatically with sensitivity and specificity of 100% and 80%, respectively [10]. Chan et al. evaluated the performance of the following algorithms for solving the glaucoma classification problem [13]: Probabilistic Neural Network (PNN), Naive Bayes Classification (NBC), k-Nearest Neighbor algorithm (k-NN), Gaussian Mixture Model (GMM), Takagi-Sugeno Fuzzy Model (TSF), Decision Tree (DT), Support Vector Machine (SVM), Linear Discriminant Analysis (LDA), Quadratic Discriminant Analysis (QDA), Parzen window, mixture of Gaussian and mixture of generalized Gaussian with STATPAC indexes [14] mean deviation, pattern standard deviation, and corrected pattern standard deviation. They found that automated classifiers showed improved performance over the best indexes from STATPAC.

Topographic images of patients' optic nerve heads were obtained using a scanning laser ophthalmoscope. Feedforward Artificial Neural Network (ANN) was designed to discriminate the glaucoma image and normal images with an accuracy of 88.9% and a sensitivity (correct abnormals) of 84.4% [15]. It was shown that the GDx software-generated parameters have limited ability for glaucoma detection [16,17]. Techniques such as relative surface height [18] and sectoral-based analysis [16] yielded better results than GDx parameters.

Glaucoma diagnosis is an important topic and much research has been dedicated to automate this process. However, the achievement of outstanding results in a laboratory environment does not yet benefit people. This research guides the way for the design and development of physical problem solutions that benefit society. To bring about these benefits, this solution must be reliable, else it is impossible to achieve the theoretical classification results. Furthermore, under no circumstances should it be possible for the system to harm a patient. Therefore we require the physical problem solution to be as safe as possible.

Reliability and safety are two high-level system requirements, which impact on the design approach for the glaucoma detection system. We propose to use digital fundus images as input to the detection system, because this data can be obtained in a cost-effective way. Furthermore, it is easy to integrate such a system into a digital processing chain. Such processing chains can be realized with inexpensive general-purpose processing components. In more abstract terms, we propose to apply the universal machine [19] to the problem of glaucoma detection. What makes these machines universal is the fact that they offer an almost infinite state space. Unfortunately, there are no physical limits when things go wrong and there are many opportunities to make errors. To be specific, every command to the processing machine can be wrong. Matters get worse when a number of independent processing entities are networked, because the communication between these processing entities opens up a meta level of problems. In particular, deadlocks and lifelocks occur when independent processing entities are combined without sufficient precautions and care to avoid the pitfalls of parallel processing. Therefore, the parallel combination of multiple universal processing machines makes it hard to build reliable and safe physical problem solutions. To give an indication of the problem, in the practical part of this chapter we propose to use a network of ten independent processing entities to realize the glaucoma detection system. With finite resources, it is impossible to check the complete un-abstracted state space of this system.

In this chapter we argue that only a well-structured and formal design method can lead to a system that meets these high-level requirements. We propose a design method called *systems engineering* for the design of an automated glaucoma classification system. This methodology structures the design work and thereby allows the people involved to focus on their particular task. One area where we go beyond systems engineering methodology is system specification. We use formal models to state the systems' functionality in a mathematically precise way. Thereby, we avoid ambiguities and misunderstandings between engineering and management groups. Furthermore, the formal method provides a way to deal with the state space of the system. We define all message sequences that constitute a reliable and safe operation of the system. Our thesis is that this formal model-driven design approach leads to reliable and safe problem solutions that work in the physical world.

In the next section we introduce systems engineering and discuss the structuring powers of this methodology. The subsequent structure of this text follows, at least to some extent, the so-called *systems engineering meta* model.

3.2   SYSTEMS ENGINEERING

Systems engineering is a methodical, disciplined approach for the design, realization, technical management, operations, and retirement of a system [20]. Systems engineering takes into account all steps necessary to create a system. This leads to trustworthy systems, because negligence in any of the design steps leads to weaker and therefore less trustworthy systems. For a large class of systems these design steps are requirements capturing, specification definition, implementation, and testing [21, Chapter 1]. Progress from one step to another is only made when all predefined conditions are met. Therefore, the work groups involved in the individual design steps can focus on their task.

Systems engineering can be applied to a wide range of engineering problems. For example, Diez et al. used the systems engineering methodology to develop computer-supported learning systems [22]. Palanisamy and Selvan propose a novel method for identifying relevant subspaces for data mining using fuzzy entropy and perform clustering [23]. Their presented theories and algorithms were evaluated through experiments on a collection of benchmark data sets. Empirical results have shown that this method outperforms several other clustering algorithms. Their design strategy follows systems engineering principles. Qian and Tang argue that with a strengthening buyer's market, retailers have begun to lead product development by introducing their own private label products [24]. The success of such a new product launch relies on transmission of demand information along a supply chain. The authors analyze these phenomena by modeling vertical information transmission in supply chains.

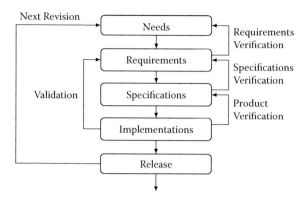

FIGURE 3.1   The systems engineering lifecycle model.

This approach follows the systems thought, where formal modeling leads to a deeper understanding of the system.

For the design of the glaucoma classification system we followed the classical systems engineering design approach. Figure 3.1 shows the systems engineering life-cycle model which was used to structure the design of the glaucoma classification system. The introduction of this chapter establishes the need for such a classification system. In the next section we discuss requirements capturing. These requirements answer the question, "What system do we have to build?" Once the requirements are established, we move on to the specification refinement where we answer the question, "How do we build the system?" The answer is based on formal models for parallel processing systems.

3.2.1   Requirements

Requirements discussions are usually done in the committees; domain-level experts come together and discuss the system properties. Therefore, field-specific research work and the associated mathematical models constitute some of the system require-ments. These requirements define what the system is expected to achieve and they should be obtained as a result of informed discussion. Analyzing field-specific research answers questions about the work context. To be specific, it answers the questions about what can be achieved and what are the most promising approaches to solve a problem in practice.

For the automated glaucoma classification system, we structure the requirements analysis in accordance with the block diagram shown in Figure 3.2. The block dia-gram details a classical test setup for classification systems. There are the fundus images as data input followed by feature extraction and classifier for automated diag-nosis. The quality of the extracted features is assessed with Student's t-test [25], which basically gives an indication that the features are fit; that is, they have the ability to differentiate glaucoma fundus images from normal ones. Once we have established that the features are fit, we move on and test a whole range of classifiers and classifier configurations. After these tests we are in a position to select the most suitable clas-sification method for the implementation of the glaucoma classification system.

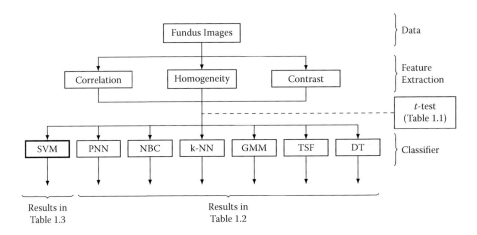

FIGURE 3.2   Block diagram.

3.2.2 DATA

Figure 3.3 shows a normal and a glaucoma fundus image. By simply looking at the pictures, trained human brains (ophthalmologists) can differentiate them. However, this task is much more complex for machines. Machine classification algorithms can only handle a small number of features.

3.2.2.1 Texture Features

It is not possible for state-of-the-art classification algorithms to process complete fundus images, because the algorithms lack perspective. That means these algorithms do not know where to look for discriminate information. Therefore, a feature extraction step is necessary which helps the classification algorithms to focus on their task. For the glaucoma classification task we extracted texture features from the fundus images. In this section we discuss correlation, homogeneity, and contrast, as indicated in Figure 3.2.

The discussion of the texture features starts with defining a Gray Level Co-occurrence Matrix (GLCM). Tan et al. have defined the GLCM for an $m \times n$ image I as follows [26]:

$$C_d(i,j) = \left| \left\{ \begin{array}{l} (p,q),\ (p+\Delta x, q+\Delta y): I(p,q) = i, \\ I(p+\Delta x, q+\Delta y) = j \end{array} \right\} \right| \tag{3.1}$$

where $(p, q), (p + \Delta x, q + \Delta y) \in m \times n$, $d = (\Delta x, \Delta y)$ and $|...|$ denotes the set cardinality. The probability of a pixel with a gray level value i having a pixel with a gray level value j at a $(\Delta x, \Delta y)$ distance away in an image is

$$P_d(i,j) = \frac{C_d(i,j)}{\sum_{<i>} \sum_{<j>} C_d(i,j)} \tag{3.2}$$

where $\sum_{<i>}$ is the sum over all possible i.

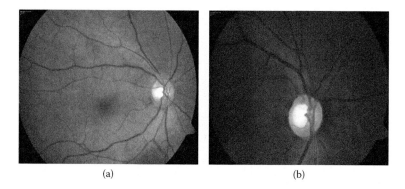

(a)   (b)

FIGURE 3.3   (a) Normal retina; (b) glaucoma retina. (Please see color insert.)

From this GLCM we can extract the three features of interest. The first of these features is contrast:

$$f_2 = \sum_{<i>} \sum_{<j>} (i - j)^2 P_d(i, j) \tag{3.3}$$

The second feature is correlation:

$$f_3 = \sum_{<i>} \sum_{<j>} \frac{(i - \mu_i)(j - \mu_j)}{\sqrt{(\sigma_i^2)(\sigma_j^2)}} P_d(i, j) \tag{3.4}$$

where μ_i and μ_j are means and σ_i and σ_j are standard deviations of $P_d(i)$ and $P_d(j)$, respectively. Finally we define homogeneity:

$$f_4 = \sum_{<i>} \sum_{<j>} \frac{P_d(i, j)}{1 + (i, j)^2} \tag{3.5}$$

3.2.2.2 Student's *t*-Test

Student's *t*-test uses variances to decide whether the *means*, which were evaluated independently for each class of input parameters, are different. The result of this test is the so-called *p-value*. A low *p*-value indicates that the means of individual classes are independent. Therefore, a low *p*-value is desired for classification problems (i.e., the result is statistically significant). In other words, a low *p*-value gives some certainty that it is possible to differentiate the individual classes with automated classifiers.

Table 3.1 shows the *t*-test results for the three features that were extracted from the fundus images. The table documents very low *p*-values for all features. That means that these features have the ability to discriminate between fundus images taken from normal and glaucoma-affected eyes. More specifically, the contrast increases for glaucoma. This increase is reasonable, because the optic disc, which is indicated

TABLE 3.1

Comparison of Different Classification Methods

Features	Normal	Glaucoma	p-Value
Contrast	46.91 ± 29.62	92.97 ± 36.3	< 0.0001
Homogeneity	0.579 ± 0.052	0.639 ± 0.055	< 0.0001
Correlation	0.98 ± 0.014	0.951 ± 0.029	< 0.0001

by a bright spot, is enlarged for glaucoma. Furthermore, the retina (excluding the optic disc) appears to be darker, as shown in Figure 3.3. Therefore, the contrast between these two regions is high. However, within these regions the homogeneity for glaucoma is higher. Figure 3.3(a) documents a normal retina with all the fine capillaries that structure the picture. These structures are quite literally connected or correlated. This causes the correlation for normal fundus images to be higher than for glaucoma fundus images.

After having established the feature quality, the next step is to find the best classification system. We approach this problem by testing a range of classifiers. More specifically, we follow the block diagram, shown in Figure 3.2, and discuss DT, TSF, GMM, k-NN, NBC, PNN, and SVM in the next sections.

3.2.2.3 Decision Trees (DT)

Tree-based classifiers are important in pattern recognition and have been well studied [27,28]. A decision tree is a decision-making device that assigns a probability to each of the possible choices based on the context of the decision [29]: $P(f \mid h)$, where f is an element of the future vocabulary (the set of choices) and h is a history (the context of the decision). This probability $P(f \mid h)$ is determined by asking a sequence of questions $q_1, q_2, \ldots q_n$ about the context, where the ith question asked is uniquely determined by the answers to the $i - 1$ previous questions.

DT has been used for the classification of proteins identified by mass spectrometry of blood serum samples from people with and without lung cancer [30].

3.2.2.4 Takagi-Sugeno Fuzzy Model (TSF)

The TSF is a universal approximator of the continuous real functions that are defined in a closed and bounded subset of P^n. That means that for each $\varepsilon < 0$ and for each continuous function g there exists a TSF such that $|g(x) - y(x)| < \varepsilon$ where $y(x)$ is the overall output of the TSF. Some definitions and notation will be useful in the sequel. More details can be found in [31]. We denote the arbitrary Dynamical System as S and we can define some operations in the systems' space.

3.2.2.5 Gaussian Mixture Model (GMM)

GMMs have been widely used in many areas, such as pattern recognition and classification. Their use has been especially successful in speaker identification and verification [32,33]. In GMM models, a probability density function is expressed as a linear combination (with weights w_i) of N multidimensional Gaussian basis functions. Each of these basis functions is specified by its mean value μ_i and its covariance matrix Σ_i; both can be derived from the input signal. For a single observation, x, the probability density function of a given GMM model, λ, is calculated as follows:

$$p(x \mid \lambda) = \sum_{i=1}^{N} w_i g(s \mid \mu_i, \Sigma_i) \tag{3.6}$$

The probability density function of a single Gaussian component of D dimensions is defined as

$$g(x \mid \mu_i, \Sigma_i) = \frac{1}{\sqrt{(2\pi)^D |\Sigma_i|}} e^{\left[-\frac{1}{2}(x-\mu_i)'\Sigma_i^{-1}(x-\mu_i) \right]} \tag{3.7}$$

where ($'$) denotes the vector transpose. The solution, to determine the parameters of the GMM, uses the Maximum Likelihood (ML) parameter estimation criterion. The model parameters are estimated through training; the goal is to maximize the likelihood of the observations using the so-called *Expectation-Maximization (E-M)* algorithm [34].

Usually, the initial estimates of the parameters are obtained from a sample of the training data using a simpler procedure, such as K-means [35]. The K-means procedure starts with randomly chosen initial means and assumed unit variances for the covariance matrix. This method has been adopted in this work.

3.2.2.6 Support Vector Machine (SVM)

SVMs were initially designed for two-class problems. But shortly after the initial postulation of the algorithm, they have been extended to multiclass problems. The SVM operation searches for a hyperplane, which acts as a decision surface that separates positive and negative values from each other with maximum margin [36,37]. This involves orienting the separating hyperplane perpendicular to the shortest line separating the convex hulls of the training data for every class, and locating it midway along this line. Let the separating hyperplane be given by $x \cdot w + b = 0$, where w is its normal.

Kernel functions can be used to extend the solution to nonlinear boundary problems [38]. The polynomial and Radial Basis Function (RBF) kernels are commonly used. With the use of kernels, an explicit transformation of the data to the feature space is not necessary. We performed an initial search for the SVM parameters by using a "grid search" approach as suggested by Hsu [39].

3.2.2.7 k-Nearest Neighbor (k-NN)

The k-NN method performs the classification of unknown data by relating the unknown data to known data according to some distance or similarity criteria [40]. The data is classified by a majority vote of its neighbors. A data is assigned a class that is the most common among its k nearest neighbors. If k is one, then the sample is assigned to the class of its nearest neighbor. Thus the contribution of the near samples is much more than that of the far samples. The neighbors should be taken from a set of samples (data) for which correct classification is known. This set of neighbors can be considered as the training data for the classifier.

3.2.2.8   Naive Bayes Classification (NBC)

Bayesian classifiers are statistical classifiers based on Bayes' theorem. Bayesian classification is very simple and it shows high accuracy and speed when applied to large databases. It works on one assumption: The effect of an attribute value on a given class is independent of the values of the other attributes. This assumption is called class conditional independence. Bayesian classification can predict class membership probabilities, such as the probability that a given tuple belongs to a particular class [41]. NBC predicts that the tuple X belongs to the class C_i. Using the formula

$$P\left(\frac{C_i}{X}\right) = \frac{P(\frac{C_i}{X}) \times P(C_i)}{P(X)} \tag{3.8}$$

where $P(C_i/X)$ is maximum posteriori hypothesis for the class C_i.

3.2.2.9   Probabilistic Neural Network (PNN)

PNN is a special type of neural network that learns to approximate the Probability Density Function (PDF) of the training data. It is a kind of two-layer radial basis network suitable for classification problems. When an input is presented, the first layer (radial basis layer) computes distances from the input vector to the training input vectors and produces a distance vector whose elements indicate how close the input is to a training input. The second layer (competitive layer) sums these contributions for each class of inputs to produce a vector of probabilities as its net output. Then the complete transfer function on the output of the second layer picks the maximum of these probabilities, and assigns a class label 1 for that class and a 0 for the other classes.

3.2.2.10   Classification Results

We close the requirements discussion by presenting the performance measurements for the individual classification algorithms. The performance was measured by using a two-step approach. First, the classifiers were trained with the texture features, which were extracted from a training set of fundus images. Next, the classifiers were tested with feature vectors from a test set of fundus images. Training and test sets were mutually exclusive. Table 3.1 shows the texture features of normal and glaucoma images.

We have used True Negative (TN), False Negative (FN), True Positive (TP), False Positive (FP), Accuracy, Positive Predictive Value (PPV), Sensitivity, and Specificity to analyze the classification results. Table 3.2 documents the scores, which were achieved by the individual classifiers, for the analysis parameters. The table is arranged such that the classifier with the lowest classification accuracy comes first. From there onward classification results get better; DT is shown in the last row, which indicates that with 88.9% DT is the best classifier in this table.

Table 3.3 discusses the classification results of different SVM configurations. With a classification accuracy of 74.1% the linear kernel shows the weakest performance. However, the different kernel configurations have a great impact on the classification accuracy—to be specific, the polynomial kernel with order 3 has the highest classification accuracy. Indeed the classification accuracy of 90.7% is higher than all the other classifiers that were tested.

TABLE 3.2
Comparison of Different Classification Methods

Classifiers	TN	FN	TP	FP	Accuracy	PPV	Sensi	Speci
GMM	7	3	6	2	70.4	77.9	66.7	74.1
NBC	6	2	7	3	72.2	76	77.8	66.7
PNN	9	2	7	0	85.2	95.8	74.1	96.3
k-NN	9	2	7	0	85.2	95.8	74.1	96.3
TSF	8	2	7	1	87	93.9	81.5	92.6
DT	9	2	7	0	88.9	96.3	81.5	96.3

TABLE 3.3
Comparison of Different SVM Configurations

SVM	TN	FN	TP	FP	Accuracy	PPV	Sensi	Speci
Linear Kernel	6	2	7	3	74.1	78.1	77.8	70.4
Polynomial Kernel with order 1	6	2	7	3	74.1	78.1	77.8	704
RBF Kernel	7	2	7	2	75.9	80.7	77.8	74.1
Polynomial Kernel with order 2	7	2	7	2	75.9	80.7	77.8	74.1
Polynomial Kernel with order 3	9	1	8	0	90.7	96.7	85.2	69.3

Tables 3.2 and 3.3 clearly show that the SVM classifier with polynomial kernel of order 3 outperformed all other classifiers; therefore we require our system design to incorporate exactly this classification method. In this requirements section we demonstrated solid research work on feature extraction and classifier testing. This research work forms the basis for the subsequent specification phase.

3.2.3 SPECIFICATION

In the specification phase we describe what system we want to build. The task for the specification phase is to answer the question of how to build the system. The second question is concerned with the mechanics of the system and therefore the answer must be much more precise. Indeed a specification should have mathematical precision, because it is used by both management and engineering teams. In other words, a specification bridges two domains and therefore requires a strong inner logic and precision to prevent misinterpretations by one or the other group.

3.2.3.1 Formal Model

To establish the mathematical precision for the specification we have used formal methods. We have chosen Communicating Sequential Processes (CSP) to model the glaucoma classification system. CSP is a process algebra for describing patterns of interaction within parallel systems. The process algebra itself is an elegant, mathematical method that includes a set of proof tools. The theory of CSP is supported by extensive literature [42,43].

We adopt a top-down approach to describe the CSP model of the glaucoma classification system. Figure 3.4 shows the process network for *MAIN*, which is the top layer of the model. The process network consists of three processes: *FE, SVMS,* and *RX*. These processes are connected via channels *f* and *result*.

Before we define the *MAIN* process with the process algebra, shown in Figure 3.4, we declare all channels for the model.

$$\textbf{channel } model : \{1..4\}$$

$$\textbf{channel } f : \{2..4\}.\{1..4\}$$

$$\textbf{channel } result : \{1..4\} \tag{3.9}$$

$$\textbf{channel } glcm : \{2..4\}$$

$$\textbf{channel } fi$$

Equation 3.10 defines that the parallel combination of *FE, SVMS,* and *RX* forms the *MAIN* process. The processes involved in the parallel combination must agree on messages sent over *f* and *result*. In other words, the parallel combination enforces the rules for information exchange between the individual processes.

$$MAIN = RX \underset{\{|result|\}}{\|} \left(SVMS \underset{\{|f|\}}{\|} FE \right) \tag{3.10}$$

The *FE* process itself is a process network that consists of five different processes. Figure 3.5 shows how these processes interact.

Equation 3.11 defines the parallel combination of *I, GLCM* and the feature extraction processes *F*. The parallel operator enforces the correct information exchange between the individual processes. The *F* processes do not exchange any information; therefore they are combined using the interleave operator (|||).

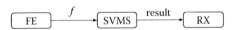

FIGURE 3.4 *MAIN* process network.

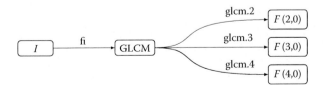

FIGURE 3.5 Feature extract (*FE*) process network.

$$FE = I \underset{\{|fi|\}}{\|} \left(GLCM \underset{\{|glcm|\}}{\|} \left(\||_{x \in \{2..4\}} \, F(x,0) \right) \right) \tag{3.11}$$

The I process represents the fundus images, such as the ones shown in Figure 3.3, which are communicated over the fi channel. The functionality of this process is modeled as a straight loop that exhibits an infinite sequence of fi events, that is, an infinite stream of fundus images.

$$I = fi \to I \tag{3.12}$$

$GLCM$ models the process that executes the GLCM extraction, as defined in Equation 3.1. The functionality is modeled as a loop that takes in an event fi and produces three events: $glcm.2$, $glcm.3$, and $glcm.4$. These three events represent the GLCM matrix, which is sent to the three individual feature extraction methods. The CSP model of $GLCM$ is shown in the following equation:

$$GLCM = fi \to glcm.2 \to glcm.3 \to glcm.4 \to GLCM \tag{3.13}$$

Equation 3.14 defines the blueprint of the $F(this, cnt)$ processes. This process has two parameters, where $this \in \{2, 3, 4\}$ indicates which of the three feature extraction methods it is and cnt is an internal counting variable. The feature extraction methods are mathematically defined in Equations 3.2 and 3.3.

$$F(this,cnt) = glcm.this \to f.this.cnt + 1 \to F(this,(cnt + 1)mod4) \tag{3.14}$$

The second process shown in Figure 3.4 is $SVMS$. This process network models the parallel implementation of four SVM classification engines. Figure 3.6 shows the four individual SVM processes which receive model information from an M process.

Equation 3.15 defines parallel combination of M and the four SVM processes. The four SVM processes receive model information from M via the $model$ channel; therefore the parallel operator enforces that the processes agree on the events communicated by this channel. However, the SVM processes do not communicate among themselves; therefore they are combined using the interleave operator.

$$SVMS = M \underset{\{|model|\}}{\|} \left(\||_{x \in \{1..4\}} \, SVM(x,2) \right) \tag{3.15}$$

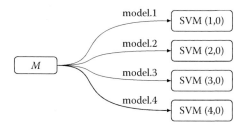

FIGURE 3.6 $SVMS$ process network.

The *M* model is straightforward. Equation 3.16 defines that the *M* process gives out a sequence of *model* events targeted at the four individual *SVM* processes.

$$M = model.1 \rightarrow model.2 \rightarrow model.3 \rightarrow model.4 \rightarrow M \qquad (3.16)$$

The *SVM(this, cnt)* processes have two parameters, where *this* ∈{1, 2, 3, 4} indicates the SVM number and *cnt* is an internal counting variable to keep track of the received feature values. Equation 3.17 defines that when all feature values are received, the feature vector ($[f.2.this, f.3.this, f.4.this]^T$) is combined with the model data (*model.this*) to form *result.this*.

$$SVM(this, cnt) =$$

$$\textbf{\textit{if}} (5 = cnt)\textbf{\textit{then}}$$

$$model.this \rightarrow result.this \rightarrow SVM(this, 2) \qquad (3.17)$$

$$\textbf{\textit{else}}$$

$$f.cnt.this \rightarrow SVM(this, cnt + 1)$$

The final process, shown in Figure 3.4, is *RX*. The functionality of this process is again straightforward; it consumes all *result.x*, where $x \in \{1,2,3,4\}$. In Equation 3.18 this functionality is realized with an indexed external choice (□).

$$RX = \square_{x \in \{1..4\}} result.x \rightarrow RX \qquad (3.18)$$

We used two automated model checkers, ProB [44] and FDR [45], to establish beyond reasonable doubt that the CSP model is deadlock and livelock free. In practice, the statement "established beyond reasonable doubt" comes down to simply checking whether our thoughts about the system are in line with the model. Therefore, checking the model really means checking our thoughts about the system. A successful model check does not mean that our thoughts were correct; there can always be shortcuts and lazy thinking. But we established another level of certainty that our ideas about the communication within the system can be realized.

3.3   DISCUSSION

The art of abstraction leads to rather simple formal models. The glaucoma classification system under discussion is no exception. The whole system can be modeled with only ten atomic processes, which are combined to form a sophisticated communication system. The *MAIN* process reflects this combination and models the important aspects of the communication functionality. The model makes no claim for completeness; it does not even represent the functionality of the system (i.e., no information processing is modeled). However, the CSP representation gives a rather good and deep insight into the communication within the system. This communication is normally difficult to communicate and even more difficult to model, because communication assumes an underlying architecture. This architecture is usually created during the implementation phase, so for ordinary designs it is only possible to reason about data communication postmortem, that is, when the implementation has been done. However, a postmortem defeats the purpose of a discussion, because the usual input from the management section boils down to the question, "Is it working?" Naturally, systems get implemented and in some way tested; therefore the inevitable answer to this question is, "Yes, the system is working." However, the question that we need to ask is, "Is the system performance reliable and safe?" Without a formal model it is even difficult to define what is meant by reliability and safety. In contrast, with a formal model we require the implementation to function according to the formally specified functionality. With CSP we can go one step further: by using a well-tested process-oriented framework, we can be reasonably sure that assumptions, made by the axioms of the process algebra, hold also for the implementation. The reason for this certainty comes from the fact that these assumptions are rather simple and therefore are easy to verify. In the case of CSP these assumptions revolve around the channel concept. A CSP style channel transfers data if and only if both sender and receiver are ready for the transfer. A communication partner has to wait when it is the only one ready for a data transfer. As long as this simple channel concept holds, the statements proven for the formal model will also hold for the implementation, under the assumption that the formal model was translated correctly and no programming errors were made. At first glance these two restrictions seem to draw the whole concept into question, because nobody can guarantee that there are no programming and translation errors. However, the nature of CSP style frameworks is such that either the communication goes wrong with deadlock/livelock situations or the system is lively, that is, there is meaningful communication going on. To define what meaningful communication is, we can go back to the formal model itself and define failure and test cases. Failure cases define correct fault behavior—for example, what happens if there is incorrect input to the system or one of the communication channels is cut. In terms of safety, such tests are very valuable, because they sharpen the awareness of both design and management teams for safety critical issues. The second group of tests are the so-called *use cases*. Usually designers focus on this type of test, because such tests answer the question, "Is it working?" In other words, use cases test whether the system produces the expected output or result from well-defined inputs. Again in most cases this is rather trivial, because the whole implementation process was governed by this type of tests. Unknown data sets, unexpected use cases, and outright failure cases constitute challenges for safety critical systems.

We aim to meet the requirements for safety critical systems by extending the systems engineering design methodology with formal modeling. Systems engineering gives us the framework for conducting the project. It helps us to establish the project mechanics, such as management and engineering processes. Formal modeling, on the other hand, gives a rigid basis for discussing the system specification. With formal models it is possible for both management and engineering groups to discuss, on a rather deep level, the communication within the system and what kind of security and safety implications a particular communication setup has.

3.4 CONCLUSION

The structure of this chapter follows the systems engineering design methodology. The introduction establishes the *need* for an automated glaucoma classification system based on fundus images. This need is established by referring to relevant studies that show how much suffering this disease brings. In the requirements phase we find out how to go about the task of building such a system. Different features have to be extracted from fundus images and their performance must be analyzed. We have chosen Student's *t*-test for this analysis and found that texture features perform well. The bulk of the requirements phase was dedicated to finding the best classification system that discriminates fundus images with from fundus images without signs of glaucoma. To do this, we have tested seven different classifiers and found that SVM outperforms the other six. Hence we established a clear requirement: the glaucoma classification system must use SVM. The specification section describes how these requirements are translated into a formal specification. One of the innovations of this chapter is the use of formal methods, in particular the process algebra CSP, to model the specifications. We establish that the CSP model is functional, reliable, and safe. In the discussion section we argue that these properties can be preserved in the implementation when it is based on a process-oriented framework.

The implementation as such was not described in this chapter for two reasons. First, size constraints: describing the implementation in a meaningful way takes careful explanations, which tend to occupy lots of page space. The second reason comes from the fact that implementations are very domain specific. This means that an implementation of such a decision-making system is always based on a particular hardware/software architecture. There is a multitude of such hardware/software architecture in existence and once an architecture was chosen the implementation is an almost mechanical process. From this perspective, a real shortcoming of this chapter is the lack of a discussion on the selection of a suitable hardware/software architecture. However, such a discussion would blur the focus of this chapter—that is, it would lead away from systems engineering and formal models.

Future work is plentiful, because the art of engineering transforms research ideas into physical problem solutions that help people. Therefore, fundamental reasoning about the process that turns ideas or research results into physical systems is an interesting and worthwhile topic. Frameworks are important to structure the thought process, which leaves more creativity to tackle real challenges within the system design. Modeling enables us to reason about the system in an abstract way, and through the steps of refinement we finally arrive at the implementation. By preserving established properties, such as functionality, reliability, and safety, even through the process of refinement we can be reasonably sure that the final implementation also contains these properties.

3.5 ACRONYMS

AI	Artificial Intelligence
ANN	Artificial Neural Network
CSP	Communicating Sequential Processes
DT	Decision Tree
E-M	Expectation-Maximization
FN	False Negative
FP	False Positive
GLCM	Gray Level Co-occurrence Matrix
GMM	Gaussian Mixture Model
HRT	Heidelberg Retinal Tomography
IOP	Intraocular Pressure
k-NN	k-Nearest Neighbor algorithm
LDA	Linear Discriminant Analysis
ML	Maximum Likelihood
NBC	Naive Bayes Classification
OCT	Optical Coherence Tomography
PDF	Probability Density Function
PNN	Probabilistic Neural Network
PPV	Positive Predictive Value
QDA	Quadratic Discriminant Analysis
RBF	Radial Basis Function
SVM	Support Vector Machine
TN	True Negative
TP	True Positive
TSF	Takagi-Sugeno Fuzzy model

REFERENCES

1. R. A. Hitchings and G. L. Spaeth. "The optic disc in glaucoma II: correlation of the appearance of the optic disc with the visual field". In: *British Journal of Ophthalmology* 61.2 (1977), pp. 107–113.
2. S. Resnikoff, D. Pascolini, D. Etya'ale, I. Kocur, R. Pararajasegaram, G. P. Pokharel, and S. P. Mariotti. "Global data on visual impairment in the year 2002." In: *Bulletin of the World Health Organization* 82 (Nov. 2004), pp. 844–851.
3. X. Song, K. Song, and Y. Chen. "A computer-based diagnosis system for early glaucoma screening." In: *Conf Proc IEEE Eng Med Biol Soc* 6 (2005).
4. U. R. Acharya, W. L. Yun, E. Y. Ng, W. Yu, and J. S. Suri. "Imaging systems of human eye: a review." In: *J. Med. Syst.* 32 (4 2008), pp. 301–315.
5. M. M. Hermann, I. Theofylaktopoulos, N. Bangard, C. Jonescu-Cuypers, S. Coburger, and M. Diestelhorst. "Optic nerve head morphometry in healthy adults using confocal laser scanning tomography." In: *British Journal of Ophthalmology* 88.6 (2004), pp. 761–765.

6. M. Hermann, D. Garway-Heath, C. Jonescu-Cuypers, R. Burk, J. Jonas, C. Mardin, J. Funk, and M. Diestelhorst. "Interobserver variability in confocal optic nerve analysis (HRT)." In: *International Ophthalmology* 26 (4 2005), pp. 143–149.

7. G. J. Jaffe and J. Caprioli. "Optical coherence tomography to detect and manage retinal disease and glaucoma." In: *American Journal of Ophthalmology* 137.1 (2004), pp. 156–169.

8. W. L. Yun, U. R. Acharya, Y. Venkatesh, C. Chee, L. C. Min, and E. Ng. "Identification of different stages of diabetic retinopathy using retinal optical images." In: *Information Sciences* 178.1 (2008), pp. 106–121.

9. U. R. Acharya, C. K. Chua, E. Y. Ng, W. Yu, and C. Chee. "Application of higher order spectra for the identification of diabetes retinopathy stages." In: *J. Med. Syst.* 32 (6 2008), pp. 481–488.

10. J. Nayak, U. R. Acharya, P. S. Bhat, N. Shetty, and T.-C. Lim. "Automated diagnosis of glaucoma using digital fundus images." In: *J. Med. Syst.* 33 (5 2009), pp. 337–346.

11. M. Ulieru, O. Cuzzani, S. H. Rubin, and M. G. Ceruti. "Application of soft computing methods to the diagnosis and prediction of glaucoma." In: *Proc IEEE Int Conf Syst Man Cybern.* 2000, pp. 3641–3645.

12. B Losch. "Application of fuzzy sets to the diagnosis of glaucoma." In: *Engineering in Medicine and Biology Society, 1996. Bridging Disciplines for Biomedicine. Proceedings of the 18th Annual International Conference of the IEEE.* 1996, pp. 1550–1552.

13. K. Chan, T.-W. Lee, M. H. Goldbaum, R. N. Weinreb, and T. J. Sejnowski. "Comparison of machine learning and traditional classifiers in glaucoma diagnosis." In: *IEEE Transactions on Biomedical Engineering.* 2002, pp. 963–974.

14. P. H. Artes, N. O'Leary, D. M. Hutchison, L. Heckler, G. P. Sharpe, M. T. Nicolela, and B. C. Chauhan. "Properties of the Statpac visual field index." In: *Investigative Ophthalmology & Visual Science* 52.7 (2011), pp. 4030–4038.

15. C. M. Parfitt, F. S. Mikelberg, and N. V. Swindale. "The detection of glaucoma using an artificial neural network." In: *IEEE 17th Annual Conference Engineering in Medicine and Biology Society.* 1995, pp. 847–848.

16. F. A. Medeiros and R. Susanna. "Comparison of algorithms for detection of localised nerve fiber layer defects using scanning laser polarimetry." In: *British Journal of Ophthalmology* 87.4 (2003), pp. 413–419.

17. M. J. Greaney, D. C. Hoffman, D. F. Garway-Heath, M. Nakla, A. L. Coleman, and J. Caprioli. "Comparison of optic nerve imaging methods to distinguish normal eyes from those with glaucoma." In: *Investigative Ophthalmology & Visual Science* 43.1 (2002), pp. 140–145.

18. J Carpioli. "Measurement of relative nerve fiber layer surface height in glaucoma." In: *Ophthalmology* 96 (1989), pp. 633–641.

19. A. M. Turing. "On computable numbers, with an application to the Entscheidungsproblem." In: *Proceedings of the London Mathematical Society.* 2nd ser. 42 (1936), pp. 230–265.

20. NASA. *Systems Engineering Handbook.* NASA, 1995.

21. Systems Management College Department of Defense. *System Engineering Fundamentals.* DoD, 2001.

22. D. Diez, C. Fernandez, and D. J. Manuel. "A systems engineering analysis method for the development of reusable computer-supported learning systems." In: *Interdisciplinary Journal of Knowledge and Learning Objects* 4 (2008), pp. 243–257.

23. C. Palanisamy and S. Selvan. "Efficient subspace clustering for higher dimensional data using fuzzy entropy." In: *Journal of Systems Science and Systems Engineering* 18.1 (2009), pp. 95–110.

24. Y. Qian and X. Tang. "Information transmission in launching a new private label product." In: *Journal of Systems Science and Systems Engineering* 18.1 (2009), pp. 111–127.

25. C. A. Boneau. "The effects of violations of assumptions underlying the t test." In: *Psychological Bulletin* 57.1 (1960), pp. 49–64.
26. J.-H. Tan, E. Ng, U. R. Acharya, and C. Chee. "Study of normal ocular thermogram using textural parameters." In: *Infrared Physics & Technology* 53.2 (2010), pp. 120–126.
27. S.-H. Cha. "A genetic algorithm for constructing compact binary decision trees." In: *Journal of Pattern Recognition Research* 4.1 (2009), pp. 1–13.
28. J. R. Quinlan. "Induction of decision trees." In: *Mach. Learn* 1 (1986), pp. 81–106.
29. D. M. Magerman. "Statistical decision-tree models for parsing." In: *Proceedings of the 33rd annual meeting on Association for Computational Linguistics*. ACL '95. Cambridge, Massachusetts: Association for Computational Linguistics, 1995, pp. 276–283.
30. M. K. Markey, G. D. Tourassi, and C. E. Floyd. "Decision tree classification of proteins identified by mass spectrometry of blood serum samples from people with and without lung cancer." In: *Proteomics* 3.9 (2003).
31. T. Takagi and M. Sugeno. "Fuzzy identification of systems and its applications for modeling and control." In: *IEEE Transactions on Systems, Man, and Cybernetics* (1999).
32. D. Reynolds, T. Quatieri, and R. Dunn. "Speaker Verification Using Adapted Gaussian Mixture Models." In: *Digital Signal Processing* 10 (Jan. 2000), 19–41(23).
33. C. Seo, K. Y. Lee, and J. Lee. "GMM based on local PCA for speaker identification." In: *Electronics Letters* 37.24 (2001), pp. 1486–1488.
34. J. Bilmes. *A Gentle Tutorial on the EM Algorithm and Its Application to Parameter Estimation for Gaussian Mixture and Hidden Markov Models*. 1997.
35. T. Kanungo, D. M. Mount, N. S. Netanyahu, C. D. Piatko, R. Silverman, and A. Y. Wu. "An efficient k-means clustering algorithm: analysis and implementation." In: *IEEE Transactions on Pattern Analysis and Machine Intelligence* 24.7 (2002), pp. 881–892.
36. V. N. Vapnik. *The Nature of Statistical Learning Theory*. New York: Springer-Verlag New York, Inc., 1995.
37. V. N. Vapnik. *Estimation of Dependences Based on Empirical Data: Springer Series in Statistics (Springer Series in Statistics)*. Secaucus, NJ: Springer-Verlag New York, Inc., 1982.
38. N. Cristianini and J. Shawe-Taylor. *An Introduction to Support Vector Machines and Other Kernel-based Learning Methods*. 1st ed. Cambridge University Press, 2000.
39. C. W. Hsu, C. C. Chang, and C. J. Lin. *A Practical Guide to Support Vector Classification*. Tech. rep. Taipei: National Taiwan University, 2003.
40. J. Han and M. Kamber. *Data Mining: Concepts and Techniques*. The Morgan Kaufmann series in data management systems. Morgan Kaufmann, 2001.
41. P. Domingos and M. Pazzani. "On the optimality of the simple Bayesian classifier under zero-one loss." In: *Machine Learning* 29 (2 1997), pp. 103–130.
42. C. A. R. Hoare. "Communicating sequential processes." In: *Commun. ACM* 21.8 (1978), pp. 666–677.
43. C. A. R. Hoare. *Communicating Sequential Processes*. Upper Saddle River, NJ: Prentice Hall, 1978.
44. M. Leuschel and M. Butler. "ProB: An automated analysis toolset for the B method." In: *Journal Software Tools for Technology Transfer* (2008).
45. *Failures-Divergence Refinement: FDR Manual*. Formal Systems (Europe) Ltd. 26 Temple Street, Oxford OX4 1JS, England, 1997.

4 Computer-Aided Assessment of Optic Nerve

Cheng-Kai Lu, Tong Boon Tang, Augustinus Laude, Baljean Dhillon, and Alan F. Murray

CONTENTS

4.1 INTRODUCTION

Retinal fundus images provide a rich source of diagnostic information not only for eye-specific diseases and conditions (e.g., glaucoma and myopia) but also for certain systemic diseases (e.g., diabetes) [1]. Tasks such as manually detecting and quantifying lesions in the human retina (e.g., exudates and parapapillary atrophy (PPA), illustrated in Figure 4.1) are time consuming for clinicians and may be prone to human error.

That is why, in ophthalmology, the automatic detection of the optic nerve (e.g., optic disc [OD] and PPA) is of considerable interest for computer-aided diagnosis. Automated image processing techniques hitherto have been employed to develop tools for early detection of glaucoma and diabetes, by identifying specific changes in the optic nerve or in the retina [2].

4.2 IMAGE ACQUISITION

Retinal images presented in this chapter were drawn from a subsample of the Lothian Birth Cohort (LBC) 1936 study [3]. The participants comprise surviving members of the Scottish Mental Survey of 1947 ($n = 70,805$) who were born in 1936 and presently inhabit the Lothian region of Scotland, UK. Three hundred and twelve of them were successfully traced and had their retinal photos taken at the Wellcome Trust Clinical Research Facility, Western General Hospital, NHS Lothian, Scotland. The research complied with the Declaration of Helsinki and was approved by the Lothian (Scotland A) Research Ethics Committee.

4.3 PREPROCESSING

Preprocessing is an essential step because segmentation of biomedical images is an arduous task often complicated by sampling artifacts and noise. In this section, we

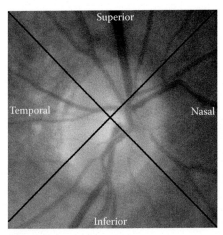
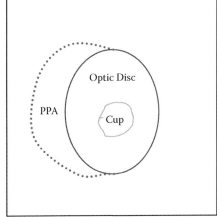

FIGURE 4.1 A retinal fundus image of a right eye shown on the left-hand side. Annotations describe the four different zones of a retina. The temporal and nasal zones are flipped for a left eye. A sketch map, shown on the right-hand side, illustrates the position of optic nerve areas, such as the optic disk (OD), optic cup (Cup), and parapapillary atrophy (PPA). (Please see color insert.)

briefly introduce the basic binary morphology and a few types of two-dimensional image filter.

4.3.1 BINARY MORPHOLOGICAL OPERATION

While we will not use mathematical morphology in the rest of this chapter, it is an essential tool for shape-based image processing, particularly for filtering purposes. Therefore we will introduce it here briefly. The term *morphological* has been widely used in many scientific fields such as material science, biology, and computational linguistics; all describe different objects. To discriminate itself from these, morphological image processing is usually called *mathematical morphology* (MM). MM was initially developed for "binary" image and was then extended to gray-scale images and functions.

In binary morphology, an image is regarded as a subset of the integer grid ($\mathbf{Z}^d$) or a Euclidean space ($\mathbf{R}^d$), for some dimension d. The fundamental concept in binary morphology is the use of a simple "structuring element" (also known as a kernel) to investigate if a predefined shape fits or misses the shapes found in an image. Two examples of commonly used kernels, marked as B, are shown as follows:

 A. Let $E = Z^2$; B is a 3 x 3 square given by $B =\{(-1,-1), (-1,0), (-1,1), (0,-1),$
  $(0,0), (0,1), (1,-1), (1,0), (1,1)\}$.
 B. Let $E = Z^2$; B is a cross given by $B =\{(-1,0), (0,-1), (0,0), (0,1), (1,0)\}$.

4.3.1.1 Binary Operators

The four key binary morphology operators [4] are erosion, dilation, closing, and opening. In a binary image, erosion "thins" the black pixels and dilation "smears" the black pixels (see Figure 4.2). These two basic operators are mutually coupled, as an erosion of the black pixels is equivalent to a dilation of the white pixels. In addition, they are translation invariant and strongly related to Minkowski addition.

4.3.1.1.1 Erosion

Let E be $\mathbf{R}^d$ or $\mathbf{Z}^d$, and A is a binary image in E. Erosion is defined by

$$A \ominus B = \{z \in E \mid B_z \subseteq A\} \tag{4.1}$$

where B_z is the translation of B by the vector z, for instance

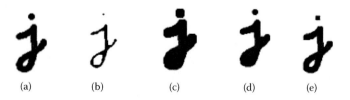

  (a)   (b)   (c)   (d)   (e)

FIGURE 4.2 Binary image morphology: (a) original image; (b) erosion; (c) dilation; (d) closing; (e) opening. The kernel for all examples is a 7 × 7 square. Due to different sequence of basic morphological operations, the void in the lower part of the character *j* remains clear after opening but is filled with dark pixels by closing.

$$B_z = \{b + z \mid b \in B\}, \forall_z \in E \tag{4.2}$$

When the kernel B has a center (e.g., B is a square or a disk), and this center is located on the origin of E, the erosion of A by B can be comprehended as the locus of points reached by the center of B when B moves inside A. (See Figure 4.2(b).)

4.3.1.1.2 Dilation
Dilation, the opposite of the erosion, of A by the kernel B is defined by

$$A \oplus B = \bigcup_{b \in B} A_b = B \oplus A = \bigcup_{a \in A} B_a \tag{4.3}$$

If B has a center on the origin, then the dilation of A by B can be comprehended as the locus of the points covered by B when the center of B moves inside A. (See Figure 4.2(c).)

4.3.1.1.3 Closing
The closing of A by B starts with a dilation of A by B, followed by an erosion of the resulting structure by B:

$$A \bullet B = (A \oplus B) \ominus B \tag{4.4}$$

The closing is also the complement of the locus of translations of the symmetric of the kernel *outside* the image A. Therefore, the closing can also be derived from $A \bullet B = (A^C \circ B^C)^C$, where $(A^C \circ B^C)^C$ denotes the complement of $(A^C \circ B^C)$ relative to E. (See Figure 4.2(d).)

4.3.1.1.4 Opening
The opening of A by B is obtained from the erosion of A by B, followed by dilation of the resulting image by B; therefore the mathematical equation is denoted as follows:

$$A \circ B = (A \ominus B) \oplus B \tag{4.5}$$

The opening is also given by $A \circ B = \bigcup_{B_x \subseteq A} B_x$, which means that it is the locus of translations of the kernel B *inside* the image A. (See Figure 4.2e.)

4.3.2 IMAGE FILTERING

Image filtering allows one to emphasize certain features or remove adverse effects on images [4]. A few types of image filtering are described here; all use a two-dimensional (2D) filter.

4.3.2.1 Average and Median Filter
Both the Average Filter (AF) and the Median Filter (MF) can be used to eliminate noise from an image. First, an AF is a filter of linear class that can smooth an image.

The basic idea behind the filter is that for any element of the image, an average of the current pixel and its neighborhood is computed. Next, the MF does similar, but instead of computing the average, it takes the median. The median is obtained by sequencing all the values from low to high and then selecting the value in the center. If there are two values in the center, the average of these two is calculated. To differentiate those two filters, we instilled the salt-and-pepper noise on the original image. (See Figure 4.3(b).) A MF gives a better result as salt-and-pepper noise is completely eliminated. (See Figure 4.4.) With an average filter, the color values of all noise pixels are taken into consideration in the mean calculation. In contrast, when taking the median, you only select the color value of one or two pixels that have the least random fluctuations; however, similar to AF, the MF might blur the object boundary.

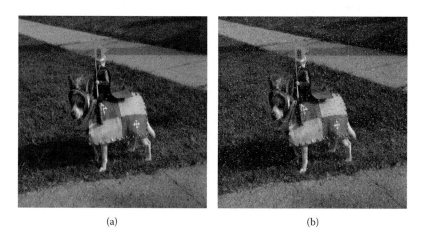

(a)   (b)

FIGURE 4.3   (a) Original image. (b) Original image with instilled salt and pepper noise.

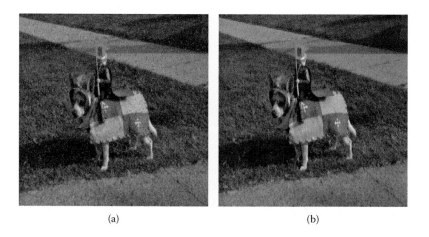

(a)   (b)

FIGURE 4.4   (a) The image after average filtering. (b) The image after median filter.

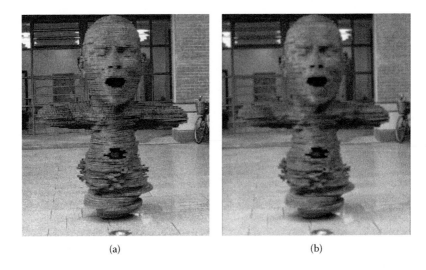

(a)   (b)

FIGURE 4.5 (a) Original image. (b) Image after convolution filtering. (Please see color insert.)

4.3.2.2 Linear Filter with Convolution

The image filter with convolution is another commonly used filter. The convolution is a neighborhood operation in which each output pixel is the weighted sum of neighboring input pixels. The matrix of weights is called the convolution kernel. To compute the output pixels, the convolution kernel is first rotated 180° about its center element; then each weight in the rotated convolution kernel is multiplied with the pixel of the image and the products are summed together, as we scan the rotated convolution kernel over the entire image. An example application of convolution filter to blur the image is shown in Figure 4.5.

4.4   FEATURE EXTRACTION

In this section, we briefly discuss some useful segmentation approaches to detect object boundary and identify the targeted region in the image.

4.4.1   ACTIVE CONTOURS (SNAKES)

Snake [5] is a framework to depict an object outline in a possibly noisy 2D/3D image. It models the outline in the form of a smooth curve that can deform under the influence of forces. The forces are a sum of the internal energy within the current contour and the external energy outside the current contour derived from the image data. The internal and external energy are minimized such that the snake will fit desired features or locate a target boundary within an image. Snakes are now extensively applied in various computer vision and image processing applications comprising segmentation, edge detection, motion tracking, and shape modeling.

The snake is an "active" model and is most ideally initialized near the object boundary. While in each iteration it always minimizes its energy function and is moved toward the prominent contour; therefore, it always presents a dynamic behavior. As the snake evolves by minimizing energy, often terms such as *wriggle* and *slither* are used to describe the process.

A simple elastic snake in the image is thus defined by a set of n points

$$V_j = (x_j, y_j), \text{ where } j = 0, 1, 2,..., (n-1) \tag{4.6}$$

The energy function of the snake can be defined as

$$E_{snake} = \int_0^1 E_{snake}(v(s))ds = \int_0^1 E_{internal}(v(s)) + E_{image}(v(s)) + E_{con}(v(s))ds \tag{4.7}$$

where $E_{internal}$ denotes the internal energy of the snake because of the curvature, E_{image} represents the image forces acting on the snake, and E_{con} serves as an external constraint force introduced by the user.

An internal elastic energy term ($E_{internal}$)

$$E_{internal} = E_{cont} + E_{curv} = \left(\alpha(s) \left\| \frac{dv}{ds}(s) \right\|^2 + \beta(s) \left\| \frac{d^2\overline{v}}{ds^2}(s) \right\|^2 \right) / 2 \tag{4.8}$$

where E_{cont} represents the energy of the snake contour and E_{curv} represents the energy of the snake curvature. The first-order term and second-order term makes the snake deform like a membrane and like a thin plate, respectively. The bigger the value of $\alpha(s)$, the more sensitive the energy function is to the amount of stretch. Likewise, bigger values of $\beta(s)$ will raise the internal energy of the snake as it evolves more rapidly into curvature, whereas small values of $\beta(s)$ will make the energy function less responsive in forming a curvature in the snake. The combination of smaller $\alpha(s)$ and $\beta(s)$ permits a more detailed modeling of the snake shape, at the expense of a longer computation time.

An external edge-based energy term ($E_{external}$)

$$E_{external} = E_{image} + E_{con} = W_{line}E_{line} + W_{edge}E_{edge} + W_{term}E_{term} \tag{4.9}$$

where $E_{external}$ represents the external energy deforming on the snake, E_{image} represents the image acting on snakes and E_{con} serves as an external constraint force introduced by the user. In addition, E_{line}, E_{edge}, and E_{term} denote line functional, edge functional, and terminations, respectively. By adjusting the weights, W_{line}, W_{edge} and W_{term}, to suitable values, the key features in the image may be extracted.

Figure 4.6(a) depicts an example application segmenting an orange color anchor. The red arrows represent the attractive forces toward anchor points, $a(i)$, as well as the repulsive forces. Figure 4.6(b) shows another example where the snake is employed to track a person's lip.

There are two major difficulties in the implementation of snakes. First, the initial contour must, in general, be close to the actual object boundary; otherwise it will generate an incorrect result. Next, snakes have a fundamental difficulty progressing into contour concavities.

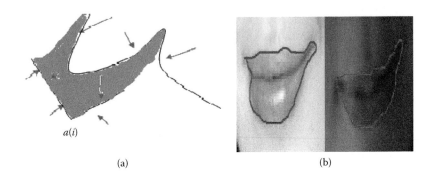

$a(i)$

(a)   (b)

FIGURE 4.6   (a) The sketch map of the motion of segmenting anchor by snakes. (b) The lips segmentation by the snake. (Please see color insert.)

4.4.2 CHAN-VESE (C-V) MODELS

The C-V model [6] is a type of snake that can trace the outline of an object from an image by minimizing an energy function associated with the current object contour. It was proposed by Tony Chan and Luminita Vese to segment objects in an image by using a combination of techniques of curve evolution, level sets, and Mumford-Shah functional for applications such as shape recognition, edge detection, and image segmentation. The C-V model can detect the contours of objects with or without gradient, unlike the original active contour model. Moreover, the model uses a level set formulation, allowing interior contours to be segmented automatically and the initial curve to be anywhere in the image.

Let Ω be a bounded open subset of $\mathbf{R}^2$ and C be an evolving curve denoting the boundary of the open subset ω of Ω, with $\partial\omega$. The direction N stands for propagating in normal direction (see Figure 4.7). In addition, let $u_0: \Omega \rightarrow \mathbf{R}$ be a given image that is formed by two regions with roughly piecewise-constant intensities. In the level set method, the curve C is represented implicitly by the zero level set of a Lipschitz function $\varphi: \Omega \rightarrow \mathbf{R}$. Therefore,

$$\begin{cases} C = \partial\omega = \{(x,y) \in \Omega : \varphi(x,y) = 0\} \\ Inside(C) = \omega = \{(x,y) \in \Omega : \varphi(x,y) > 0\} \\ Outside(C) = \Omega \setminus \overline{\omega} = \{(x,y) \in \Omega : \varphi(x,y) < 0\} \end{cases} \qquad (4.10)$$

Here, x and y are image coordinates on a given image u_0.

The energy function of the image μ_0 can be defined as

$$F(c_1, c_2, C) = \mu \cdot L(C) + v \cdot a(in(C)) = \lambda_1 \int_{in(C)} |\mu_0(x,y) - c_1|^2 dxdy$$

$$+ \lambda_2 \int_{out(C)} |\mu_0(x,y) - c_2|^2 dxdy \qquad (4.11)$$

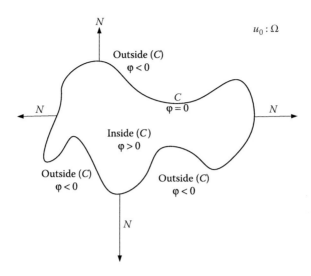

FIGURE 4.7   Curve $C = \{(x,y) : \varphi(x,y)=0\}$ propagating in all normal directions until it reaches the resting points ($\varphi=0$). (Adapted from Chan T.F. and Vese L.A. Active contours without edges. *IEEE Trans Image Process* 2001;10:266–277 © 2001 IEEE.)

where c_1, c_2 are the constants, depending on C, $L(C)$ is length of the curve C, and a is the area of the inside region, respectively. Other parameters μ, v, λ_1, λ_2 are positive fixed constants. Between the two regions on the image u_0, the boundary of the object could be detected by the zero-level curve where $\varphi(x, y) = 0$.

4.4.3   Seeded Region Growing

Seeded region growing technique [7] involves the selection of initial seed points, which is not limited to pixel-based but also allows pure and simple region-based selection. This method of image segmentation inspects adjacent pixels of initial "seed points" and then decides whether the neighboring pixels should be added to the region, beginning with the points of lowest priority. The process is iterated on using an approach similar to those used in generic data clustering algorithms. The seeded region growing algorithm is described briefly below.

4.4.3.1   Primary Concept of Seed Points

The foremost step in seeded region growing is to determine a set of initial seed points. The selection is based on criteria defined by attributes of the target regions in the image such as the brightest pixel or pixels in a certain range of gray level. The initial region starts with the exact location of these initial seeds and then adds adjacent points as new seeds, beginning with the points of lowest priority of region membership criterion. The priority is defined by a distance function; it could be, for instance, variance, color, gray level texture, motion, geometric properties, and pixel average intensity. The distance of each pixel to a contiguous region is defined by

$$R(x, \delta_i) = [I(x) - mean_{j \in \delta_i}(I(j))] \qquad (4.12)$$

where $I(x)$ is the gray image value of the point $x \in \delta$ and δ_i is the region labeled i.

All the information embedded within the image should be exploited to achieve the optimal result. For instance, one could study the histogram of the image and hence might identify a suitable threshold value of intensity. This threshold value could be then used to restrain the inclusion of undesired pixels into the region of membership.

The pros and cons of seeded region growing are summarized in Table 4.1.

4.4.3.2 Essential Issue about Seeded Region Growing

There are two main concepts about seeded region growing:

1. Selecting the correct initial seed points is extremely important; however, the selection is bound to vary from person to person or be diverse for different applications.
2. The more information (e.g., average intensity or variance of gray level image, color, and texture) about the image we have, the better the results we could achieve.

4.4.4 IMAGE DATA FUSION

4.4.4.1 Definition

Image data fusion generates a single image from a set of input images. The fused image could provide more comprehensive information for machine or man perception. Multimodality fusing data can enhance the reliability of perception by exploiting mutual information and further improve the data fusion result by offering supplementary information.

TABLE 4.1
The Pros and Cons of Seeded Region Growing Method

Pros	Cons
Simple concept and easy to be implemented	Time consuming
Multiple criteria are allowed	May not discriminate shadings in the image
Correctly discriminates the regions that have the same properties	Variation of intensity may result in oversized segmentation
Performs well in certain noise	
Provides good segmentation results when edges on original images are visibly clear	

4.4.4.2   Objectives of Image Fusion Schemes

The purpose of using image fusion schemes is to extract all essential information from the source images without introducing additional artifacts. Such objective could be achieved through producing a unified format of images that is more appropriate for computerized image processing such as feature extraction, object recognition, and segmentation. For medical applications, image fusion schemes are essential for enhancing information, and allow a better comprehension of the image datasets for clinical diagnosis.

4.5   AUTO-DETECTION OF PPA

In this section, we report the development of a system for the automatic detection of parapillary atrophy (PPA). We will first explain the key features of PPA and subsequently outline a strategy using the aforementioned image processing techniques to detect the PPA.

4.5.1   FEATURE SELECTIONS

There are three main features of the optic nerve observed from the fundus image (see Figure 4.8):

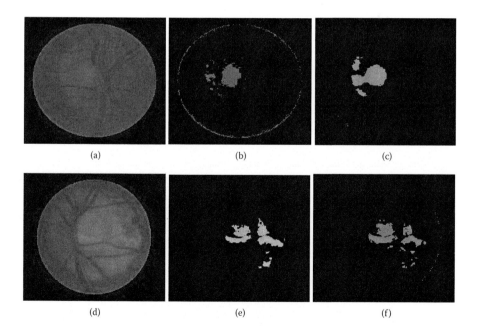

(a)	(b)	(c)
(d)	(e)	(f)

FIGURE 4.8   First row (a), (b), (c): Example images with no PPA. Second row (d), (e), (f): Example images with PPA. First column (a), (d): raw image in blue channel. Second column (b), (e): top 11% brightest spots in green channel. Third column (c), (f): top 11% brightest spots in blue channel.

1. Optic cup roughly takes up the top brightest 8% of all pixels in the case of images in the absence of PPA (see Figure 4.8b and c).
2. Optic cup and some parts of PPA takes up approximately the top brightest 11% of all pixels in the case of images in the presence of PPA (see Figure 4.8e and f).
3. PPA region often appears more obvious in blue channel and green channel, but not in all cases; therefore, the technique of image data fusion could be applied in this application to improve the detection rate.

Based on the features A, B, and C, the PPA detecting system could be designed, and its flow chart is shown in Figure 4.9. It begins with the determination of a region of interest (ROI), an area that is always bigger than the combined region of OD and PPA. Then, the First Guess (FG) procedure works on the image in the blue channel to calculate the difference of four equally divided subregions to make a preliminary determination if PPA is present. Next, our algorithm configures automatically the initial setting for the modified Chan-Vese algorithm, based on the results obtained from the FG procedure

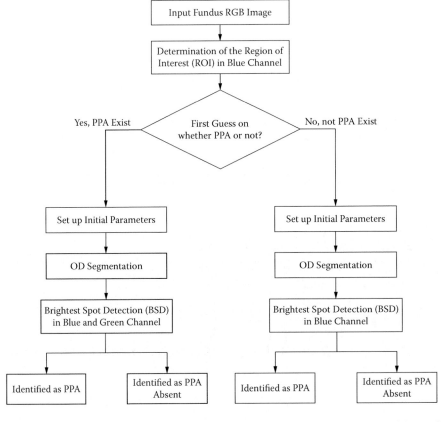

FIGURE 4.9 Flow chart for the detection of PPA using Modified Chan-Vese algorithm and Brightest Spot Detection.

and the histogram of intensity value in each subregion. The result from the modified Chan-Vese algorithm generates an estimated OD region, which is subsequently covered by a mask created by Brightest Spot Detection (BSD) procedure; at this stage, BSD detects the presence of the brightest spot outside the OD mask only in the blue channel if the initial guess was no PPA; otherwise BSD detects the presence of the brightest spot in both the blue and green channels. If the BSD detects the brightest spot in any of the channels, our PPA detection system will classify it as an image with PPA.

4.5.2 EXPERIMENTAL RESULTS

To evaluate the performance of the system, our software was tested on 102 randomly selected retinal fundus images, including fifty-nine images with PPAs, from the Lothian Birth Cohort database. Figure 4.10 shows three example detection results: (a) image without PPA (in blue channel), (b) image with PPA in green channel and (c) blue channel, respectively. The detection rate is 79.41%. To further assess the performance, we determined the specificity and sensitivity of the system under test. Sensitivity, defined as the number of true positives (TP) divided by the sum of TP and false negatives (FN), indicates how well a test is able to identify actual positives. Specificity, defined as the number of true negatives (TN) divided by the sum of TN and false positives (FP), indicates how well a test is able to correctly identify negatives. Based on the results, our system was able to achieve a specificity and sensitivity of 0.75 and 0.86, respectively.

4.6 QUANTIFICATION OF OPTIC NERVE FEATURES

Optic nerve features (e.g., OD and PPA) in the retina have been associated with eye diseases and certain eye conditions. A novel approach to automatically segment and quantify the OD and PPA has been proposed in [10]. The methodology exploits both the red and blue channels of the color image to maximize information extraction of features (PPA) while keeping interference (blood vessels) to a minimum. A combination of several techniques, including a scanning filter, thresholding, region growing, as well as a modified Chan-Vese (C-V) model with a shape constraint, is used to segment and quantify the OD and PPA.

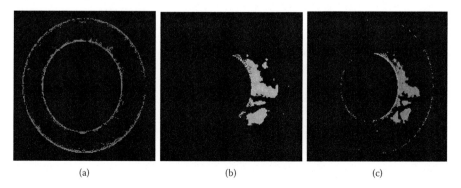

(a)   (b)   (c)

FIGURE 4.10 (a) An example result in the blue channel in the case when the fundus image has no PPA; (b) and (c): Example results in the case when the fundus image has PPA, in the green channel and blue channel, respectively.

4.6.1   OD EXTRACTION

As the OD region appears to be more or less an ellipse, Tang's model [9], which integrated the C-V model with an elliptical shape restraint, has been adopted to segment
the OD region. Tang proposed a modified C-V model, which included an elliptical
shape restraint imposed on the zero-level set of the Lipschitz function in the C-V
model. Therefore, a new "fitting energy" function E is then

$$\inf\left\{E[c_1, c_2, \varphi \mid u_0]\right\} = \alpha \int_{\Omega} (u_0 - c_1)^2 H(\varphi) + (1 - \alpha) \int_{\Omega} (u_0 - c_2)^2 (1 - H(\varphi)) \quad (4.13)$$

subject to

$$\varphi = 1 - \left[\left((x - x_0)\cos\theta + (y - y_0)\sin\theta \right)^2 / a^2 \right.$$
$$\left. + \left(-(x - x_0)\sin\theta + (y - y_0)\cos\theta \right)^2 / b^2 \right]^{1/2} \quad (4.14)$$

where Lipschitz function $\varphi: \Omega \to R$ of R_2, $\alpha > 0$ are fixed parameters and H(·) is
the Heaviside function. In addition, x_0, y_0, θ, major axis (a), minor axis (b) are the
parameters of the ellipse when $\varphi = 0$. The evolutions related to the Euler-Lagrange
equations are

$$\frac{da(t)}{dt} = -\int_{\Omega} \left[\alpha(u_0 - c_1)^2 - (1 - \alpha)(u_0 - c_2)^2 \right] \delta(\varphi) A(1/a^3) dxdy \quad (4.15)$$

$$\frac{db(t)}{dt} = -\int_{\Omega} \left[\alpha(u_0 - c_1)^2 - (1 - \alpha)(u_0 - c_2)^2 \right] \delta(\varphi) B^2(1/b^3) dxdy \quad (4.16)$$

$$\frac{dx_0(t)}{dt} = -\int_{\Omega} \left[\alpha(u_0 - c_1)^2 - (1 - \alpha)(u_0 - c_2)^2 \right] \delta(\varphi) L dxdy \quad (4.17)$$

$$\frac{dy_o(t)}{dt} = -\int_{\Omega} \left[\alpha(u_0 - c_1)^2 - (1 - \alpha)(u_0 - c_2)^2 \right] \delta(\varphi) M dxdy \quad (4.18)$$

$$\frac{d\theta(t)}{dt} = -\int_{\Omega} \left[\alpha(u_0 - c_1)^2 - (1 - \alpha)(u_0 - c_2)^2 \right] \delta(\varphi) N dxdy \quad (4.19)$$

Here, $\delta(\varphi)$ is the Dirac function and

$$c_1 = \left(\int_{\Omega} u_0 H(\varphi) dxdy \right) / \left(\int_{\Omega} H(\varphi) dxdy \right)$$

$$c_2 = \left(\int_\Omega u_0 (1 - H(\varphi)) dx dy \right) / \left(\int_\Omega (1 - H(\varphi)) dx dy \right)$$

$$A = (x - x_0)\cos\theta + (y - y_0)\sin\theta$$

$$B = -(x - x_0)\sin\theta + (y - y_0)\sin\theta$$

$$L = A\cos\theta/a^2 - B\sin\theta/b^2$$

$$M = A\sin\theta/a^2 + B\cos\theta/b^2$$

$$N = AB[1/b^2 - 1/a^2]$$

with

$$\varphi_0(x,y) = 1 - (\sqrt{(x - x_c)^2 + (y - y_c)^2})/r$$

where $r > 0$ is a constant; therefore, the steady solution of equations (4.14)–(4.19) at time T is as follows:

$$1 = \left[((x - x_0(T))\cos(\theta(T)) + (y - y_0(T))\sin(\theta(T)))^2 / (a(T))^2 \right.$$
$$\left. + (-(x - x_0(T))\sin(\theta(T)) + (y - y_0(T))\cos(\theta(T)))^2 / (b(T))^2 \right]^{1/2} \qquad (4.20)$$

An example of the OD segmentation using Tang's model is shown in Figure 4.11.

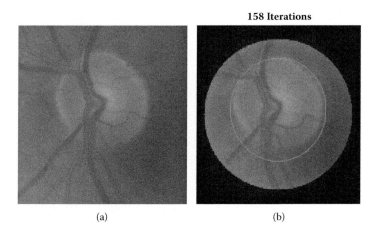

(a)   (b)

FIGURE 4.11   (a) Original fundus image. (b) A segmentation result of the optic disk using Tang's model. (Please see color insert.)

4.6.2　PPA Extraction

4.6.2.1　Methodology

The proposed algorithm [10] combined a collection of image processing techniques (Figure 4.12). Fundus images were initially preprocessed in two channels of the RGB space to reduce the interference of blood vessels and to better distinguish the regions of OD and PPA. The OD region could be reliably detected in the red channel as it appeared brighter than the rest of the image, while the blood vessels appeared least influential. The region consisting of both the OD and the PPA (hereafter referred to as the region of OD-plus-PPA) was also found to be most well defined in the blue channel. Consequently, the region of OD-plus-PPA was first segmented by a modified C-V model in the blue channel. Then, a variant of the C-V model with a shape restraint was applied to segment the OD region in the red channel. In this case, the restraint was based on an ellipse reflecting the actual shape of an OD. Removing the OD region from the region of OD-plus-PPA produced the first-order estimation of the PPA region. Moving back to the blue channel, the segmented image was then equally divided into four zones automatically.

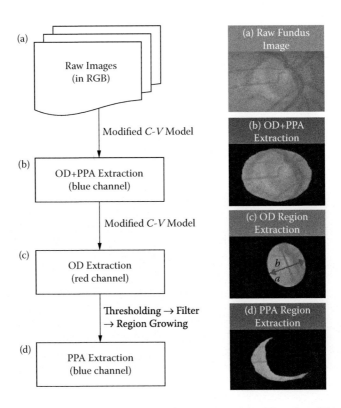

FIGURE 4.12　Flow chart shows the extraction of the PPA and the OD region. (Please see color insert.)

Based on the auto-set thresholds acquired from each zone, the image was then filtered to reduce the influence of crossing vessels and artifacts. Finally, the PPA was extracted by using a multiseed region growing method.

The following describes the details of each implemented model/filter.

4.6.2.1.1 Segmentation with Modified C-V Model

The C-V model could be used to segment the OD-plus-PPA region. However, the PPA region may sometimes appear in an irregular shape, so we had to modify slightly the rules for the evolution of the C-V model. The set of starting C-V model points, also known as the initial mask, was arranged to be in an ellipse as per normal. However, the model was then allowed to deform freely as it edged closer to the boundary of OD-plus-PPA in the subsequent iterations. This allowed the model to produce an enclosed but not necessarily elliptical shape, which was always bigger than the exact region of the OD-plus-PPA.

Next, Tang's C-V model was exploited to detect the OD region. To accurately segment the OD, we introduced two modifications to the model. First, equation (4.15) was restored to its original form (of an ellipse):

$$\frac{da(t)}{dt} = -\int_{\Omega}[\alpha(u_0 - c_1)^2 - (1-\alpha)(u_0 - c_2)^2]\delta(\varphi)A^2(1/a^3)\,dx\,dy \qquad (4.21)$$

Next, we introduced a new way to automatically detect the center of OD for more accurate segmentation. First, we divided the image into four subregions. Then we adopted the approach used in Tang's model to estimate the initial mask center (x_0, y_0). The initial function in the equation was chosen as

$$\varphi_0(x,y) = 1 - (\sqrt{(x-x_0)^2 + (y-y_0)^2})/R \qquad (4.22)$$

Here, R is the estimated radius of the OD and can be defined as

$$R = \min\{\min\{x_0/2, (w-x_0)/2\}, \min\{y_0/2, (h-y_0)/2\}\} \qquad (4.23)$$

where w and h are the width and height of the image, respectively.

Then, our algorithm calculated automatically the offset, f_x and f_y, of the initial mask center, based on the histogram of intensity value of each of the four regions. The updated initial mask center is thus:

$$(x_0', y_0') = (x_0 + f_x, y_0 + f_y) \qquad (4.24)$$

4.6.2.1.2 Auto-Set of Thresholds and Scanning Filter

To eliminate the unwanted pixels in the oversized OD-plus-PPA region, we acquired threshold values from the histogram of intensity values in the four subregions. In this context, the threshold was set by the brightest 30% of all pixels in each region. This produced a better-defined OD-plus-PPA region. We then subtracted the OD region and obtained the first order estimation of the PPA region as illustrated in Figure 4.12(f).

The PPA region is a nonhomogeneous region divided into multiple sections by a few crossing blood vessels. We therefore proposed the use of a scanning [1 × 3] filter to create a path through the vessels for the following region growing model to reach different sections of the PPA.

4.6.2.1.3   Multi-Initial Seed Region Growing

From the knowledge established in Section 4.4.3, setting both the right initial seed and distance function is one of the most important steps in PPA extraction. Our algorithm automatically placed one initial seed in each of the four subregions and set an optimal distance function for each subregion. Each seed was then allowed to grow until the regional threshold distance set by the equation has been met. Finally, we combined the results at all four subregions to produce an integrated PPA region. By combining the techniques listed above, our methodology permitted the full use of both global and local information for PPA and OD segmentation.

4.6.3   EXPERIMENTAL RESULTS

A total of ninety-four color fundus images of sixty-six subjects with PPA, including eighteen faint images, were randomly selected for test. Without knowing the segmentation results from the proposed tool, the human assessor (AL) provided the ground estimate of the OD and the PPA regions in the images. Subsequently, the area enclosed by the ground estimate was counted pixel by pixel with a commercial software package, Photoshop (Adobe Systems Inc., San Jose, CA), to quantify the size of each region. This was repeated with the segmentation results from the tool.

Figure 4.13 shows six samples from the segmentation results of the proposed tool. The first column depicts the results obtained from good-quality images while the second column depicts the results from poor-quality images. The ground estimate is drawn on the black solid line. The results of the estimated PPA and OD regions are enclosed by the spots and triangles, respectively. Meanwhile, Figure 4.14(a) compares the OD area size (in arbitrary pixel unit) based on the ground estimate and the estimated OD area size by the proposed tool in the ninety-four trials, with a line of best fit. Figure 4.14(b) shows a similar graph but for the PPA area size estimation.

The results suggest that the proposed algorithm or estimation model was able to detect the general boundary of OD and PPA. However, it tended to terminate the snake evolution prematurely on all good-quality images; hence the results appeared to underestimate the actual size. This is less consistent in the case of poor-quality images where the intensity variation/resolution in defining the boundary of OD is limited. Figure 4.13(d) shows a good example when the model missed the mark by pushing the boundary into the scleral rim. Overall, it appears that most of the estimation results in the ninety-four trials are underestimated. This is confirmed by the gradients (both <1) of the best-fit lines in Figure 4.14(a) and Figure 4.14(b). We therefore calibrated our estimation model by using these values as scaling factors. The final estimation results are plotted in Figure 4.14(c) and Figure 4.14(d). As shown, a correlation coefficient of 0.98 (max = 1) is achieved in the size estimation of both the OD and PPA regions. This suggests that our estimation is not stochastic but fairly consistent with the ground estimate defined by an ophthalmologist (i.e., the best-fit line is defined by the equation $y = x$).

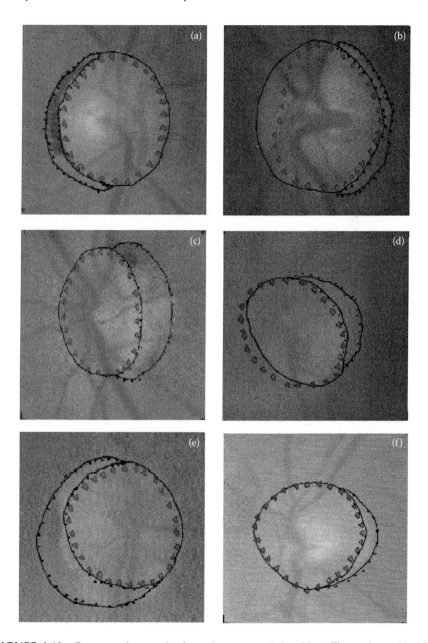

FIGURE 4.13 Segmentation results from the proposed algorithm. First column (a), (c), (e): Results from good-quality images. Second column (b), (d), (f): Results from poor-quality images. The ground estimate is drawn on the black solid line while the estimated PPA and OD regions are enclosed by the spots and the triangles, respectively. (Please see color insert.)

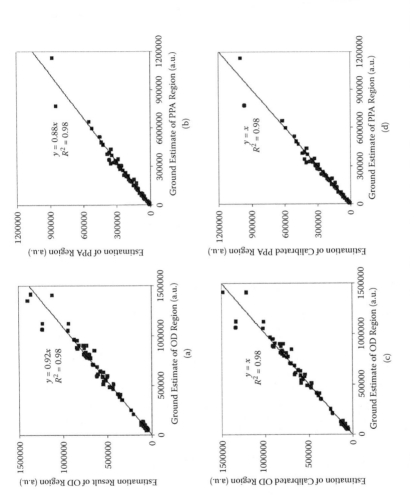

FIGURE 4.14 The correlation between the ground estimate (*x*-axis) and the results obtained by the proposed tool (*y*-axis) in quantifying the size of each region, in arbitrary pixel unit. First column (a), (b): direct estimation results from the tool; second column (c), (d): estimation results of the OD and PPA regions after calibration such that $y = x$. The correlation coefficient was found to be 0.98 in all cases. (Please see color insert.)

TABLE 4.2

The Statistical Data of Results of PPA and OD Segmentation in 94 Trials

Results	Before Calibration		After Calibration	
	PPA	OD	PPA	OD
Mean accuracy (%)	88.2	90.0	93.8	94.0
Standard deviation	5.85	6.20	5.26	5.88
Correlation coefficient, R^2	0.98	0.98	0.98	0.98

4.6.4 VALIDATION WITH GROUND ESTIMATE

In this section, we calculated the mean accuracy (M.A.) to validate our estimation model, which is given by

$$M.A. = \left(1 - \frac{\sum_{i=1}^{n}\left(\frac{S_a - S_e}{S_a}\right)}{n} \right) \times 100\% \qquad (4.25)$$

where S_a represents the actual size (ground estimate) of PPA or OD, while S_e represents the estimated size (by our model) of PPA or OD. The numerical value n is the total number of images analyzed in our experiment. Prior to calibration, our estimation model achieved a mean accuracy level of 90.0% (S.D. = 6.20) and 88.2% (S.D. = 5.85), in defining the size of OD and PPA, respectively. With the same set of color fundus images, our estimation model after calibration achieved a mean accuracy level of 94.0% (S.D. = 5.88) and 93.8% (S.D. = 5.26). Table 4.2 summarizes the estimation results.

4.7 DISCUSSION AND FUTURE DIRECTIONS

The automatic detection and the quantification of the OD in fundus images are particularly important tasks in retinal image analysis for two reasons: First, the OD has similar attributes to the PPA, both in terms of contrast and brightness, making their boundary detection a difficult task. Second, the OD is often seen as a landmark that can be used for a coarse localization of area of interest in retinal images, reducing the search space during the preprocessing stage.

In this work, we exploited a dual-channel approach with a modified C-V model to measure the size of PPA and the OD individually. The proposed algorithm particularly aims to address the aforementioned challenges on how to maximize information extraction of features (OD/PPA) while keeping interference (blood vessels) to a minimum. Our experimental results with a very wide variety of fundus images showed that the proposed algorithm not only was robust for automatic PPA shape detection and area quantification but also could provide the transverse and conjugate diameter of the OD as well as PPA-to-OD ratio, which may be useful in early detection and grading of eye conditions such as glaucoma.

In comparison to the works by other groups, there are three main merits of the proposed tool. First, our software tool could measure the PPA region automatically in two-dimensional color fundus images. This is the first tool which could achieve that without any human intervention. In the previous studies, investigators were required to manually measure the PPA region in either 2D images [11–17] or 3D images [18] which were constructed by a specially written computer planimetry program. (*Note:* direct images of the objects are preferred by the ophthalmologists.) Second, the proposed tool could not only detect the OD region and estimate its size but also provide readings of its transverse and conjugate diameter—two commonly used parameters in retinal image analysis. Using this tool, we could potentially further derive the normalized PPA size (i.e., the ratio between the PPA and the OD size) to explore its association with different eye diseases or conditions and establish a better understanding about the significance of the PPA development. Third, this tool has been automated, which means that not only could it reduce the dependence on the human assessor and thus avoid problems associated with human errors such as fatigue, it could also be more cost-effective for larger-scale population-based screening.

There remain some limitations within our method, however: First, our software stopped at undesired points upon encountering irregular dark pixels prior to the OD boundary in good-quality images and less consistently in poor-quality images. This results in underestimation of the actual size. Second, the proposed algorithm estimates the sizes of OD and PPA regions, providing a means to measure the extent of PPA. It would be ideal if the software could also define the absolute shapes allowing the patterns in PPA progression to be studied in different eye conditions. One possible way to address the above limitations would be to take into consideration additional local information (e.g., texture and variance of gray level image) and further exploit the image fusion from multiple channels.

4.8 CONCLUSION

This chapter first introduces image processing techniques applicable for color fundus images. Subsequently, a practical example of object detection and segmentation is presented. In this case, the object is the region of parapillary atrophy (PPA) in the retina. As discussed, the accurate segmentation of the optic disk (OD) is important as it may affect the detection rate and the quantification of the PPA. The algorithm or estimation model described in Section 4.6.2 after calibration achieved a mean accuracy of level 94.0% (S.D. = 5.88) and 93.8% (S.D. = 5.26) in defining the size of OD and PPA, respectively compared with the "gold standard" of an experienced human assessor (AL). Our model also showed high reliability in estimating the size, with correlation coefficient reaching 0.98 for both cases (OD and PPA). Moreover, our method could also provide researchers and ophthalmologists additional information, namely transverse and conjugate diameter of the OD as well as the sizes and the ratio between the OD and PPA. Further work to test out this method on a larger sample set is indicated, in an effort to develop automated screening systems for diagnosis of eye conditions associated with PPA in the community.

REFERENCES

1. Damms, T., and Dannheim, F. Sensitivity and specificity of optic disc parameters in chronic glaucoma. *Invest. Ophthalmol. Vis. Sci.* 1993; 34:2246–2250.
2. Walter, T., Klein, J.-C., Massin, P., and Erginay, A. A contribution of image processing to the diagnosis of diabetic retinopathy—Detection of exudates in color fundus images of the human retina. *IEEE Trans. Med. Imaging.* 2002; 21:1236–1243.
3. Deary, I.J., Gow, A.J., Taylor, M.D., et al. The Lothian Birth Cohort 1936: A study to examine influences on cognitive ageing from age 11 to age 70 and beyond," *BMC Geriatr.*, 2007; 7:28.
4. Gonzalez, R.C., Woods, R.E., and Eddins, S.L. *Digital image processing using MATLAB.* Upper Saddle River, NJ: Prentice Hall, 2004.
5. Kass, M., Witkin, A., and Terzopoulos, D. Snakes: Active contour models. *Int. J. Computer Vis.,* 1987; 1:321–331.
6. Chan, T.F., and Vese, L.A. Active contours without edges. *IEEE Trans. Image Processing,* 2001; 10:266–277.
7. Adams, R., and Bischof, L. Seeded region growing. *IEEE Trans. Pattern Analysis Machine Intelligence,* 1994; 16:641–647.
8. Lu, C.-K., Tang, T.B., Laude, A., Deary, I.J., Dhillon, B., and Murray, A.F. Automatic parapapillary atrophy shape detection and quantification in color fundus images, *IEEE Biomedical Circuits Systems Conf, 3–5th November 2010,* Paphos, Cyprus, pp. 86–89.
9. Tang, Y., Li, X., von Freyberg, A., and Goch, G. Automatic segmentation of the papilla in a fundus image based on the C-V model and a shape restraint. *Proc. 18th Int. Conf. Pattern Recognition,* 2006; 183–186, Piscataway, NJ: IEEE Press.
10. Lu, C.-K., Tang, T.B., Laude, A., Deary, I.J., Dhillon, B., and Murray, A.F. Quantification of parapapillary atrophy and optic disc, *Invest. Ophthalmol. Vis. Sci.,* 2011; 52:4671–4677.
11. Healey, P.R., Mitchell, P., Gilbert, C.E., et al. The inheritance of peripapillary atrophy. *Invest Ophthalmol. Vis. Sci.,* 2007; 48:2529–2534.
12. Tezel, G., Kolker, A.E., Kass, M.A., et al. Parapapillary chorioretinal atrophy in patients with ocular hypertension. I. An evaluation as a predictive factor for the development of glaucomatous damage. *Arch. Ophthalmol.,* 1997; 115:1503–1508.
13. Honrubia, F., and Calonge, B. Evaluation of the nerve fiber layer and peripapillary atrophy in ocular hypertension. *International Ophthalmol.,* 1989; 13:57–62.
14. Xu, L., Wang, Y., Yang, H., and Jonas, J.B. Differences in parapapillary atrophy between glaucomatous and normal eyes: the Beijing Eye Study. *Am. J. Ophthalmol.,* 2007; 144:541–546.
15. Uhm, K.B., Lee, D.Y., Kim, J.T., and Hong, C. Peripapillary atrophy in normal and primary open-angle glaucoma. *Korean J. Ophthalmol,* 1998; 12:37–50.
16. Laemmer, R., Horn, F.K., Viestenz, A., Link, B., Juenemann, A.G., and Mardin, C.Y. Measurement of autofluorescence in the parapapillary atrophic zone in patients with ocular hypertension. *Graefe's Arch. Clin. Exp. Ophthalmol.,* 2007; 245:51–58.
17. Kolář, R., Laemmer, R., Jan, J., and Mardin, C.Y. The segmentation of zones with increased autofluorescence in the zone of parapapillary atrophy. *Physiol. Meas.,* 2009; 30:505–516.
18. Uchida, H., Ugurlu, S., and Caprioli, J. Increasing peripapillary atrophy is associated with progressive glaucoma. *Ophthalmology,* 1998; 105:1541–1545.

5 A Survey of Instruments for Eye Diagnostics with Special Emphasis on Glaucoma Detection

Teik-Cheng Lim, U. Rajendra Acharya,
and Subhagata Chattopadhyay

CONTENTS

5.1 INTRODUCTION

Glaucoma is a form of ophthalmic disorder where the optic nerve suffers permanent damage, leading to progressive loss of vision and, if left untreated, blindness [1]. The progression is irreversible in nature, emphasizing the importance of adopting serious screening procedures to prevent blindness [2]. The pathophysiology of this disorder is the blockade of aqueous humor flow leading to a condition known as *ocular hypertension* [3]. Progressive increment of the stagnant aqueous humor level puts pressure on the optic nerve and it is then damaged, causing blindness [3]. Loss of optic nerve denotes the loss of retinal ganglion cells producing optic neuropathy [3]. There are two main types of glaucoma—*open angle* and *closed angle*. Open-angle type progresses with a slower pace; closed angle is much faster [4]. However, open-angle glaucoma is considered more dangerous than closed angle, because it is often asymptomatic, while the latter causes eye pain [4]. With open-angle glaucoma, the patient fails to recognize that there is a problem prior to losing his or her vision due to permanent damage of the optic nerve.

The incidence of glaucoma is age dependent. Older people suffer more than the young population [5]. It forms the second most common form of age-related blindness in the world, after cataracts [6]. Glaucoma is much more serious than cataracts due to its irreversibility. As a consequence of this irreversibility, timely diagnosis is crucial in damage control and good management of the glaucomatous condition. This chapter describes various instruments used for the screening and diagnosis of glaucoma. The following instruments are surveyed in individual sections:

Tonometers

- Air-puff tonometers
- Applanation tonometers
- Impression tonometers
- Rebound tonometers
- Pneumatonometer
- Dynamic contour tonometers (DCT)
- Optical coherence tomography (OCT) tonometers

Gonioscopes

- Koeppe gonioscopes
- Goldmann gonioscopes
- Zeiss gonioscopes

Imaging techniques

- Optical coherence tomography
- Scanning laser polarimetry
- Scanning laser ophthalmoscopy

Corneal pachymetry

5.2 TONOMETERS

Tonometers are instruments for measuring intraocular pressure (the fluid pressure in the eye).

5.2.1 Air-Puff or Noncontact Tonometers

Air-puff tonometers obtain intraocular pressure by measuring the cornea deflection as a consequence of air-puff, that is, a sudden shot of pressurized air to the eye (see Figure 5.1). The Pulsair tonometer has a compressor, which is connected to a hand-held air gun. When held perpendicularly to and at a correct distance from the cornea, the Keeler Pulsair tonometer releases an air impulse. This Pulsair tonometer obtains the required pressure for depressing the cornea within a circular area of diameter 3 mm [7,8]. A similar air-puffing working principle applies to the Reichert tonometer [9,10].

5.2.2 Applanation Tonometers

Applanation tonometers obtain intraocular tension by measuring the required pressure for flattening a small region of the cornea (Figures 5.2 and 5.3). These include the Goldmann tonometer [11,12], which measures the pressure for flattening a circular area of diameter 3.06 mm, the Maklakov tonometer [13,14], the Perkins tonometer [15,16], and the tonomat tonometer [17,18]. The Goldmann tonometer is the most commonly used tonometer for measuring intraocular pressure and it is considered the gold standard, because results of newly developed tonometers are compared with it. (In some literature and patents, the Maklakov tonometer is classified under impression tonometer.)

5.2.3 Impression Tonometers

Impression tonometers obtain intraocular pressure by applying pressure directly on the eyeball. They measure the indentation depth via application of a predetermined force. An example of an impression tonometer is the Schiotz tonometer [19,20], which uses a plunger to gently press the patient's cornea. The intraocular pressure is implied from the applied force for flattening the cornea. Impression tonometers are also called indentation tonometers. See Figures 5.4 and 5.5.

5.2.4 Rebound Tonometer

A rebound tonometer has an induction coil to magnetize a metal probe with a polymer tip. Upon magnetization, the probe hits the cornea and then bounces back. As the probe moves back into the device, an induction current is generated. The intraocular

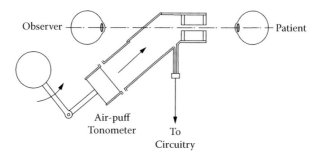

FIGURE 5.1 A non-contact tonometer. (Adapted from N. Suzuki, M. Nakao, and T. Miwa, Non-contact type tonometer. U.S. 6537215 B2 (2002), showing the air-puff mechanism.)

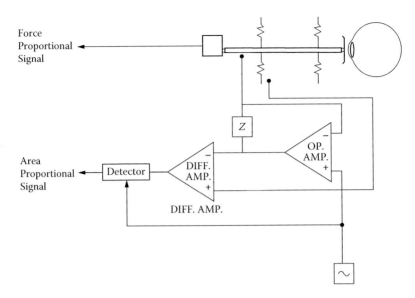

FIGURE 5.2 A typical applanation tonometer, showing some circuitry. (Adapted from G.J. Eilers, Automatic applanation tonometer. U.S. Patent US4621644, 1986.)

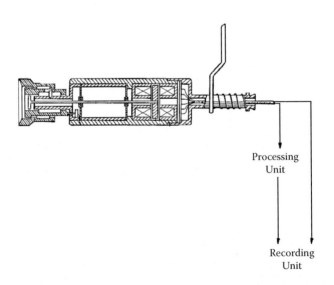

FIGURE 5.3 Another applanation tonometer, showing the mechanical parts. (Adapted from M.P. Kozon, N.V. Kudashov, J.I. Sakharov, S.N. Fedorov, Applanation tonometer. U.S. Patent 4766904, 1988.)

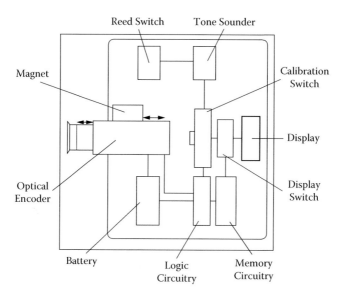

FIGURE 5.4   An impression or indentation tonometer. Shown here is the circuitry. (Adapted from C.R. Munnerlyn and T.N. Clapham, Indentation tonometer. U.S. Patent 4192317, 1980.)

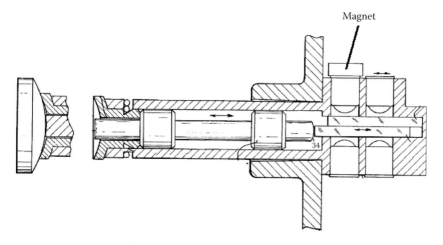

FIGURE 5.5   An impression or indentation tonometer. Shown here are the mechanical parts. (Adapted from C.R. Munnerlyn and T.N. Clapham, Indentation tonometer. U.S. Patent 4192317, 1980.)

pressure is calculated from the generated induction current [21] (Figure 5.6). A commercialized rebound tonometer is the Icare® tonometer [22].

5.2.5 PNEUMATONOMETER

In a pneumatonometer, an accurately regulated flow of clean air enters a piston, which floats on an air bearing. A fenestrated membrane at the end of the piston is subjected to forces from the airflow and the cornea. The intraocular pressure is obtained at force equilibrium [23,24]. As shown in Figure 5.7, P1 is air pressure within the probe, P2 is the intraocular pressure, A_T is the total airflow entering the

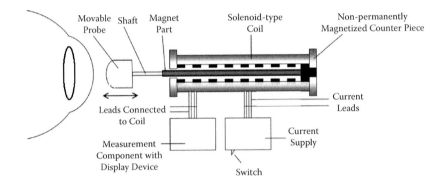

FIGURE 5.6 A rebound tonometer invention. (Adapted from A. Kontiola, Apparatus for measuring intraocular pressure. U.S. Patent 6093147, 2000).

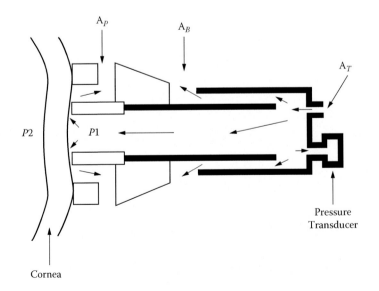

FIGURE 5.7 Schematic of a pneumatonometer. (Adapted from Morgan et al. [24].)

probe, A_B is proportion of airflow escaping from the "air bearing," and A_P is proportion of airflow escaping from the probe head [24].

5.2.6 DYNAMIC CONTOUR TONOMETER

The dynamic contour tonometer (DCT) [25,26] applies the concept of contour matching rather than flattening a region of the cornea. In this way, the influence of cornea modulus is reduced. At present, the PASCAL tonometer is the only commercial tonometer based on DCT. An embedded pressure sensor in its tonometer tip, with concave radius of curvature 1.05 cm, touches the cornea with a force equivalent to one gram weight (Figure 5.8). The force is kept constant when the tip scans across the cornea through an electrical feedback; that is, it moves forward toward the cornea when a drop in force is detected and retracts away from the cornea when the detected force is higher than one gram weight. The cornea convex radius of curvature approximates 1.05 cm when the intraocular pressure matches the pressure of the tonometer tip.

Figure 5.9 shows a setup of a DCT comparative study, with (1) dynamic contour tonometer (DCT) base station, (2) DCT recharge unit, (3) DCT pressure-sensitive tip, (4) Goldmann applanation tonometry tip holder mounted at a slitlamp, (5) human cadaver eye, anterior chamber filled with 20% dextran, (6) eye holder with moisturized gauze, (7) pressure transducer, (8) manometric device, (9–11) tubing system filled with balanced salt solution, (9) reference tube open to atmospheric pressure, (10) bottle with isotonic sodium chloride solution, variable height, (11) stopcocks with syringes to bleed air bubbles from the tubing system. CCW 3-6 indicates that items labeled 3, 4, 5, and 6 were rotated 90° during the actual measurements of intraocular pressure with all of the instruments but are shown in the displayed orientation for simplicity of diagram [27].

5.2.7 OCT TONOMETERS

The Optical Coherence Tomography (OCT) tonometer is a type of noncontact tonometer currently in the development stage. Unlike the usual OCT used for

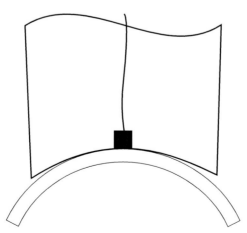

FIGURE 5.8   Close-up view of DCT.

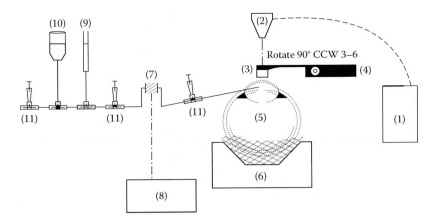

FIGURE 5.9 Dynamic contour tonometry apparatus. (Adapted from [27].)

obtaining detailed retina images in other areas of ophthalmology or any other biological tissues, the OCT tonometer obtains the change in cornea curvature resulting
from application of air pressure or sound wave. The working mechanism of the OCT
tonometer is the same as that for the general OCT, which is presented later.

5.3 GONIOSCOPY

The gonioscope is used for checking the anterior chamber of the eye [28–30].
The physical property measured is the iridocorneal angle via mirror(s) or prism
(Figure 5.10). In this way, ophthalmologists can check whether the drainage angle
is open or closed. Buildup of intraocular pressure occurs for closed drainage angle.

5.3.1 Koeppe Gonioscopy

The Koeppe goniolens is placed directly onto the patient's cornea with a lubricating
fluid to prevent damage on the cornea's surface. The patient must lie down during the
Koeppe gonioscopy procedure.

5.3.2 Goldmann Gonioscopy

The Goldmann gonioscope uses a mirror to direct light from the iridocorneal angle
to the ophthalmologist's view. The patient can sit upright during the Goldmann gonioscopy procedure.

5.3.3 Zeiss Gonioscopy

The Zeiss gonioscope uses prisms instead of mirror for directing light. The
four prisms enable all four quadrants of the patient's iridocorneal angle to be
visualized.

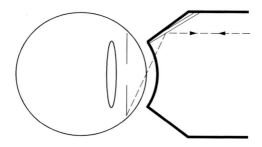

FIGURE 5.10   Schematic of a typical gonioscope.

5.4   IMAGING TECHNIQUES

5.4.1   OPTICAL COHERENCE TOMOGRAPHY

Optical coherence tomography is an optical technique for constructing three-dimensional images of biological tissues [31–33]. Unlike the OCT tonometry, which is in the development stage, the general OCT is an established medical imaging technique. The OCT technique has gained attention due to its attractive attributes:

1. No harmful radiation
2. No requirement for sample preparation—measurement can be done on life subjects, i.e., *in vivo*
3. Instant imaging

The working mechanism of OCT is on the basis of optical coherence. The beam coming out from a low coherent light source is split into two parts, one of which is reflected from the tissue to be imaged while the other is reflected by a reference mirror. In this way, scattered light from the tissue is left out. During scanning, interference of recombined light allows a three-dimensional image to be constructed. Shown in Figure 5.11 is a typical single point OCT setup, which can perform imaging of tissues up to a depth of 0.3 cm. Other types of OCT include the full-field OCT, Fourier-domain OCT, and swept-source OCT.

5.4.2   SCANNING LASER POLARIMETRY

Scanning laser polarimetry (SLP) adopts polarized laser to obtain the thickness of the retinal nerve fiber layer (RNFL) to detect glaucoma. Specifically, SLP provides RNFL measurements via obtaining the polarized change (i.e., retardation) that occurs when a beam of light comes across materials with birefringent (double refraction) properties, such as RNFL. The birefringent property in RNFL is due to the parallel array of microtubules inside the axon bundles.

The polarized light in SLP is split into two parts before entering the eye. Thereafter the polarized light is projected on the surface of the retina and double crosses the RNFL. A phase shift (or retardation) occurs when the two parts of the split light travel at different speeds. Theoretically, the extent of retardation is in proportion to the thickness of the RNFL. This theory has been confirmed by

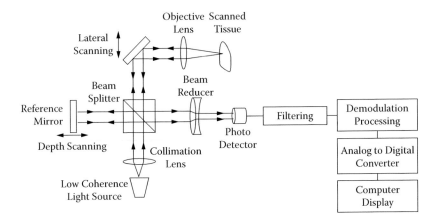

FIGURE 5.11 A typical setup of an OCT.

microscopic measurements of RNFL thickness [34,35]. Figure 5.12 shows a setup for a high-resolution low-noise optical polarimeter.

5.4.3 SCANNING LASER OPHTHALMOSCOPY

Scanning laser ophthalmoscopy (SLO) is based on confocal laser scanning microscopy (Figure 5.13) for examining the eye tissues such as cornea and retina. Since the SLO is used for imaging the retina, a number of eye diseases can be detected using SLO:

1. Macular degeneration
2. Glaucoma
3. Other retina degeneration

Figures 5.14 and 5.15 show some patented scanning laser ophthalmoscopes.

The SLO uses mirrors that can scan the region of interest of the retina both horizontally and vertically, in order to construct raster images that can be viewed from the computer screen or TV monitor. Although SLO has its advantages in that it allows real-time imaging, the SLO suffers from optical aberrations including reflections from the cornea and eye astigmatism. To address this shortcoming, the Adaptive Optics SLO was developed to observe a distinct layer of interest at microscopic level. A typical setup of the Adaptive Optics SLO is shown in Figure 5.16.

5.5 CORNEAL PACHYMETRY

Corneal pachymetry refers to a group of diagnostic techniques (including ultrasound, confocal microscopy, optical biometry, OCT, etc.) for measuring the corneal thickness.

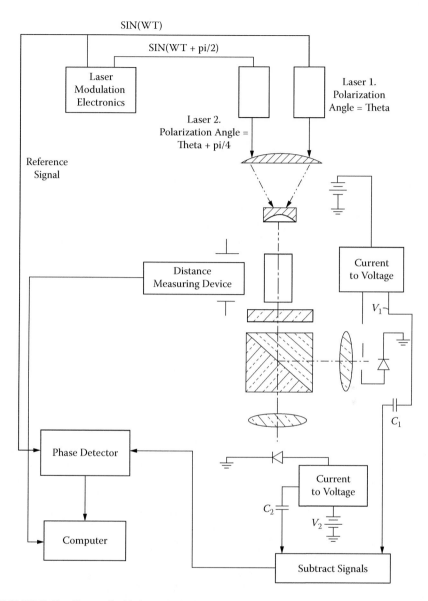

FIGURE 5.12 Setup of a high-resolution low-noise optical polarimeter. (Adapted from J.D. Bergman, High-resolution low-noise optical polarimeter, US Patent 5,477,327, 1995.)

An investigation by the Ocular Hypertension Study (OHTS) in 2002 found that corneal pachymetry, in combination with established intraocular pressure measurement techniques, is able to accurately detect the early stage of glaucoma. Resulting from this report and later studies, corneal pachymetry is widely adopted by researchers and clinicians to detect early-stage glaucoma.

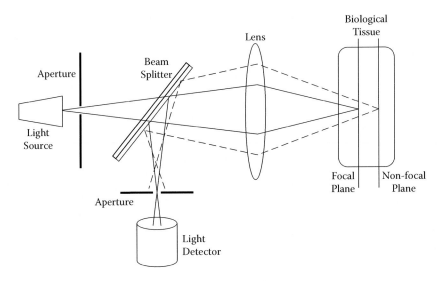

FIGURE 5.13   Working principle of confocal microscopy, which the SLO is based upon.

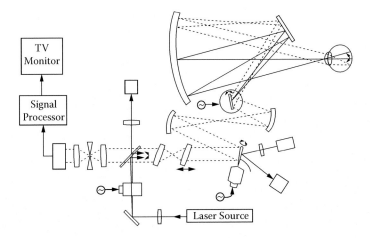

FIGURE 5.14   A scanning laser ophthalmoscope. (Adapted from K. Kobayashi, US Patent 5,430,509, 1995.)

5.6   CONCLUSIONS

Various techniques for diagnosis of glaucoma have been surveyed. They are broadly categorized under the mechanical techniques (or IOP measurement techniques) by tonometry, the optical techniques (or iridocorneal angle observation techniques) by gonioscopy, and the imaging techniques. Corneal pachymetry measures central cornea thickness because the apparent IOP measurement is overestimated by cornea of higher thickness, higher curvature, and higher elastic modulus.

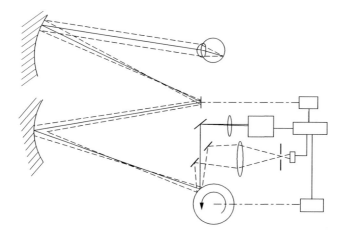

FIGURE 5.15 A scanning laser ophthalmoscope. (Adapted from A. Manivannan and P.F. Sharp, US Patent 6,099,127, 2000.)

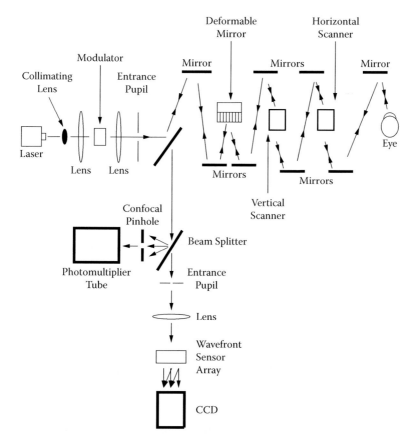

FIGURE 5.16 A typical Adaptive Optics SLO setup.

REFERENCES

1. R.P. Finger, D.G. Kupitz, F.G. Holz, B. Balasubramaniam, R.V. Ramani, E.L. Lamoureux, and E. Fenwick, The impact of the severity of vision loss on vision-related quality of life in India—An evaluation of the IND-VFQ-33, *Invest. Ophthalmol. Vis. Sci.*, DOI: 10.1167/iovs.11-7388 (2011).
2. H. Taylor, Glaucoma screening in the real world, *Ophthalmology* 118(5), 1008 (2011).
3. Y. Bai, D. Sivori, S.B. Woo, K.E. Neet, S.F. Lerner, and U. Saragovi, During glaucoma α2-macroglobulin accumulates in aqueous humor, and binds to nerve growth factor neutralizing neuroprotection, *Invest. Ophthalmol. Vis. Sci.*, DOI: 10.1167/iovs.10-6691 (2011).
4. N. MacReady, Study identifies glaucoma progression risk factors, *Arch. Ophthalmol.*, 129, 562–568 (2011).
5. W. Song, L. Shan, F. Cheng, P. Fan, L. Zhang, W. Qu, Q. Zhang, and H. Yuan, Prevalence of glaucoma in a rural Northern China adult population: A population-based survey in Kailu Country, Inner Mongolia, *Ophthalmology*, DOI: 10.1016/j.ophtha.2011.02.050 (2011).
6. http://www.who.int/bulletin/volumes/82/11/en/844.pdf [last accessed on 04/07/2011].
7. L. Bonomi, S. Baravelli, C. Cobbe and L. Tomazzoli, Evaluation of Keeler Pulsair non-contact tonometry: Reliability and reproducibility, *Graefe's Arch. Clin. Exp. Ophthalmol.* 229, 210–212 (1991).
8. T.A. Armstrong, Evaluation of the Tono-Pen and the Pulsair tonometers, *Am. J. Ophthalmol.* 109, 716–720 (1990).
9. B. Brown and D. Darin, Comparison of Keeler and Reichert non-contact tonometers, *Clin. Expt. Optometry* 72, 98–101 (1989).
10. J. Jorge, J.A. Díaz-Rey, J.M. González-Méijome, J.B. Almeida, and M.A. Parafita, Clinical performance of the Reichert AT550: A new non-contact tonometer, *Ophthalmic and Physiological Optics* 22, 560–564 (2002).
11. H. Goldmann and T. Schmidt, Über Applanationstonometrie, *Ophthalmologica* 134, 221–242 (1957).
12. M.J. Moseley, N.M. Evans, and A.R. Fielder, Comparison of a new non-contact tonometer with Goldmann applanation, *Eye* (London) 3, 332–337 (1989).
13. A. Posner, An evaluation of the Maklakov applanation tonometer, *Eye, Ear, Nose & Throat Monthly* 41, 377–378 (1962).
14. W.G. Kett, Tonometry: A case for the Maklakov tonometer, *Aust. J. Optometry* 33, 107–108 (1961).
15. B.R. Hammond and P. Bhattacherjee, Calibration of the Alcon applanation pneumatonograph and Perkins tonometer for use in rabbits and cats, *Curr. Eye Res.* 3, 1155–1159 (1984).
16. J. Wallace and H.G. Lovell, Perkins hand-held applanation tonometer: A clinical evaluation, *British Med. J.* 52, 568–572 (1968).
17. A. Posner and R. Inglima, The tonomat applanation tonometer, *Eye, Ear, Nose & Throat Monthly* 46, 996–1000 (1967).
18. A. Posner and R. Inglima, The tonomat applanation tonometer: A comparison with the Goldmann applanation tonometer and the applanometer, *Eye, Ear, Nose & Throat Monthly* 48, 189–194 (1969).
19. M.F. Armaly, Schiotz tonometer calibration and applanation tonometry, *Arch. Ophthalmol.* 64, 426–432 (1960).
20. R.A. Moses, Theory of the Schiotz tonometer and its empirical calibration, *Trans. Am. Ophthalmol. Soc.* 69, 494–562 (1971).
21. L.N. Davies, H. Bartlett, E.A.H. Mallen, and J.S. Wolffsohn, Clinical evaluation of rebound tonometer, *Acta Ophthalmologica* 84, 206–209 (2006).

22. C. Garcia-Resua, J.M. Gonzalez-Meijome, J. Gilino, and E.Y.P. Vilar, Accuracy of the new Icare rebound tonometer vs. other portable tonometers in healthy eyes, *Optometry and Visual Science* 83, 102–107 (2006).
23. S. Wittenberg, Evaluation of the pneuma-tonometer, *Am. J. Optom. Physiol. Opt.* 55, 337–347 (1978).
24. A.J. Morgan, J. Harper, S.L. Hosking, and B. Gilmartin. The effect of corneal thickness and corneal curvature on pneumatonometer measurements, *Curr. Eye Res.* 25, 107–112 (2002).
25. H.E. Kanngiesser, C. Kniestedt, and Y. Robert, Dynamic contour tonometry: Presentation of a new tonometer, *J. Glaucoma* 14, 344–350 (2005).
26. O.S. Punjabi, C. Kniestedt, R.L. Stamper, and S.C. Lin, Dynamic contour tonometry: Principle and use, *Clin. Exp. Ophthalmol.* 34, 837–840 (2006).
27. C. Kniestedt, M. Nee, and R.L. Stamper, Dynamic contour tonometry: A comparative study on human cadaver eyes, *Acta Ophthalmol.* 122, 1287–1293 (2004).
28. J. Rourke, M. Lal, and W. Kalwat, Weightless Koeppe gonioscopy, *Arch. Ophthalmol.* 99, 1646 (1981).
29. R.N. Shaffer and R.L. Tour, A comparative study of gonioscopic methods, *Trans. Am. Ophthalmol. Soc.* 53, 189–208 (1955).
30. P.L. Kaufman, M.W. Neider, and W.H. Pankonin, Slitlamp mount for Zeiss gonioscopy lens, *Arch. Ophthalmol.* 99, 1455 (1981).
31. J.G. Fujimoto, Optical coherence tomography, Comptes Rendus de l'Académie des Sciences—Series IV, *Physics* 2, 1099–1111 (2001).
32. A.F. Fercher, W. Drexler, C.K. Hitzenberger, and T. Lasser, Optical coherence tomography—principles and applications, *Rep. Prog. Phys.* 66, 239–303 (2003).
33. A.G. Podoleanu, Optical coherence tomography, *British Journal of Radiology* 78, 976–988 (2005).
34. R.N. Weinreb, A.W. Dreher, A. Coleman, H. Quigley, B. Shaw, and K. Reiter, Histopathologic validation of Fourier-ellipsometry measurements of retinal nerve fiber layer thickness, *Arch. Ophthalmol.* 108, 557–560 (1990).
35. J.E. Morgan, A. Waldock, G. Jeffrey, and A. Cowey. Retinal nerve fiber layer polarimetry: Histological and clinical comparison, *Br. J. Ophthalmol.* 82, 684–690 (1998).

6 Imaging Modalities and Medical Applications in the Ocular Surface

A. Petznick, W. Lan, S. Y. Lee, and L. Tong

CONTENTS

6.1 INTRODUCTION

Ocular surface diseases refer to pathological conditions involving the anterior layers of the eye such as microbial infections, allergies, or scarring diseases. Collectively, these are very prevalent in Asia and the rest of the world, causing morbidity and blindness (Whitcher, Srinivasan et al. 2001; Lam, Houang et al. 2002). Ocular surface diseases present with various clinical signs that can be visualized by a medical practitioner in an ophthalmic clinic. However, many of these signs are either subtle or difficult to quantify, and a clinician often needs to know if these signs are improving or worsening so that appropriate treatment can be administered (Behrens, Doyle et al. 2006; DEWS 2007a).

In multifactorial conditions such as dry eye disease or dysfunctional tear syndrome, there is no single gold standard diagnostic criterion (DEWS 2007c). Therefore, imaging modalities can contribute immensely to the diagnosis and management of ocular surface diseases. A recent article discussed the newer diagnostic methods used in dry eye disease, and many of the methods mentioned require imaging (Yokoi, Komuro et al. 2005). An article on tear film assessment using noninvasive methods has also been published (Yokoi and Komuro 2004). In the latter article, imaging modalities such as videomeniscometry, interferometry, and laser meibometry have been described.

A previous review on anterior segment imaging has introduced important concepts such as how resolution can affect image quality, and how digital slit-lamp photography can be used to document clinical signs such as conjunctival hyperemia (Wolffsohn and Peterson 2006). The paper also discussed techniques such as the Scheimpflug technique and corneal topography, which, in the interest of space, will not be elaborated upon in this chapter. Much of the published literature on ocular imaging has focused on posterior segment anatomy, anterior segment structures relevant to glaucoma, and orbital details with computed tomography or magnetic resonance (Malhotra, Minja et al. 2011). Since this chapter is concerned with ocular surface imaging, these techniques will not be discussed. Moreover, imaging can be used to study tear fluid dynamics and wavefront aberrations (Maeda 2011); wavefront aberrations are a mathematical description of the optical imperfection of the eye. Imaging may be useful in patients with dry eye or patients undergoing custom refractive surgery, where the result of the imaging is taken into consideration for the medical treatment decision.

The outcomes of any clinical tools used, especially imaging tools, should be properly documented. Such documentation facilitates interpretation of whether the test result is normal or abnormal. Such an approach is more objective than traditional recordings or manual drawings, which are less reproducible and less precise.

In inflammatory diseases of the cornea—for example, Mooren's ulcer (Kafkala, Choi et al. 2006), which causes a painful inflammatory melt of the cornea—color imaging of the cornea may be used to record the progression of the disease. When there is an obvious progression, a clinical decision may be made to increase or commence more aggressive immunosuppression (Wakefield and Robinson 1987). During the examination of a patient who underwent a surgical procedure, such as Descemet's stripping endothelial keratoplasty (Ghaznawi and Chen 2010), anterior segment optical coherence tomography (ASOCT) can be used to record the position of the graft within the anterior chamber. This is crucial, because the transparency of the cornea depends on the adherence or apposition of the implanted corneal endothelium against the host or recipient cornea. Only when the implant is positioned correctly can the pump function of the endothelium keep the cornea dehydrated and transparent (Bourne 2010).

The clinical utility of any imaging modality is not solely about its technical performance. In practice, it is also about factors such as convenience, cost–benefit ratio, ease of interpretation of the results, availability of the tool, likelihood of adverse effects, and time required to perform the test (Shen and Hwang 2010). In some countries, health delivery may depend on electronic referrals by optometrists to other health care services (Cameron, Ahmed et al. 2009). Since images can be transmitted digitally, imaging may play a bigger role in the future. In this chapter, we explore the clinical utility of some imaging tools available for the assessment of ocular surface diseases (see summary in Table 6.1). Toward the end of this chapter, we also briefly describe the use of imaging in the study of ocular surface that may enable us

TABLE 6.1
Clinical Use and Limitations of Imaging Modalities

Imaging Modality	Clinical Use	Advantages	Limitations
Topography-based imaging	Evaluation of corneal radius and thickness Screening and diagnosis of keratoconus Assessment of tear film quality	Noninvasive, objective measurement Highly accurate for tear breakup time	Costly equipment
Angiography	Observation of blood flow in ocular surface	Visualization and differentiation of blood flow *Indocyanine-green angiography* No leakage from normal blood vessels, which enables thorough examination *Fluorescein angiography* Quick visualization of changes in blood perfusion	Invasiveness due to intravenous administration of dyes with discomfort for patients Possible allergic reaction *Indocyanine-green angiography* Possible allergic reaction to iodine *Fluorescein angiography* Fast leakage from normal blood vessels, which reduces necessary examination times
Confocal microscopy (CM)	*In vivo* clinical imaging of ocular surface structures and optical sectioning of human eye	*In vivo* usage High magnification and resolution Detailed visualization of cornea, conjunctiva and meibomian glands	Possible discomfort to patients Costly equipment
Meibomian gland imaging	Visualization of meibomian gland embedded in the eyelids Diagnosis of MGD	*Meibography* Mounting onto slit-lamp biomicroscope Affordable equipment	*Meibography* Decreased image quality due to overexposure or reflection Eversion of eyelid with discomfort to patients

(Continued)

TABLE 6.1 (CONTINUED)
Clinical Use and Limitations of Imaging Modalities

Imaging Modality	Clinical Use	Advantages	Limitations
		Meibography using confocal microscopy	*Meibography using confocal microscopy*
		High magnification	Invasive as objective touches the eyelid with possible discomfort to patients
		Detailed imaging of glandular ducts and acinar cells	Costly equipment
Tear interferometry	Diagnosis of abnormal tear film	Noninvasive	Constant temperature and humidity required
		Fast measurement	Costly equipment
		Detailed assessment of tear film quality	
Anterior segment optical coherence tomography	Diagnosis of abnormalities in cornea and tear film	Noninvasive	Constant temperature and humidity required for tear film evaluation
			External analysis tools
			Costly equipment
Ocular thermography	Measurement of ocular surface temperature	Noninvasive	External analysis tools
	Diagnosis of tear abnormalities using tear evaporation	Fast measurement	Costly equipment
		Calculation of tear evaporation	

to understand basic pathology of diseases. For example, epifluorescence intravital microscopy in murine cornea can be used to examine the migration of corneal dendritic cells (Lee, Rosenbaum et al. 2010). This type of imaging may shed light on immune responses in diseases and may even have implications for human ocular imaging in future (Spencer, Lee et al. 2008). Another type of study involves the evaluation of corneal nerves (Richter, Slowik et al. 1997; Guthoff, Wienss et al. 2005; Erdelyi, Kraak et al. 2007; Stachs, Zhivov et al. 2007). This is relevant in investigating diseases such as dry eye induced by corneal refractive surgery, where damage to the corneal nerves plays an important role.

6.2 DIGITAL PHOTOGRAPHY OF THE CORNEA AND CONJUNCTIVA

Documentation of the eye using photography is an essential component in eye care clinics. It enables the eye care clinician to refer to previous recordings of superficial corneal lesions or abnormalities embedded in the cornea such as vascularization, lipid and calcium deposits, spreading of corneal nerves, or lesions in the Descemet's membrane or endothelium. These images may be crucial in making comprehensive decisions on the presenting eye disease. For example, the size of a corneal abscess and the distance of this abscess from the central visual axis are important considerations for its management (Gokhale 2008). Other types of imaging, such as confocal microscopy, may play a similar role in the documentation of lesions, such as lesions in fungal and amebic keratitis (Labbe, Khammari et al. 2009; Kumar, Cruzat et al. 2010). These methods, as well as *ex vivo* methods of examining infected tissue, such as multiphoton fluorescence and second harmonic generation microscopy (Tan, Sun et al. 2007), will be discussed in another section. For research purposes, documentation of the morphology of lesions may also shed information on prognosis. For instance, a photographic imaging that reveals a pterygium lesion with a fleshy appearance may imply that it is more likely to recur after surgical excision than in the case of a more atrophic lesion (Tan, Chee et al. 1997).

Certain auxiliary procedures, such as the use of fluorescein and other dyes, provide additional clinical information. For example, the recording of corneal fluorescein dye staining and conjunctival rose bengal dye staining are excellent means of describing the severity of dry eye (DEWS 2007c). Some of these imaging techniques require hardware modifications that are commonly available. For instance, visualization of fluorescein staining patterns of the cornea must be performed using a cobalt blue filter and light with appropriate exciting wavelength. The clinical classification of dry eye severity is in part determined by the location of the corneal epitheliopathy (Behrens, Doyle et al. 2006). A central corneal staining would reflect a more severe dry eye condition than inferior corneal staining.

Dry eye disease is perhaps the most common ocular surface disease encountered in eye care clinics today (DEWS 2007a; DEWS 2007b). The management of this condition includes lifestyle modification, omega-3 supplements, removal of aggravating factors, moisture occlusion eyewear, ocular lubricants, immunosuppressive therapy, doxycycline, punctual occlusive therapy, autologous plasma tear therapy, and surgical modalities such as tarsorrhaphy (DEWS 2007a; DEWS 2007b). It is essential to establish the level or severity of dry eye as this determines the type of therapy recommended to the patient (Behrens, Doyle et al. 2006). For example, presence of no or minimal corneal epithelial staining may only require environmental advice such as lowering of the height of computer monitor, use of humidifier, and use of ocular lubricant. When the staining intensity is more severe or involves the visual axis, more aggressive therapy including nonpreserved lubricants, ointments, moisture occlusion eyewear, punctual occlusion, or topical cyclosporine (an immunosuppressive agent) eyedrops may be necessary.

There are many ways imaging may help clinicians. Dry eye is a multifactorial disease and there may not always be an agreement between symptoms (the patients' complaints) and clinical signs, such as tear production determined with the Schirmer's test (Fuentes-Paez, Herreras et al. 2011). The reasons for these discordances are complex. In cases where corneal neuropathy is deteriorating, the patient's symptoms may actually improve (DEWS 2007c). In such a scenario, the patient's symptoms alone may not be sufficient for monitoring the effects of the given treatment. Here, objective imaging of the corneal epitheliopathy is vital and enables the clinician to advise the patient on whether the corneal epithelial damage has improved (reduced staining) or worsened (increased staining).

Imaging of corneal staining is not without obstacles. First, some nasal corneal fluorescein dye staining may occur in asymptomatic subjects, but this is not necessarily a sign of dry eye. Second, many symptomatic dry eye patients (categorized as level 1 disease in the dry eye workshop classification) may present without any corneal staining, suggesting that staining may be more valuable for the monitoring of severity rather than detection of mild dry eye.

Although clinicians are often able to visualize minute amounts of corneal epithelial staining using the slit-lamp microscope with high-power binocular eyepiece objective lenses, very often these details escape proper documentation by digital imaging. This may be due to the difficulty in finding the optimal focusing point of the instrument, lack of sufficient resolution or sensitivity of the charge-coupled device (CCD) chip. Sometimes poor imaging quality may also be a consequence of insufficient communication between the clinician who manages the patient and the ophthalmic imaging technician tasked to acquire the images.

Another important sign of dry eye is the reduction of fluorescein tear breakup time (DEWS 2007c), indicating instability of the tear film. Determination of tear breakup time requires prior instillation of fluorescein dye into the eye and is defined as the time taken for a dry spot to appear on the cornea after eye opening. It is possible for an astute technician to image the tear film breaking up, but the pattern observed will clearly depend on the exact time of image acquisition. For proper documentation of tear breakup, it is more appropriate to use videography instead of a single image. However, this may not be feasible as storage requirements of videos are extensive and may increase the cost of this measurement dramatically. One has to note that there are other variables in this test which may affect the tear breakup time, including the volume and concentration of the fluorescein dye instilled into the eye. As long as these parameters have not been universally agreed upon, videos of patients cannot be compared between different research centers. Even so, these modalities are useful for clinical monitoring of individual patients longitudinally and for comparison of patients imaged with the same methodology. In addition to tear breakup time, other phenomena can also be recorded by videography. For example, tear spreading pattern as well as the presence of moving debris on the tear layer can be documented.

Dry eye disease can also be associated with redundant conjunctival folds called conjunctivochalasis (Yokoi, Komuro et al. 2005). Unfortunately, there is no published imaging system that documents the presence and severity of this condition.

Detailed anatomical structures of the eye can be studied, but this usually requires imaging tools that are more elaborate than slit-lamp camera. For instance, a handheld version of a confocal microscope may be used to visualize epithelial and goblet cells in the conjunctiva, accessory lacrimal gland cells, lacrimal ducts, and superficial layers of the sclera (Wells, Wakely et al. 2006). This technique is even able to track individual erythrocytes moving in conjunctival vessels. In the limbal area, the rete ridges and the probable corneal limbal progenitor/stem cells can also be evaluated. In another section of this chapter, we will discuss the use of confocal imaging in greater detail.

6.3   DIGITAL PHOTOGRAPHY OF THE EYELID

Imaging of the eyelid is an ideal method to document the appearance of certain diseases, such as blepharitis, eyelid tumors, eyelid mal-positioning, eyelid retraction, and eyelid ptosis. Meibomian gland dysfunction (MGD), a type of posterior blepharitis, is defined as a chronic diffuse abnormality of the meibomian glands, commonly characterized by terminal duct obstruction and/or qualitative/quantitative changes in the glandular secretion (Nichols 2011). It may result in alteration of the tear film, symptoms of eye irritation, clinically apparent inflammation and ocular surface disease (Nelson, Shimazaki et al. 2011). In MGD, image documentation should include the position of the Marx's line or mucocutaneous junction of the lid margin, the scalloping and notching of the lid borders, telangiectatic vessels, and the rounding of the posterior lid margin. Additional helpful information for the diagnosis of MGD includes pouting, occlusion of the orifices by plugs, irregularity, and abnormal shape of the meibomian gland orifices. Imaging can also be useful in recording abnormal coloring of the meibomian gland secretions, so-called meibum. To illustrate the characteristics and ease of meibum flow, images may be taken before and after manual expression of the glands. Collarettes around the base of eyelashes and lid crusting, both signs of blepharitis, or misdirection and loss of eyelashes are important signs to note as well.

One major limitation of slit-lamp imaging of meibomian gland features is the relatively subjective nature of interpretation. For example, the recorded sign may need to be graded into levels of severity based on standard pictures, which today is not universally agreed upon.

In slit-lamp microscopy and imaging based on a camera attached to the slit lamp, the magnification of the device is not sufficient to visualize important entities such as the Demodex mite, a common organism residing on eyelashes and related glands including meibomian glands (Liu, Sheha et al. 2010). The number of such mites has been shown to correlate with the severity of MGD, the presence of corneal infiltrates, and tear film instability evidenced by a decreased tear breakup time. However, most dissecting microscopes and laboratory direct microscopes, which are usually not available in eye care clinics, can easily be utilized to recognize and image the presence of Demodex mites on, for example, eyelashes. The feasibility of testing for Demodex mites and monitoring the parasitic load depends on the ability to transport specimens, such as epilated eyelashes, from the clinic to a technician in a laboratory who can then image the actual mites.

Demodex mite infestation is treated by repeatedly applying tea-tree oil preparations onto the eyelids which requires proper counseling of the patient and training of the eye care clinician or nurse (Liu, Sheha et al. 2010). Such preparations may cause burning and stinging when used inappropriately or when exposed directly to the conjunctiva or cornea and it is therefore essential that a firm diagnosis is made before commencement of this special treatment. The parasitic load is important to monitor as Lee et al. (2010) found that a higher number of parasites on eyelashes positively correlated with the frequency of ocular discomfort. Even after treatment has commenced, it is recommended to periodically determine the number of mites per eyelash using imaging—for example, three weeks after initial treatment and less frequently thereafter.

Many of these types of lid imaging mentioned above employ rather common equipment. However, more specialized equipment may be necessary if one aims to document the loss or hypertrophy of meibomian glands. This will be discussed in detail in the section on meibography.

6.4 TOPOGRAPHY-BASED IMAGING

Corneal topography was first introduced in the late 1800s to evaluate the curvature of the cornea across its entire surface. The cornea is responsible for two-thirds of the refractive power of the human eye and its refractive power is determined by its curvature. The corneal radius is not constant, and it increases (becomes flatter) toward the periphery, resulting in a gradual change of refractive power through different portions of the cornea.

The topographic modeling system (TMS) is one of the two most widely used computer-assisted video-photokeratographies. The other system is the EyeSys Corneal Analysis System (Morrow and Stein 1992). EyeSys uses a larger placido disk and longer working distances while TMS employs a small, cone-type placido disk method, with smaller object size and shorter working distance. Placido ring patterns are projected onto the front of the eye and the reflected image is captured with a CCD camera. The exact location of each of the mire of the placido pattern is then determined and converted into curvature measurements at each point. The measurement units can be presented in millimeter (mm) and diopter (D). The following section describes the clinical applications of this form of topography.

The system has been widely used in the detection and diagnosis of keratoconus, a non-inflammatory disease characterized by gradual progressive steepening and thinning of the cornea. Thinning usually starts in the central, slightly inferior part of the cornea, causing the cornea to become cone shaped. This may lead to corneal scarring and loss of vision if left unmanaged.

Topography using TMS is also an integral part in the assessment of patient suitability for refractive surgery. Adverse events may occur if surgeons operate on a cornea with undetected keratoconus. These include escalated progression of thinning or ectasia, and unpredictable visual outcomes. Mapping of the anterior and posterior corneal curvature as well as thickness measurements enable early detection and monitoring of the progression of keratoconus. The system also computes indices that may be helpful in the diagnosis of keratoconus. These indices include surface regularity index (SRI), a measure of local regularity of the cornea within the central 4.5 mm diameter (Wilson and Klyce 1991), and surface asymmetry index (SAI), a measure of corneal power differences between points on the same placido ring (Dingeldein, Klyce et al. 1989).

Video-photokeratography, such as TMS, may also be valuable for the evaluation of tear film characteristics in dry eye. In normal conditions, the tear film acts as a protective layer of the cornea and provides a smooth optical surface. The air/tear interface is primarily responsible for the refraction of light through the visual axis. Studies and clinical investigations in dry eye research have mainly focused on the integrity of the tear film. However, it is important to understand that information gained from these conventional dry eye tests often does not reflect quality of vision. Visual disturbances in dry eye patients may be related to optical imperfections (aberrations) that may have been induced by instability of the tear film (Goto, Ishida et al. 2006). The tear stability analysis system (TSAS) incorporated in TMS has been employed to evaluate the regularity and dynamics of the air/tear interface which were shown to be directly affected by distribution of the tear film (Liu and Pflugfelder 1999; Ozkan, Bozkurt et al. 2001; Goto, Ishida et al. 2006; Gumus, Crockett et al. 2011). Conventionally, testing of the visual function in dry eye patients includes assessment of visual acuity and decay of the inter-blink visual acuity (Goto, Ishida et al. 2006). These tests, however, rely primarily on patient feedback. SRI and SAI values computed by the TMS system present a good indicator for the quality of the optical surface and vision, and may thus be a more objective measure compared to conventional visual function methods. The SRI and SAI values have been used for the evaluation of dry eye treatments (Kojima, Ishida et al. 2004). Kojima et al. (2004) showed that SRI and SAI values in dry eye patients were significantly greater than in control patients and decreased following punctal plug insertion.

Generally, evaporation or breakup of the tear film may cause disturbances to the optical surface quality and visual performance. During eye opening, TMS together with TSAS is able to noninvasively collect information on tear film breakup times, which is then reported as TMS-TBUT (Goto, Ishida et al. 2006). In this context, TMS-TBUT is defined as the time taken for the TMS image to degrade or blur; longer TMS-TBUT indicates a more stable tear film while shorter TMS-TBUT may indicate the presence of dry eye. TSAS was found to be highly sensitive and more effective in the measurement of tear breakup times than non-imaging-based assessments (Goto, Zheng et al. 2003; Goto, Zheng et al. 2004).

The TSAS system has several advantages over traditional means to measure tear film breakup time and may find increased application in eye care clinics in the near future. It has the capability to record ten continuous corneal topography maps in 10 seconds, providing a suitable method for the measurement of the dynamic nature of the tear film breakup time. Additionally, there is no need to instill fluorescein dye into the eye. Fluorescein is used to visualize the tear film and tear film breakup time, but it has been shown to artificially increase the measurement depending on the volume of fluorescein instilled into the eye (Johnson and Murphy 2005).

6.5 ANGIOGRAPHY

The use of indocyanine green angiography (ICG-A) to evaluate blood flow has been practiced for over half a century. Indocyanine dye increases the contrast between blood flow patterns and background tissues. In ophthalmology, ICG-A was employed to visualize choroidal blood vessels in the posterior segment of the eye (Shields, Shields et al. 1995; Diallo, Kuhn et al. 2009). However, ICG-A is currently not commonly used for the assessment of the anterior segment of the eye.

In 2001, ICG-A was first used to observe changes in the conjunctival and episcleral vasculature of the anterior segment of the eye (Alsagoff, Chew et al. 2001). To perform this technique, a preparation containing indocyanine green was injected intravenously. When imaged through a camera fitted with an 830-nm barrier filter, the episcleral vessels were seen approximately 16 to 25 seconds after dye administration (Chan, Chew et al. 2001).

Angiography was used to visualize the vasculature in pterygium (Chan, Chew et al. 2001; Tayanc, Akova et al. 2003), a fibrovascular tissue that grows centripetally from the conjunctiva to the cornea, and conjunctival graft, a tissue placed on the area of the removed pterygium. Using ICG-A, early signs of perfusion were noted after a week of pterygium excision in a study conducted by Chan et al. (2001). In the majority of patients undergoing pterygium excision with conjunctival grafting, vascular patterns of the graft itself were recognized at approximately 1 to 2 months postsurgery, which may explain why grafts were viable (Chan, Chew et al. 2001; Tayanc, Akova et al. 2003).

Changes in conjunctival vasculature can also be observed using ICG-A following trabeculectomy, a surgical procedure to control intraocular pressure in glaucoma by creating a passageway between the posterior chamber of the eye and the subconjunctival space. The procedure involves a creation of a conjunctival/scleral flap (Moster and Azuara-Blanco 2003), also named bleb, that triggers inflammation and changes of the vasculature. The dye injected for ICG-A evaluation binds to plasma proteins and should not leak from undamaged vessels (Aydin, Akova et al. 2000; Chan, Chew et al. 2001), allowing for observation of vascular changes (Alsagoff, Chew et al. 2001). During inflammation, blood vessels dilate and become more permeable, and the amount of leakage from these vessels may thus be used as a measure of inflammation. Inflammation of the conjunctival flap may be used as a predictor of excessive scarring and consequent failure of this surgery. However, more clinical studies need to be conducted to prove that angiography is a good technique for predicting success or failure of this type of surgery.

Anterior fluorescein angiography (FA) is another method that visualizes blood vessels. This method is seldom used, as leakage of fluorescein from blood vessels with subsequent loss of vascular outlines occurs rapidly (Meyer and Watson 1987). Fluorescein consists of small molecules that easily leak from normal blood vessels (Aydin, Akova et al. 2000; Chan, Chew et al. 2001). Nevertheless, it may still be useful for observation of the limbal blood vessel arcades (Kuckelkorn, Remky et al. 1997). For example, this methodology may be employed in conditions such as severe chemical injury that result in limbal ischemia with consequent loss of stem cells (Wagoner 1997), and conjunctivalization of the cornea, scarring, and even blindness. In such cases, where the severity of limbal ischemia is clinically difficult to ascertain, this technique may be useful.

A major disadvantage of angiography-based imaging is that the dye has to be administered intravenously. This of course causes discomfort to the patient. Furthermore, unlike other imaging techniques where diagnostic drug is not necessary, trained medical or nursing personnel is mandatory for the administration of the dye, which increases operational cost. Insertion of an intravenous cannula into patients may also be complicated by venous thrombosis. Adverse reactions to dye in the bloodstream may occur, such as anaphylactic shock. Other adverse reactions include nausea or allergic reactions to the iodine present in ICG solutions. In conclusion, the complex nature of this type of imaging and the high risks involved during usage are likely to prevent widespread adoption in clinical practice.

6.6   CONFOCAL MICROSCOPY

In vivo examinations have the advantage to allow for real-time direct observations, while *in vitro* studies perform examinations on biopsy tissue. Performing biopsies is invasive and may induce the release of inflammatory metabolites that may not be present in the original condition of the eye (Jester, Petroll et al. 1992; Wolffsohn and Peterson 2006).

The technology of clinical examination on the human eye followed a progression from the invention of slit-lamp biomicroscopy to the more sophisticated microscopy such as specular microscopy and later confocal microscopy (CM). CM is a system for high-resolution clinical imaging and optical sectioning of the human eye *in vivo* (Bohnke and Masters 1999). It comprises tandem scanning confocal microscopy, slit scanning microscopy, and laser scanning microscopy (Niederer and McGhee 2010). They are built on the principle that both illumination and detection systems are focused on the same point, hence the term *confocal*. Returning out-of-focus light cannot enter the observing pinhole, producing a narrow depth of view (Jalbert, Stapleton et al. 2003). The technical aspects and operational details of the CM have been extensively covered in previous reviews (Bohnke and Masters 1999; Masters and Bohnke 2001). It should be noted that the use of CM requires contact of the eye with an external lens, usually with topical administration of anesthesia and gel coupling in between the two surfaces, presenting a certain level of discomfort to the patient (Reinhard and Larkin 2006). CM use may also result in corneal abrasions and transfer of infections if the lens is not disinfected properly (Niederer and McGhee 2010). However, compared to slit-lamp biomicroscopy and specular microscopy, CM provides much higher magnification and resolution (transverse and axial), rendering it a very useful clinical tool for the imaging of diseased cornea (Furrer, Mayer et al. 1997; Petroll, Cavanagh et al. 1998).

Confocal imaging allows for exciting, novel fields of medical applications. One of the most common medical applications of CM is the detection of infectious diseases (e.g., Acanthameba and fungal keratitis), corneal degenerations and dystrophies, as well as the examination of the tissue effects associated with contact lens wear and photorefractive keratectomy (PRK) (Petroll, Cavanagh et al. 1998; Masters and Bohnke 2001; Jalbert, Stapleton et al. 2003). The presence of Demodex mites, found to be related to MGD, has been observed using CM (Messmer, Torres Suarez et al. 2005). With advances in its technology, the clinical indications of CM will continue to expand. The *in vivo* fiberoptic confocal imaging (FOCI) probe is capable of producing high-quality images of ocular surface structures such as the conjunctival goblet cells, accessory lacrimal glands, and even erythrocytes in conjunctival vessels (Wells, Wakely et al. 2006).

One key feature of CM is its ability to observe corneal stromal nerves and sub-basal nerve plexus (Niederer and McGhee 2010). The cornea is the most richly innervated structure in the human body (Oliveira-Soto and Efron 2003), responsible for various physiological functions including corneal sensation and wound healing (Cruzat, Pavan-Langston et al. 2010). CM can detect changes in corneal nerve morphology and density, reflecting corneal health and disease. Corneal nerves are found to appear swollen in Acanthameba keratitis (Pfister, Cameron et al. 1996). The sub-basal nerve plexus was shown to be thickened and more prominent in keratoconus (Ucakhan, Kanpolat et al. 2006). Sub-basal nerve plexus density was decreased in keratitis (Rosenberg, Tervo et al. 2002), after refractive surgery (Jones, Leech et al. 2002; Erie 2003), as well as in subjects with dry eye and Sjögren's syndrome (Benitez-Del-Castillo, Acosta et al. 2007). In contrast, another study found increased corneal nerve density in a subgroup of Sjögren's syndrome (Zhang, Chen et al. 2005). CM can also serve as a method of detecting early-stage type I diabetes by observing changes in corneal nerve tortuosity and density, and possibly play an important role in monitoring systemic diseases involving peripheral neuropathy (Rosenberg, Tervo et al. 2000; Mehra, Tavakoli et al. 2007).

Langerhans cells have also been seen in the basal epithelium of the cornea using CM (Zhivov, Stave et al. 2005; Mastropasqua, Nubile et al. 2006). They possess a dendritic-like morphology and are responsible for presenting antigens for eliciting immune responses (Niederer and McGhee 2010). Any increase in tissue Langerhans cells suggests increased inflammation or activation of innate immunity. Proliferation of Langerhans cells is associated with adenoviral keratoconjunctivitis (Niederer and McGhee 2010), other infectious keratitis (Altinors, Akca et al. 2006), contact lens wear (Erdelyi, Kraak et al. 2007), and ophthalmic surgery including PRK (Erie 2003). The inflammatory cell count after pterygium excision may have special importance (Zhivov, Beck et al. 2009), as inflammation post-surgery could possibly have an influence on pterygium recurrence rate.

A recent study utilized CM to investigate conjunctival-associated lymphoid tissue (CALT) in rabbit (Liang, Baudouin et al. 2010), which is known to contribute to immune responses in eye. CALT structures were also observed in human patients (Knop and Knop 2000; Liang, Baudouin et al. 2010).

Although CM presents an excellent analysis tool and may help to detect many pathologies, the purchasing costs are extremely high, which restricts its use to specialized eye centers. In summary, CM presents new possibilities in medical applications and for the understanding of ocular diseases, and certainly there will be more applications to be explored in the near future.

6.7 MEIBOMIAN GLAND IMAGING

Meibography is the only method available to observe the meibomian glands. Meibomian glands are large, tubuloacinar structures embedded within the tarsal plate of the eyelids. The glands consist of branched round shaped acini that contain acinar epithelial cells. The acinar cells secrete lipids into the ocular surface system and form a superficial lipid layer of the tear film which acts to reduce tear evaporation. There are about thirty-two glands in the upper eyelid and twenty-five glands in the lower eyelid (Korb, Greiner et al. 1998).

Early attempts to obtain information on the glandular morphology were made in a rabbit model by Jester et al. (Jester, Rife et al. 1982) and in human by Robin et al. (Robin, Jester et al. 1985). The turning over (eversion) of the individual eyelids enabled visualization of the meibomian glands using a transilluminating light probe that is directly applied to the skin (Robin, Jester et al. 1985; Nichols, Berntsen et al. 2005; Yokoi, Komuro et al. 2007; Matsumoto, Sato et al. 2008).

Today, meibography can be performed using a noncontact system. Figure 6.1 shows representative images of a normal and abnormal distribution of meibomian glands in the eyelid. The main advantage of this noninvasive type of meibography is that it reduces discomfort to the patient induced by the application of the probe (Arita, Itoh et al. 2009). Images of the glands in the upper and lower eyelids can be

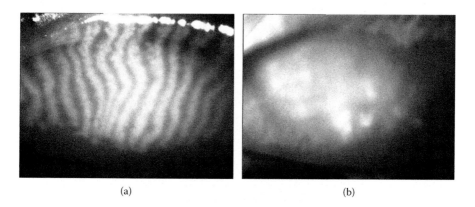

(a)   (b)

FIGURE 6.1 Meibography. Imaging of the meibomian gland is used to diagnose normal or abnormal conditions. (a) A representative image of a normal eyelid with healthy meibomian gland morphology. In infrared meibography, white areas represent glandular structures. (b) An abnormal meibography image and late stage of meibomian gland dysfunction. Glandular structures are lost, and such loss is clinically associated with the lack of meibum released to the ocular surface and consequently leads to dry eye syndrome.

captured using an infrared transmitting filter and infrared video camera, which can be mounted on a slit-lamp microscope (Arita, Itoh et al. 2008; Arita, Itoh et al. 2009). Meibography can detect and document morphological changes, such as dropouts, shortening, dilation, and distortion of the meibomian glands (Arita, Itoh et al. 2008; Arita, Itoh et al. 2009). Studies have shown that meibography can successfully be utilized to classify morphological changes associated with aging and MGD, a major cause for evaporative dry eye (Arita, Itoh et al. 2008; Arita, Itoh et al. 2009; Arita, Itoh et al. 2009; Arita, Itoh et al. 2010; Ibrahim, Matsumoto et al. 2010; Nichols 2011). Meibomian glands from patients with MGD have enlarged acini and subsequently decreased density of acini compared to normal subjects (Matsumoto, Sato et al. 2008). Changes in expressibility of the glands occur in MGD; meibum becomes more viscous and yellow-white instead of clear transparent (Matsumoto, Sato et al. 2008). In advanced stages of MGD, the glands may become permanently occluded and atrophied. Meibomian gland shortening (Arita, Itoh et al. 2009) and a higher meibomian gland dropout rate (Arita, Itoh et al. 2009; Ibrahim, Matsumoto et al. 2010) were observed in patients suffering from MGD compared to normal subjects. Together, this type of meibography would be an extremely valuable tool to any clinical practice.

A highly sophisticated methodology to visualize meibomian gland structures can be performed using CM (Matsumoto, Sato et al. 2008). An example of an image taken with CM is presented in Figure 6.2. In this methodology, the objective of the microscope (an immersion lens covered by a polymethylmethacrylate cap) was applanated directly onto the skin of the everted eyelid. Patients usually did not experience discomfort, as the procedure was performed after application of topical anesthetic to the eye. Captured images were then used to calculate the mean diameter and density of acinar cells (Matsumoto, Sato et al. 2008). Additionally, the laser scanning CM detected thickening of meibum, fibrosis of the gland, and the presence of inflammatory cells which is commonly seen in MGD (Matsumoto, Shigeno et al. 2009). A study evaluating the effectiveness of anti-inflammatory treatments found that the density of inflammatory cells decreased significantly in patients with obstructive MGD over a twelve-week period (Matsumoto, Shigeno et al. 2009).

In future, an imaging technique that allows visualization of the meibomian gland without eversion of the eyelids would be ideal and help to encourage a larger number of clinicians to routinely inspect the health of meibomian glands.

6.8 TEAR INTERFEROMETRY

Tear interferometry has been developed in an effort to measure the thickness of the tear film (Doane 1989; Prydal, Artal et al. 1992; Prydal and Campbell 1992). Optical reflections caused by the two surfaces, air/tear film and tear film/cornea, are captured and the tear film thickness is subsequently calculated (Danjo, Lee et al. 1994; King-Smith, Fink et al. 2000; Hosaka, Kawamorita et al. 2011). This method enabled the measurement of the tear film thickness in normal subjects. However, studies reported differing results on the tear film thickness, ranging from 3 μm (King-Smith, Fink et al. 2000), 6 μm (Hosaka, Kawamorita et al. 2011) to 45 μm (Prydal, Artal

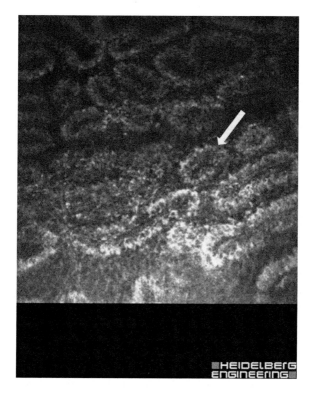

FIGURE 6.2   Meibomian gland imaging using *in vivo* laser confocal microscopy. This is the typical appearance of meibomian gland secretory units on confocal imaging. White oval rings represent normal conditions of acinar units within the meibomian gland ducts. The white arrow indicates an example of an acinar unit. This type of imaging allows for counting of acinar unit density and diameters. (Image is licensed by and reprinted with permission from the Brien Holden Vision Institute Sydney, Australia.)

et al. 1992). These variations in the value may be explained by different temperature and humidity settings used in the studies, which consequently affected the very sensitive balance of the tear film.

Early determinations of tear film thickness were mainly invasive measures, such as glass fibers (Ehlers 1965; Mishima 1965), absorbent paper (Ehlers 1965) that were directly applied to the cornea, and instillation of fluorescein dye (Mishima 1965; Lin, Graham et al. 1999). Tear interferometry, due to its noninvasive nature, has a major advantage over previous methods in the assessment for dry eye treatments. Hosaka et al. (2011) performed interferometry measurements on normal subjects and dry eye patients with and without punctal plug occlusion. It was noted that dry eye patients had a significantly thinner tear film (2.0 ± 1.5 μm) compared to normal subjects (6.0 ± 2.4 μm) and that occlusion treatment significantly improved tear film thickness (Hosaka, Kawamorita et al. 2011).

Tear film lipid layer interferometry presents another approach to evaluate tear film characteristics. This type of interferometry is also a noninvasive technique that observes

the specular reflected light from the tear film surface—the so-called lipid layer interference patterns. Images were graded manually using color-comparison tables (Yokoi,
Takehisa et al. 1996); a somewhat gray color with uniform distribution represents a
healthy tear film (grade 1), while many colors with nonuniform distribution (grade 4) or
a partially exposed corneal surface (grade 5) represent an abnormal tear film. Analysis
of lipid layer interference patterns may be applicable in the diagnostic of dry eye (Yokoi,
Takehisa et al. 1996; Ban, Ogawa et al. 2009). Using the color-comparison table, dry eye
patients who underwent hematopoietic stem cell transplantation and developed chronic
graft-versus-host disease were found to have significantly higher gradings than patients
undergoing the same procedure without side effects (Ban, Ogawa et al. 2009).

Optical interference patterns were also objectively analyzed using a computerized
system introduced by Goto et al. (2003). The interference pattern images were used
to measure the thickness of the tear film lipid layer (Goto, Zheng et al. 2003; Blackie,
Solomon et al. 2009). Decreased lipid layer thickness, indicating an abnormal tear
film, has been noted in dry eye (Blackie, Solomon et al. 2009) and in patients with
MGD (Matsumoto, Sato et al. 2008). Tear film lipid layer measurements can be
employed to evaluate the efficacy of existing and novel treatments for MGD (Olson,
Korb et al. 2003; Matsumoto, Dogru et al. 2006; Ishida, Matsumoto et al. 2008;
Carlson 2010; Grenon, Korb et al. 2010).

Overall, tear interferometry may significantly contribute to the diagnosis of dry
eye and the evaluation of the efficacy of dry eye treatments. The limited range of
commercially available instruments and the associated costs, however, may not
enable common use of this exciting technology in clinical practice.

6.9 ANTERIOR SEGMENT OPTICAL COHERENCE TOMOGRAPHY

The use of anterior segment optical coherence tomography (ASOCT) for the evaluation of the corneal epithelium, stroma, endothelium, and various other purposes in
the anterior segment of the eye has been previously described. ASOCT uses include
examination of glaucoma filtering blebs (Singh, Aung et al. 2009), corneal thickness
(Rao, Kumar et al. 2011), corneal layers after keratectomy (Ma, Tseng et al. 2009),
iris configuration (Cheung, Liu et al. 2010), and the investigation of tear meniscus
(Qiu, Gong et al. 2011). Since this chapter primarily focuses on ocular surface imaging, we will concentrate on the imaging of tear meniscus as an example of the clinical use of ASOCT.

A large quantity of tear film is contained in tear meniscus formed along the
entire eyelid margins of the upper and lower eyelids (Mishima, Gasset et al. 1966;
Holly 1985). To visualize the tear meniscus in a noninvasive fashion and to identify, for example, a reduced tear film volume in patients with aqueous-deficient dry
eye, ASOCT technology can be used (see Figure 6.3) (Shen, Li et al. 2009). The
tear meniscus height, meniscus volume, and cross-sectional area are calculated with
the help of customized analysis software (Jones, Leech et al. 2002; Bitton, Keech
et al. 2007; Chen, Shen et al. 2010). A main advantage of this method is that tear
film is captured in its natural state, with little or no reflex tearing induced, because
the patient is allowed to blink normally during measurements (except during the
moments of image acquisition when the eyelids need to be kept open).

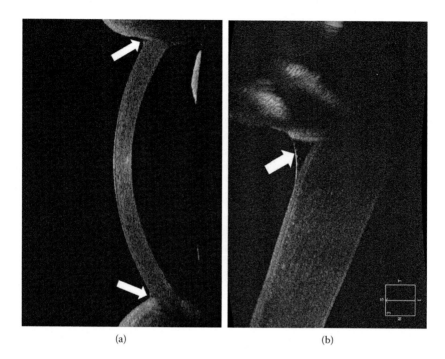

(a)   (b)

FIGURE 6.3   ASOCT for measurements of tear film meniscus. (a) A low-resolution image of the entire ocular surface showing the upper (top arrow) and lower (bottom arrow) tear film meniscus. (b) A high-resolution image of the upper tear film meniscus. Tear film menisci are indicated by the white arrows. Images can be analyzed for tear film meniscus height and tear film volume. (These images are the kind contribution of Dr. Htoon and Mr. Lee Man Xin, Singapore Eye Research Institute.)

Tear meniscus measurement has the potential to deliver valuable information for the clinician in the diagnosis and management of dry eye (Shen, Li et al. 2009; Chen, Shen et al. 2010; Ibrahim, Dogru et al. 2010). Shen et al. (2009) reported a lower tear meniscus height, a smaller radius and cross-sectional area of the upper and lower tear menisci in aqueous-deficient dry eyes compared to normal eyes, measured by customized analysis software for ASOCT images.

ASOCT imaging of tear film has also been shown to be effective in evaluating dry eye treatments. Wang et al. (2006) found that a single dose of artificial tear (35 μl) is retained in ocular surface for up to 20 minutes. Using dissolvable punctal plugs made of collagen, Chen et al. (2010) showed that the occlusion of the upper and lower eyelid puncta significantly increased the tear meniscus height and tear volume in patients with dry eye. The same study also revealed an autoregulatory mechanism in control patients (without dry eye). Authors reported on significantly decreased Schirmer's test values detected in control patients after puncta occlusion, which might be due to a possible feedback mechanism that prevented overflowing of tears (Chen, Shen et al. 2010).

The tear menisci of upper eyelids in normal patients (Wang, Aquavella et al. 2006; Chen, Shen et al. 2010), but not dry eye patients (Shen, Li et al. 2009), were found to be smaller than lower counterparts. However, it is imperative to note that the tear film is very sensitive and can change dramatically in different room temperatures and humidity levels. These parameters must be kept constant to minimize tear evaporation during ASOCT imaging (Borchman, Foulks et al. 2009). Some studies did not sufficiently limit the range of temperature and humidity in their facility (Shen, Li et al. 2009; Chen, Shen et al. 2010). It is also crucial to be consistent in taking images at approximately the same time of the day (Srinivasan, Chan et al. 2007). In the study conducted by Chen et al. (2010) and Shen et al. (2009) image acquisition was performed between 10 a.m. and 4 p.m., a time period with a steady decline of tear meniscus height (Srinivasan, Chan et al. 2007).

In summary, the use of ASOCT is of great benefit in the diagnosis of dry eye and assessment of the efficacy of dry eye treatments. It may, however, be difficult to determine tear film heights in patients presenting with conjunctivochalasis or eyelid abnormalities. Future studies should consider employing OCT instruments with higher or ultra-high resolution to overcome accuracy issues associated with pixilated, low-resolution images taken with the first generation of OCT instruments (Johnson and Murphy 2005). A previous report mentioned that in low-resolution images, the selection of tear prism boundaries (see arrows in Figure 6.3) during analysis may easily introduce inconsistencies, such as over- or underestimation of the tear meniscus (Bitton, Keech et al. 2007). Therefore, future studies conducted by research centers should focus on concordance training of their investigators to fully utilize this very promising technique.

6.10   OCULAR THERMOGRAPHY

Ocular thermography is a noninvasive procedure that detects subtle changes in ocular surface temperature using infrared technology. Dynamic thermal imaging of the eye has provided valuable data on the relationship between ocular surface temperature and tear film stability (Purslow and Wolffsohn 2007; Giraldez, Naroo et al. 2009). Purslow et al. (2007) noted that thermography essentially measures the temperature of the tear film and was mainly influenced by body temperature. Giraldez et al. (2009) found that lower ocular surface temperatures were associated with a thinner lipid layer in normal subjects. Similar to the tear film measurements using ASOCT, in the measurement of ocular surface temperature, environment temperature and its humidity are crucial and variations must to be kept to a minimum to avoid tear film disturbance (Borchman, Foulks et al. 2009; Arciniega, Wojtowicz et al. 2011).

The technique has also examined temperature changes in inflammatory or diseased eye conditions, including dry eye (Mori, Oguchi et al. 1997; Singh and Bhinder 2005; Galassi, Giambene et al. 2007; Sodi, Giambene et al. 2009). Patients with dry eye were found to have higher ocular surface temperatures (Singh and Bhinder 2005), and soon after the blink dry eye patients exhibited a more rapid temperature loss than control subjects (Mori, Oguchi et al. 1997). The tear film of patients with dry eye was shown to have increased tear evaporation rates and be less stable than that of normal subjects, which may account for the rapid temperature loss seen in dry eye (Craig, Singh et al. 2000).

In clinical practice, the importance of observing ocular surface temperature in anterior eye pathologies may be of limited use when diagnosing and managing diseases. However, new emerging analysis software that enables the calculation of tear evaporation rates from thermography images are extremely informative and would be applicable in the diagnosis of dry eye or MGD and in the evaluation of treatments (Tan, Ng et al. 2010). Ocular surface researchers will now have to establish the repeatability of these methods to monitor patients or participants in a research study.

6.11 MISCELLANEOUS IMAGING

Imaging models based on the Scheimpflug principle, such as the Pentacam, have recently emerged in imaging laboratories (Ho, Tsai et al. 2008). For ocular surface purposes, this device combines the advantages of ASOCT in producing a cross-sectional corneal image and also the topography as in TMS.

The eye, and in particular the ocular surface, is a unique structure because of its accessibility to visualization. One potential application is the investigation of immune cell interactions. For example, it is possible to label lymphocytes and then analyze the timing and the movements of lymphocytes in ocular structures after antigen presentation in animal studies (Becker, Crespo et al. 2001; Spencer, Lee et al. 2008; Lee, Rosenbaum et al. 2010). In any other organs, it may not be possible to study these interactions in real time; in some cases, this may require sacrifice of animals at different time points after the commencement of experiment. Epifluorescence videomicroscopy was used to record continuous movement of dendritic cell processes in the cornea, and this provided valuable insight not only on the distribution of dendritic cells in the cornea but also on the response of the dendritic cells to stimulation by cytokines such as tumor necrosis factor-alpha (Lee, Rosenbaum et al. 2010).

Imaging techniques are used in many situations *in vitro* in ocular surface science. One of the commonly used techniques is immunofluorescence imaging of corneal tissue. For example, the loss of tight junction proteins as a response to desiccation has been documented in this way (Pflugfelder, Farley et al. 2005). Another method of examination is high-voltage electron microscopy on corneal tissue (Binder, Rock et al. 1991). In this technique, it was possible to visualize epithelial anchoring fibrils between the basal lamellae of the corneal epithelial cells and the Bowman's layer. In addition, many keratocyte extracellular matrix interactions, not previously seen by conventional transmission electron microscopy, were also observed. Multiphoton imaging is also a promising new technique in the imaging of corneal fine structures (Dorostkar, Dreosti et al. 2010).

6.12 CONCLUSION

In conclusion, a number of modalities are currently used for imaging of ocular surface diseases and many more will be used in future. Certainly, the front surface of the eye is more accessible to noninvasive imaging techniques than other parts of the eye or human body. Although clinical management of many ocular surface diseases requires proper imaging for diagnosis and monitoring, there are many limitations associated with the use of such imaging (see Table 6.1). In this chapter, we have evaluated a range of imaging modalities without prioritizing our discussion based on how frequently they are used.

Certain clinical tests in dry eye are routinely performed—for example, fluorescein dye staining and fluorescein tear breakup patterns—but the clinical signs are perhaps not imaged frequently enough. In addition, many of the newer tools, such as ocular surface thermography (Kamao, Yamaguchi et al. 2011), are still very much in the research realm and the clinical indications are not clear yet.

The acceptance of many of the new tools for evaluation—for example, infrared meibography (Arita, Itoh et al. 2009)—is also currently unclear. Ocular surface clinicians should collaborate closely with imaging scientists and equipment manufacturers to develop and validate new promising technologies. Any proposed imaging modality must necessarily go through a long process before it gains approval and wide usage among clinicians, ocular researchers, and scientists. The lack of a single gold standard diagnostic modality for dry eye/MGD represents a problem in the assessment of new imaging tools. The imaging tool may not be evaluating a novel parameter (for example, an imaging system for corneal fluorescein staining) to detect dry eye/MGD, but may be potentially an improvement over non-imaging methods. The validity of this imaging modality will then have to be evaluated against conventional criteria (combination of corneal fluorescein staining, tear breakup times, questionnaire, etc.). Such comparisons are cumbersome but are currently unavoidable given the complex nature of dry eye.

Many forms of multicenter collaborations are helpful. For example, international databases with clinical information and images can be used to validate newer image analysis algorithms. If comprehensive databases exist, one can obtain sensitivity, specificity, and positive and negative predictive values of these strategies in a more efficient manner. The clinical classification of dry eye may change in the future depending on the ever-increasing understanding on the disease pathogenesis. For example, dry eye induced by laser in situ keratomileusis (LASIK) may be different from that induced by autoimmune Sjögren's syndrome. Given that idiopathic dry eye may actually have different entities in individual patients—for example, some may have primarily MGD and hyperevaporative tendencies while others may have primarily aqueous tear deficiency—imaging modalities may need to be evaluated against specific subtypes of dry eye. With increasing knowledge on the pathogenesis of ocular surface diseases, some older imaging modalities may need to be re-evaluated against the newer diagnostic criteria. Certainly, more innovative technologies will appear in image laboratories and clinics, making the decade very exciting for professionals working in ocular imaging.

REFERENCES

Alsagoff, Z., P. T. Chew, et al. (2001). Indocyanine green anterior segment angiography for studying conjunctival vascular changes after trabeculectomy. *Clin Experiment Ophthalmol* **29**(1): 22–26.
Altinors, D. D., S. Akca, et al. (2006). Smoking associated with damage to the lipid layer of the ocular surface. *Am J Ophthalmol* **141**(6): 1016–1021.

Arciniega, J. C., J. C. Wojtowicz, et al. (2011). Changes in the evaporation rate of tear film after digital expression of meibomian glands in patients with and without dry eye. *Cornea* **30**(8): 843–847.

Arita, R., K. Itoh, et al. (2008). Noncontact infrared meibography to document age-related changes of the meibomian glands in a normal population. *Ophthalmology* **115**(5): 911–915.

Arita, R., K. Itoh, et al. (2009). Noncontact meibography detects changes in meibomian glands in the aging process in a normal population and patients with meibomian gland dysfunction. *Cornea* **28**(9(S1)): S75–S79.

Arita, R., K. Itoh, et al. (2009). Proposed diagnostic criteria for obstructive meibomian gland dysfunction. *Ophthalmology* **116**(11): 2058–2063 e2051.

Arita, R., K. Itoh, et al. (2010). Proposed diagnostic criteria for seborrheic meibomian gland dysfunction. *Cornea* **29**(9): 980–984.

Aydin, P., Y. A. Akova, et al. (2000). Anterior segment indocyanine green angiography in scleral inflammation. *Eye (Lond)* **14**(Pt 2): 211–215.

Ban, Y., Y. Ogawa, et al. (2009). Tear function and lipid layer alterations in dry eye patients with chronic graft-vs-host disease. *Eye (Lond)* **23**(1): 202–208.

Becker, M. D., S. Crespo, et al. (2001). Intraocular in vivo imaging of activated T-lymphocytes expressing green-fluorescent protein after stimulation with endotoxin. *Graefes Arch Clin Exp Ophthalmol* **239**(8): 609–612.

Behrens, A., J. J. Doyle, et al. (2006). Dysfunctional tear syndrome: a Delphi approach to treatment recommendations. *Cornea* **25**(8): 900–907.

Benitez-Del-Castillo, J. M., M. C. Acosta, et al. (2007). Relation between corneal innervation with confocal microscopy and corneal sensitivity with noncontact esthesiometry in patients with dry eye. *Invest Ophthalmol Vis Sci* **48**(1): 173–181.

Binder, P. S., M. E. Rock, et al. (1991). High-voltage electron microscopy of normal human cornea. *Invest Ophthalmol Vis Sci* **32**(8): 2234–2243.

Bitton, E., A. Keech, et al. (2007). Variability of the analysis of the tear meniscus height by optical coherence tomography. *Optom Vis Sci* **84**(9): 903–908.

Blackie, C. A., J. D. Solomon, et al. (2009). The relationship between dry eye symptoms and lipid layer thickness. *Cornea* **28**(7): 789–794.

Bohnke, M. and B. R. Masters (1999). Confocal microscopy of the cornea. *Prog Retin Eye Res* **18**(5): 553–628.

Borchman, D., G. N. Foulks, et al. (2009). Factors affecting evaporation rates of tear film components measured in vitro. *Eye Contact Lens* **35**(1): 32–37.

Bourne, W. M. (2010). Corneal endothelium—past, present, and future. *Eye Contact Lens* **36**(5): 310–314.

Cameron, J. R., S. Ahmed, et al. (2009). Impact of direct electronic optometric referral with ocular imaging to a hospital eye service. *Eye (Lond)* **23**(5): 1134–1140.

Carlson, A. N. (2010). A new paradigm for treating dry eye patients. *Advanced Ocular Care*: 37–41.

Chan, C. M., P. T. Chew, et al. (2001). Vascular patterns in pterygium and conjunctival autografting: a pilot study using indocyanine green anterior segment angiography. *Br J Ophthalmol* **85**(3): 350–353.

Chen, F., M. Shen, et al. (2010). Tear meniscus volume in dry eye after punctal occlusion. *Invest Ophthalmol Vis Sci* **51**(4): 1965–1969.

Cheung, C. Y., S. Liu, et al. (2010). Dynamic analysis of iris configuration with anterior segment optical coherence tomography. *Invest Ophthalmol Vis Sci* **51**(8): 4040–4046.

Craig, J. P., I. Singh, et al. (2000). The role of tear physiology in ocular surface temperature. *Eye (Lond)* **14**(Pt 4): 635–641.

Cruzat, A., D. Pavan-Langston, et al. (2010). In vivo confocal microscopy of corneal nerves: analysis and clinical correlation. *Semin Ophthalmol* **25**(5–6): 171–177.

Danjo, Y., M. Lee, et al. (1994). Ocular surface damage and tear lactoferrin in dry eye syndrome. *Acta Ophthalmol (Copenh)* **72**(4): 433–437.

DEWS (2007a). The definition and classification of dry eye disease: report of the Definition and Classification Subcommittee of the International Dry Eye WorkShop (2007). *Ocul Surf* **5**(2): 75–92.

DEWS (2007b). The epidemiology of dry eye disease: report of the Epidemiology Subcommittee of the International Dry Eye WorkShop (2007). *Ocul Surf* **5**(2): 93–107.

DEWS (2007c). Methodologies to diagnose and monitor dry eye disease: report of the Diagnostic Methodology Subcommittee of the International Dry Eye WorkShop (2007). *Ocul Surf* **5**(2): 108–152.

Diallo, J. W., D. Kuhn, et al. (2009). [Contribution of indocyanine green angiography in sickle cell retinopathy]. *J Fr Ophtalmol* **32**(6): 430–435.

Dingeldein, S. A., S. D. Klyce, et al. (1989). Quantitative descriptors of corneal shape derived from computer-assisted analysis of photokeratographs. *Refract Corneal Surg* **5**(6): 372–378.

Doane, M. G. (1989). An instrument for in vivo tear film interferometry. *Optom Vis Sci* **66**(6): 383–388.

Dorostkar, M. M., E. Dreosti, et al. (2010). Computational processing of optical measurements of neuronal and synaptic activity in networks. *J Neurosci Methods* **188**(1): 141–150.

Ehlers, N. (1965). The precorneal film. Biomicroscopical, histological and chemical investigations. *Acta Ophthalmol Suppl*: Suppl 81:81–134.

Erdelyi, B., R. Kraak, et al. (2007). In vivo confocal laser scanning microscopy of the cornea in dry eye. *Graefes Arch Clin Exp Ophthalmol* **245**(1): 39–44.

Erie, J. C. (2003). Corneal wound healing after photorefractive keratectomy: a 3-year confocal microscopy study. *Trans Am Ophthalmol Soc* **101**: 293–333.

Fuentes-Paez, G., J. M. Herreras, et al. (2011). Lack of concordance between dry eye syndrome questionnaires and diagnostic tests. *Arch Soc Esp Oftalmol* **86**(1): 3–7.

Furrer, P., J. M. Mayer, et al. (1997). Confocal microscopy as a tool for the investigation of the anterior part of the eye. *J Ocul Pharmacol Ther* **13**(6): 559–578.

Galassi, F., B. Giambene, et al. (2007). Evaluation of ocular surface temperature and retrobulbar haemodynamics by infrared thermography and color Doppler imaging in patients with glaucoma. *Br J Ophthalmol* **91**(7): 878–881.

Ghaznawi, N. and E. S. Chen (2010). Descemet's stripping automated endothelial keratoplasty: innovations in surgical technique. *Curr Opin Ophthalmol* **21**(4): 283–287.

Giraldez, M. J., S. A. Naroo, et al. (2009). A preliminary investigation into the relationship between ocular surface temperature and lipid layer thickness. *Cont Lens Anterior Eye* **32**(4): 177–180; quiz 193, 195.

Gokhale, N. S. (2008). Medical management approach to infectious keratitis. *Indian J Ophthalmol* **56**(3): 215–220.

Goto, E., R. Ishida, et al. (2006). Optical aberrations and visual disturbances associated with dry eye. *Ocul Surf* **4**(4): 207–213.

Goto, T., X. Zheng, et al. (2003). A new method for tear film stability analysis using videokeratography. *Am J Ophthalmol* **135**(5): 607–612.

Goto, T., X. Zheng, et al. (2004). Tear film stability analysis system: introducing a new application for videokeratography. *Cornea* **23**(8 Suppl): S65–70.

Grenon, S. M., D. R. Korb, et al. (2010). A unique ocular surface interferometer (OSI) to measure and evaluate lipid layer thickness (LLT). *ARVO Meeting Abstracts* **51**.

Gumus, K., C. H. Crockett, et al. (2011). Noninvasive assessment of tear stability with the tear stability analysis system in tear dysfunction patients. *Invest Ophthalmol Vis Sci* **52**(1): 456–461.

Guthoff, R. F., H. Wienss, et al. (2005). Epithelial innervation of human cornea: a three-dimensional study using confocal laser scanning fluorescence microscopy. *Cornea* **24**(5): 608–613.

Ho, J. D., C. Y. Tsai, et al. (2008). Validity of the keratometric index: evaluation by the Pentacam rotating Scheimpflug camera. *J Cataract Refract Surg* **34**(1): 137–145.

Holly, F. J. (1985). Physical chemistry of the normal and disordered tear film. *Trans Ophthalmol Soc UK* **104**(Pt 4): 374–380.

Hosaka, E., T. Kawamorita, et al. (2011). Interferometry in the evaluation of precorneal tear film thickness in dry eye. *Am J Ophthalmol* **151**(1): 18–23 e11.

Ibrahim, O. M., M. Dogru, et al. (2010). Application of visante optical coherence tomography tear meniscus height measurement in the diagnosis of dry eye disease. *Ophthalmology* **117**(10): 1923–1929.

Ibrahim, O. M., Y. Matsumoto, et al. (2010). The efficacy, sensitivity, and specificity of in vivo laser confocal microscopy in the diagnosis of meibomian gland dysfunction. *Ophthalmology* **117**(4): 665–672.

Ishida, R., Y. Matsumoto, et al. (2008). Tear film with Orgahexa EyeMasks in patients with meibomian gland dysfunction. *Optom Vis Sci* **85**(8): 684–691.

Jalbert, I., F. Stapleton, et al. (2003). In vivo confocal microscopy of the human cornea. *Br J Ophthalmol* **87**(2): 225–236.

Jester, J. V., W. M. Petroll, et al. (1992). Comparison of in vivo and ex vivo cellular structure in rabbit eyes detected by tandem scanning microscopy. *J Microsc* **165**(Pt 1): 169–181.

Jester, J. V., L. Rife, et al. (1982). In vivo biomicroscopy and photography of meibomian glands in a rabbit model of meibomian gland dysfunction. *Invest Ophthalmol Vis Sci* **22**(5): 660–667.

Johnson, M. E. and P. J. Murphy (2005). The agreement and repeatability of tear meniscus height measurement methods. *Optom Vis Sci* **82**(12): 1030–1037.

Johnson, M. E. and P. J. Murphy (2005). The effect of instilled fluorescein solution volume on the values and repeatability of TBUT measurements. *Cornea* **24**(7): 811–817.

Jones, L., R. Leech, et al. (2002). A novel method to determine tear prism height. *Optom Vis Sci* **79**(suppl): 252.

Kafkala, C., J. Choi, et al. (2006). Mooren ulcer: an immunopathologic study. *Cornea* **25**(6): 667–673.

Kamao, T., M. Yamaguchi, et al. (2011). Screening for dry eye with newly developed ocular surface thermographer. *Am J Ophthalmol* **151**(5): 782–791.

King-Smith, P. E., B. A. Fink, et al. (2000). The thickness of the human precorneal tear film: evidence from reflection spectra. *Invest Ophthalmol Vis Sci* **41**(11): 3348–3359.

Knop, N. and E. Knop (2000). Conjunctiva-associated lymphoid tissue in the human eye. *Invest Ophthalmol Vis Sci* **41**(6): 1270–1279.

Kojima, T., R. Ishida, et al. (2004). A new noninvasive tear stability analysis system for the assessment of dry eyes. *Invest Ophthalmol Vis Sci* **45**(5): 1369–1374.

Korb, D. R., J. V. Greiner, et al. (1998). Human and rabbit lipid layer and interference pattern observations. *Adv Exp Med Biol* **438**: 305–308.

Kuckelkorn, R., A. Remky, et al. (1997). Video fluorescein angiography of the anterior eye segment in severe eye burns. *Acta Ophthalmol Scand* **75**(6): 675–680.

Kumar, R. L., A. Cruzat, et al. (2010). Current state of in vivo confocal microscopy in management of microbial keratitis. *Semin Ophthalmol* **25**(5–6): 166–170.

Labbe, A., C. Khammari, et al. (2009). Contribution of in vivo confocal microscopy to the diagnosis and management of infectious keratitis. *Ocul Surf* **7**(1): 41–52.

Lam, D. S., E. Houang, et al. (2002). Incidence and risk factors for microbial keratitis in Hong Kong: comparison with Europe and North America. *Eye (Lond)* **16**(5): 608–618.

Lee, E. J., J. T. Rosenbaum, et al. (2010). Epifluorescence intravital microscopy of murine corneal dendritic cells. *Invest Ophthalmol Vis Sci* **51**(4): 2101–2108.

Lee, S. H., Y. S. Chun, et al. (2010). The relationship between demodex and ocular discomfort. *Invest Ophthalmol Vis Sci* **51**(6): 2906–2911.

Liang, H., C. Baudouin, et al. (2010). Live conjunctiva-associated lymphoid tissue analysis in rabbit under inflammatory stimuli using in vivo confocal microscopy. *Invest Ophthalmol Vis Sci* **51**(2): 1008–1015.

Lin, M. C., A. D. Graham, et al. (1999). Measurement of post-lens tear thickness. *Invest Ophthalmol Vis Sci* **40**(12): 2833–2839.

Liu, J., H. Sheha, et al. (2010). Pathogenic role of Demodex mites in blepharitis. *Curr Opin Allergy Clin Immunol* **10**(5): 505–510.

Liu, Z. and S. C. Pflugfelder (1999). Corneal surface regularity and the effect of artificial tears in aqueous tear deficiency. *Ophthalmology* **106**(5): 939–943.

Ma, J. J., S. S. Tseng, et al. (2009). Anterior segment optical coherence tomography for transepithelial phototherapeutic keratectomy in central corneal stromal scarring. *Cornea* **28**(8): 927–929.

Maeda, N. (2011). [New diagnostic methods for imaging the anterior segment of the eye to enable treatment modalities selection]. *Nippon Ganka Gakkai Zasshi* **115**(3): 297–322; discussion 323.

Malhotra, A., F. J. Minja, et al. (2011). Ocular anatomy and cross-sectional imaging of the eye. *Semin Ultrasound CT MR* **32**(1): 2–13.

Masters, B. R. and M. Bohnke (2001). Three-dimensional confocal microscopy of the human cornea in vivo. *Ophthalmic Res* **33**(3): 125–135.

Mastropasqua, L., M. Nubile, et al. (2006). Epithelial dendritic cell distribution in normal and inflamed human cornea: in vivo confocal microscopy study. *Am J Ophthalmol* **142**(5): 736–744.

Matsumoto, Y., M. Dogru, et al. (2006). Efficacy of a new warm moist air device on tear functions of patients with simple meibomian gland dysfunction. *Cornea* **25**(6): 644–650.

Matsumoto, Y., E. A. Sato, et al. (2008). The application of in vivo laser confocal microscopy to the diagnosis and evaluation of meibomian gland dysfunction. *Mol Vis* **14**: 1263–1271.

Matsumoto, Y., Y. Shigeno, et al. (2009). The evaluation of the treatment response in obstructive meibomian gland disease by in vivo laser confocal microscopy. *Graefes Arch Clin Exp Ophthalmol* **247**(6): 821–829.

Mehra, S., M. Tavakoli, et al. (2007). Corneal confocal microscopy detects early nerve regeneration after pancreas transplantation in patients with type 1 diabetes. *Diabetes Care* **30**(10): 2608–2612.

Messmer, E. M., E. Torres Suarez, et al. (2005). [In vivo confocal microscopy in blepharitis]. *Klin Monbl Augenheilkd* **222**(11): 894–900.

Meyer, P. A. and P. G. Watson (1987). Low dose fluorescein angiography of the conjunctiva and episclera. *Br J Ophthalmol* **71**(1): 2–10.

Mishima, S. (1965). Some physiological aspects of the precorneal tear film. *Arch Ophthalmol* **73**: 233–241.

Mishima, S., A. Gasset, et al. (1966). Determination of tear volume and tear flow. *Invest Ophthalmol* **5**(3): 264–276.

Mori, A., Y. Oguchi, et al. (1997). Use of high-speed, high-resolution thermography to evaluate the tear film layer. *Am J Ophthalmol* **124**(6): 729–735.

Morrow, G. L. and R. M. Stein (1992). Evaluation of corneal topography: past, present and future trends. *Can J Ophthalmol* **27**(5): 213–225.

Moster, M. R. and A. Azuara-Blanco (2003). *Surgical management of glaucoma: trabeculectomy and glaucoma drainage devices*. New York, McGraw Hill.

Nelson, J. D., J. Shimazaki, et al. (2011). The international workshop on meibomian gland dysfunction: report of the definition and classification subcommittee. *Invest Ophthalmol Vis Sci* **52**(4): 1930–1937.

Nichols, J. J., D. A. Berntsen, et al. (2005). An assessment of grading scales for meibography images. *Cornea* **24**(4): 382–388.

Nichols, K. K. (2011). The international workshop on meibomian gland dysfunction: introduction. *Invest Ophthalmol Vis Sci* **52**(4): 1917–1921.

Niederer, R. L. and C. N. McGhee (2010). Clinical in vivo confocal microscopy of the human cornea in health and disease. *Prog Retin Eye Res* **29**(1): 30–58.

Oliveira-Soto, L. and N. Efron (2003). Morphology of corneal nerves in soft contact lens wear. A comparative study using confocal microscopy. *Ophthalmic Physiol Opt* **23**(2): 163–174.

Olson, M. C., D. R. Korb, et al. (2003). Increase in tear film lipid layer thickness following treatment with warm compresses in patients with meibomian gland dysfunction. *Eye Contact Lens* **29**(2): 96–99.

Ozkan, Y., B. Bozkurt, et al. (2001). Corneal topographical study of the effect of lacrimal punctum occlusion on corneal surface regularity in dry eye patients. *Eur J Ophthalmol* **11**(2): 116–119.

Petroll, W. M., H. D. Cavanagh, et al. (1998). Clinical confocal microscopy. *Curr Opin Ophthalmol* **9**(4): 59–65.

Pfister, D. R., J. D. Cameron, et al. (1996). Confocal microscopy findings of Acanthamoeba keratitis. *Am J Ophthalmol* **121**(2): 119–128.

Pflugfelder, S. C., W. Farley, et al. (2005). Matrix metalloproteinase-9 knockout confers resistance to corneal epithelial barrier disruption in experimental dry eye. *Am J Pathol* **166**(1): 61–71.

Prydal, J. I., P. Artal, et al. (1992). Study of human precorneal tear film thickness and structure using laser interferometry. *Invest Ophthalmol Vis Sci* **33**(6): 2006–2011.

Prydal, J. I. and F. W. Campbell (1992). Study of precorneal tear film thickness and structure by interferometry and confocal microscopy. *Invest Ophthalmol Vis Sci* **33**(6): 1996–2005.

Purslow, C. and J. Wolffsohn (2007). The relation between physical properties of the anterior eye and ocular surface temperature. *Optom Vis Sci* **84**(3): 197–201.

Qiu, X., L. Gong, et al. (2011). Age-related variations of human tear meniscus and diagnosis of dry eye with Fourier-domain anterior segment optical coherence tomography. *Cornea* **30**(5): 543–549.

Rao, H. L., A. U. Kumar, et al. (2011). Evaluation of central corneal thickness measurement with RTVue spectral domain optical coherence tomography in normal subjects. *Cornea* **30**(2): 121–126.

Reinhard, T. and D. F. P. Larkin, Eds. (2006). *Cornea and External Eye Disease*. Essentials in Ophthalmology. Germany, Springer.

Richter, A., C. Slowik, et al. (1997). [In vivo imaging of corneal innervation in the human using confocal microscopy]. *Ophthalmologe* **94**(2): 141–146.

Robin, J. B., J. V. Jester, et al. (1985). In vivo transillumination biomicroscopy and photography of meibomian gland dysfunction. A clinical study. *Ophthalmology* **92**(10): 1423–1426.

Rosenberg, M. E., T. M. Tervo, et al. (2000). Corneal structure and sensitivity in type 1 diabetes mellitus. *Invest Ophthalmol Vis Sci* **41**(10): 2915–2921.

Rosenberg, M. E., T. M. Tervo, et al. (2002). In vivo confocal microscopy after herpes keratitis. *Cornea* **21**(3): 265–269.

Shen, B. and J. Hwang (2010). The clinical utility of precision medicine: properly assessing the value of emerging diagnostic tests. *Clin Pharmacol Ther* **88**(6): 754–756.

Shen, M., J. Li, et al. (2009). Upper and lower tear menisci in the diagnosis of dry eye. *Invest Ophthalmol Vis Sci* **50**(6): 2722–2726.

Shields, C. L., J. A. Shields, et al. (1995). Patterns of indocyanine green videoangiography of choroidal tumours. *Br J Ophthalmol* **79**(3): 237–245.

Singh, G. and H. S. Bhinder (2005). Comparison of noncontact infrared and remote sensor thermometry in normal and dry eye patients. *Eur J Ophthalmol* **15**(6): 668–673.

Singh, M., T. Aung, et al. (2009). Utility of bleb imaging with anterior segment optical coherence tomography in clinical decision-making after trabeculectomy. *J Glaucoma* **18**(6): 492–495.

Sodi, A., B. Giambene, et al. (2009). Ocular surface temperature in diabetic retinopathy: a pilot study by infrared thermography. *Eur J Ophthalmol* **19**(6): 1004–1008.

Spencer, D. B., E. J. Lee, et al. (2008). In vivo imaging of the immune response in the eye. *Semin Immunopathol* **30**(2): 179–190.

Srinivasan, S., C. Chan, et al. (2007). Apparent time-dependent differences in inferior tear meniscus height in human subjects with mild dry eye symptoms. *Clin Exp Optom* **90**(5): 345–350.

Stachs, O., A. Zhivov, et al. (2007). In vivo three-dimensional confocal laser scanning microscopy of the epithelial nerve structure in the human cornea. *Graefes Arch Clin Exp Ophthalmol* **245**(4): 569–575.

Tan, D. T., S. P. Chee, et al. (1997). Effect of pterygium morphology on pterygium recurrence in a controlled trial comparing conjunctival autografting with bare sclera excision. *Arch Ophthalmol* **115**(10): 1235–1240.

Tan, H. Y., Y. Sun, et al. (2007). Multiphoton fluorescence and second harmonic generation microscopy for imaging infectious keratitis. *J Biomed Opt* **12**(2): 024013.

Tan, J. H., E. Y. Ng, et al. (2010). Evaluation of tear evaporation from ocular surface by functional infrared thermography. *Med Phys* **37**(11): 6022–6034.

Tayanc, E., Y. Akova, et al. (2003). Anterior segment indocyanine green angiography in pterygium surgery with conjunctival autograft transplantation. *Am J Ophthalmol* **135**(1): 71–75.

Ucakhan, O. O., A Kanpolat, et al. (2006). In vivo confocal microscopy findings in keratoconus. *Eye Contact Lens* **32**(4): 183–191.

Wagoner, M. D. (1997). Chemical injuries of the eye: current concepts in pathophysiology and therapy. *Surv Ophthalmol* **41**(4): 275–313.

Wakefield, D. and L. P. Robinson (1987). Cyclosporin therapy in Mooren's ulcer. *Br J Ophthalmol* **71**(6): 415–417.

Wang, J., J. Aquavella, et al. (2006). Repeated measurements of dynamic tear distribution on the ocular surface after instillation of artificial tears. *Invest Ophthalmol Vis Sci* **47**(8): 3325–3329.

Wells, A. P., L. Wakely, et al. (2006). In vivo fibreoptic confocal imaging (FOCI) of the human ocular surface. *J Anat* **208**(2): 197–203.

Whitcher, J. P., M. Srinivasan, et al. (2001). Corneal blindness: a global perspective. *Bull World Health Organ* **79**(3): 214–221.

Wilson, S. E. and S. D. Klyce (1991). Advances in the analysis of corneal topography. *Surv Ophthalmol* **35**(4): 269–277.

Wolffsohn, J. S. and R. C. Peterson (2006). Anterior ophthalmic imaging. *Clin Exp Optom* **89**(4): 205–214.

Yokoi, N. and A. Komuro (2004). Non-invasive methods of assessing the tear film. *Exp Eye Res* **78**(3): 399–407.

Yokoi, N., A. Komuro, et al. (2005). New instruments for dry eye diagnosis. *Semin Ophthalmol* **20**(2): 63–70.

Yokoi, N., A. Komuro, et al. (2005). Clinical impact of conjunctivochalasis on the ocular surface. *Cornea* **24**(8 Suppl): S24–S31.

Yokoi, N., A. Komuro, et al. (2007). A newly developed video-meibography system featuring a newly designed probe. *Jpn J Ophthalmol* **51**(1): 53–56.

Yokoi, N., Y. Takehisa, et al. (1996). Correlation of tear lipid layer interference patterns with the diagnosis and severity of dry eye. *Am J Ophthalmol* **122**(6): 818–824.

Zhang, M., J. Chen, et al. (2005). Altered corneal nerves in aqueous tear deficiency viewed by in vivo confocal microscopy. *Cornea* **24**(7): 818–824.

Zhivov, A., R. Beck, et al. (2009). Corneal and conjunctival findings after mitomycin C application in pterygium surgery: an in-vivo confocal microscopy study. *Acta Ophthalmol* **87**(2): 166–172.

Zhivov, A., J. Stave, et al. (2005). In vivo confocal microscopic evaluation of Langerhans cell density and distribution in the normal human corneal epithelium. *Graefes Arch Clin Exp Ophthalmol* **243**(10): 1056–1061.

7 Current Research on Ocular Surface Temperature

Jen Hong Tan, E. Y. K. Ng, and
U. Rajendra Acharya

CONTENTS

7.1 INTRODUCTION

Ocular surface temperature (OST) in literature primarily refers to the temperature measured at the ocular surface enclosed by palpebral fissure. Generally, the value measured at this ocular surface is regarded as the tear film surface temperature. Numerous relationships among ocular physiologies, pathologies, and this temperature were unveiled, despite the absence of sophisticated and consistent analytical methods in the field.

Dohnberg in 1975 measured ocular surface temperature by a specially adapted mercury glass and discovered that subjects who had acute iritis exhibited higher ocular surface temperature [1]. This seminal investigation paved the way for examinations on the ocular surface temperature by the use of needle-like thermometer and thermistor. However, these invasive techniques have not been used on human studies in the past three decades due to their severe disadvantages: the measured temperature was determined to be lower compared to the actual value, and such discrepancy can increase by 6°C. Also, topical anesthesia was required in some measurements and may cause trauma to the subject.

The above difficulties were overcome by the introduction of the infrared thermometer. Its use was pioneered by Mapstone [2] and Wachtmeister [3], and later inspired a number of researchers using infrared thermography to look into thermal asymmetry or anomalies in ocular surface temperature in an attempt to establish diagnostic criteria based on these asymmetries and anomalies. The investigations in this field were further advanced in the 1980s and 1990s due to the rapid improvement in the technology of infrared thermography.

7.2 INVESTIGATIONS ON OCULAR PHYSIOLOGY USING INFRARED THERMOGRAPHY

Efron et al. in the 1980s utilized the thermography to observe variation in temperature over the ocular surface and determined the temporal stability of central cornea temperature [4]. They observed the presence of a temperature apex that was slightly inferior to the geometric center of cornea, surrounded by ellipsoidal isotherms [4]. Limbus was reported to be 0.45°C warmer compared to that of the geometric center of cornea [4].

On a latter investigation on Chinese origin subjects, however, the limbus-geometric corneal center temperature difference was found to be 0.23°C~0.43°C [5]. Such observation was attributed to the lower tear volume and tear stability in Chinese eyes compared to Caucasian eyes [6–9] and hence the lower temperature at limbus in brown eyes compared to blue eyes [5].

Purslow and Wolffsohn employed infrared thermography to perform examinations on relationships between OST and physical parameters of the anterior eye such as corneal thickness, corneal topography, bulbar hyperaemia, and tear film stability. Dynamic infrared thermography [10] was used to study the aforementioned relationships. They have found that the ocular surface temperature at the time immediately after a blink was correlated to body temperature and tear film stability [10].

7.3 INVESTIGATIONS BY INFRARED THERMOGRAPHY ON OCULAR DISEASES

The earliest investigation on ocular disease using thermography was conducted on Graves' ophthalmopathy. An infrared thermal imager was used to assess left endocrinal exophthalmos and metastasis of the left orbit [11]. Statistical analysis was not performed in the study as the number of subjects in each case was too small [11]. In recent investigations, the infrared thermal imager was once again adopted to examine the inflammatory state in patients with Graves' ophthalmopathy, and the follow-up effect of methylprednisolone pulse therapy [12]. This study reported higher temperature differences in between lateral orbit and other target areas (caruncle, medial conjunctiva, lateral conjunctiva, and lower eyelid) in Graves' ophthalmopathy [12]. Furthermore, the difference in the sum of temperatures before and after treatment was found to be positively correlated to the change in clinical activity score [12].

Dry eye disease is one of the major topics in investigations of ocular surface temperature. In one study, ocular surface of dry eye patients was determined to be warmer, although by common understanding dry eye should cool and evaporate faster [14–15]. The author deduced that happened because the cooling effect was outweighed by conjunctival hyperemia associated with the disease, therefore causing an increase in surface temperature [13]. However, Craig et al. reported this otherwise [16]: they observed cooler cornea (at the corneal center) in dry eyes. They also reported a higher temperature variation factor, and mean osmolality and the temperature variation factor were found to be inversely correlated to central corneal temperature.

OST of the dry eye patient was looked into from a temporal (with respect to time) point of view. It was assumed that OST decreases exponentially immediately after the eye opens. Such decrease asymptotically approaches a constant value after some time [17], and can be modeled by the following formula:

$$T(t) = (T_o - T_\infty)e^{(-kt)} + T_\infty \qquad (7.1)$$

where T is the corneal surface temperature after the eye opens for a period of t, T_o is the temperature immediately after the eye opens, k is the temperature coefficient, and T_∞ is the corneal surface temperature at equilibrium.

The mean k value in the above expression for both normal subjects and dry eye patients was the main interest of researchers. In one study, the OST was measured using a box of 20×20 pixels, or $3.3\ mm^2$, placed at the center of cornea for a period of 30 seconds [17]. They found that, for normal blinking, the mean k value in dry eye patients (5.6 ± 2.9 per second) was significantly lower compared to that of normal control subjects (9.3 ± 5.0 per second) [17]. The k value was hence deemed to reflect tear film stability [17].

In a later study by Chang et al., the above principle was further extended to the diagnosis of dry eye. They measured OST by an encircled region, the diameter of which was 4.4 mm (22 pixels), positioned at the center of eye [18]. The study illustrated a diagnosis accuracy with a sensitivity of 79% and specificity of 75% [18]. In another study, infrared thermography was used to determine the acupuncture treatment effect on this ocular disease [19]. The middle of the cornea was reported to be cooler after the treatment [19].

Recently, a Japanese research group using a custom-made ocular surface thermographer measured the OST immediately after the opening of the eye, and in the subsequent 10 seconds they recorded the temperature once in each second [20]. In the controlled study, at the 10th second after the opening of the eye, a significant decrease in temperature of dry eyes was observed compared to normal eyes [20]. This significant decrease was found to be negatively correlated to tear breakup time [20]. Another Taiwanese research team studied both the change in temperature and the irregularity in topographical profile of temperature at the ocular surface [21]. They quantified the above factors using two parameters: temperature difference value and compact value [21]. Using these two features, they achieved a considerable discrimination between normal and dry eyes, with a sensitivity of 0.84, specificity of 0.83, and receiver operating characteristic of 0.87 [21].

Ocular surface temperature was also studied in conjunction with lipid layer thickness [22]. According to the classification system described by Guillon and Guillon [23], for a normal subject the lipid layer can be described by one of the five patterns: open marmoreal (lipid thickness 13–30 nm), closed marmoreal (lipid thickness 30–50 nm), flow or wave (lipid thickness 50–80 nm), amorphous (lipid thickness 80–90 nm), and colored fringes 1 (lipid thickness 90–140 nm). Giraldez et al. found that among the five, ocular surface was on average the warmest in subjects exhibiting lipid pattern of colored fringes 1, both before and after the blink. They further suggested positive association between a warmer ocular surface and a thicker lipid layer, though no significant correlations were observed in relation to noninvasive tear breakup time (NIBUT).

Regarding the correlation between OST and ocular blood flow by infrared thermometer, it was observed that corneal temperature was positively correlated to the ipsilateral values of end diastolic velocity (in left and right eyes, respectively) and the resistivity index (of left and right eyes, respectively). The interocular difference was indicated to be positively correlated with the difference in end diastolic velocity, and negatively correlated with resistivity index [24]. On the other hand, by infrared thermography and color Doppler imaging, Galassi et al. evaluated the OST of both patients with primary open-angle glaucoma (POAG) and normal group [46]. Compared to normal subjects, patients with primary open-angle glaucoma had lower temperatures at five anatomical points (internal and external canthus, halfway from the internal canthus and nasal limbus, center of the cornea, halfway from the temporal limbus and external canthus), and these temperatures were significantly correlated to resistivity index according to their findings [25]. The influence of retrobulbar hemodynamics on OST was highlighted in their results [25]. In another study, patients with central retinal vein occlusion (CRVO) showed warmer ocular surface compared to normal subjects, and OST in ischemic CRVO eyes was lower compared to nonischemic ones [26].

7.4   THE CHALLENGES AND RECENT ADVANCES IN THE INVESTIGATION OF OCULAR SURFACE TEMPERATURE

It can be seen from the above studies that the temperature variation on OST by infrared thermography is very useful and indicates the ocular health of the subject. Despite this, several important issues in the studying methodology remained unresolved [27]. First, each pixel in an ocular thermal image (ocular thermogram) denotes a temperature value; thus the captured ocular thermogram is deeply dissimilar with optical image captured at the respective region. The cornea-sclera boundary is indiscernible in the ocular thermogram though easily seen in optical image, and the edge of palpebral fissure is not apparent in some cases and has to be observed in conjunction with eyelashes, which exhibit far lower temperature.

The above dissimilarities have significant consequences. Unclear palpebral fissure and absence of cornea-sclera boundary in ocular thermogram deter any consistent anatomical localization. Despite this, most of the investigations on the ocular surface need consistency in anatomical localization, especially the corneal center. A variety of approaches were proposed to work around the above obstacles, but did not give the satisfactory results.

Subjective assessment was the primary measure in the beginning to look into ocular thermogram. However, as this measure does not provide quantitative data that allows further processing, and the conclusion reached might vary among examiners, it does not suffice for advanced analysis. Researchers in the 1980s and 1990s examined the ocular surface temperature based on few temperature points. They determined corneal center mostly by subjective assessment [27]. On the other hand, there were investigations that examined ocular surface temperature by getting a mean temperature over a pool of temperature values located within a box or a circle; some acquired the mean over several boxes or circular regions. The corneal center in these studies was approximated by subjective judgment.

The above approaches have provided quantitative data about the OST, but they are sensitive to local thermal fluctuation. For instance, the mean temperature over some enclosed regions was the most widely employed first-order spatial statistics, in the attempt to get a "middle" or "expected" temperature on those sites. However this single parameter is far from sufficient and comprehensive to provide insights on the physiology at ocular surface or be used for diagnosis, and there comes the second unresolved issue: a dearth of features to depict the pattern of OST [27].

This difficulty can be resolved by consistent, better-defined measures in both ocular and corneal localizations, and this would serve a great deal to facilitate investigation on OST. This can be achieved by some manual approaches and also by some automated methods. As a start, Acharya et al. proposed a semi-automated measure in which a rectangle tightly enclosing the palpebral fissure was drawn. Subsequently, the corneal center and its radius were determined by the algorithm according to the size of the palpebral fissure [28].

Tan et al. proposed the otherwise fully automated method to diagnose OST [29–31]. In their method, snake algorithm, gradient vector flow field, and genetic algorithm were combined to perform automated ocular and corneal localization (see Figure 7.1). The region of interest was delineated by snake algorithm, with the aid of gradient vector flow field, which served as the external force field acting on snake for the converge. The combination of the two gives a local optimizer, which can only correctly localize the palpebral fissure when the starting contour is placed in an appropriate location. To resolve this initialization issue, the authors proposed a target tracing function, which helps to search for the appropriate initializing position. The function was formulated in such a way that when the correct initializing position was determined, the function would give a minimum. Thus, the position-searching problem was translated into a minimizing problem, and in their case it was solved by genetic algorithm.

In addition to the above, better analytical methods are also needed to unveil relationships among surface temperature and other ocular physiologies. This concerns the second conundrum. Instead of utilizing only first-order textural analysis, computer methods in image analysis such as textural method have recently been introduced to extract subtle details in ocular thermogram [32]. Cross co-occurrence matrix [33] was used, along with first-order statistics, difference histogram, and moments to extract texture features from ocular thermogram. They have shown distinct ranges of texture parameters for normal subjects of different age groups [32]. It was found that subjects aged above thirty-five years showed significantly higher interocular difference in median, textural contrast, moment 2, and moment 3 (in absolute value) compared to their younger peers. Several relationships among features of cross co-occurrence matrix, first-order statistics, and age of subjects were observed [32]. These relationships may be helpful in the diagnosis of various ocular diseases in the future [32].

The surface temperature can also be analyzed as a whole instead of in fragments. In fact, if the surface temperature is captured and analyzed in its entirety, the obstacle posed by the indiscernible cornea-sclera boundary to some extent can be resolved. This idea was adopted in one recent investigation, which used ocular

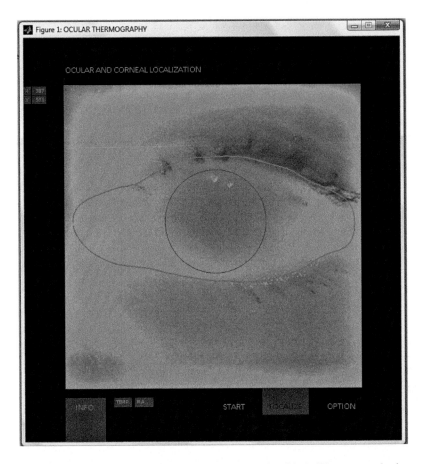

FIGURE 7.1 Ocular and corneal localization by snake algorithm. (Please see color insert.)

thermographic sequences to estimate the rate of tear evaporation from the ocular surface [34]. In this study, a region of palpebral fissure was warped into a standard form (octagon, to mimic the eye). Temperature values within that region were read and calculation was performed based on a thermodynamic model to estimate the rate of evaporation at any instant. It was determined that for elder subjects (aged above thirty-five), the rate was 55.82Wm^{-2} and 58.9Wm^{-2} for younger subjects; corneal rate of evaporation was statistically higher in elder subjects [34]. The blinking frequency was indicated to be related to the variation of evaporation rate [34].

Recently, another localization scheme to capture the entire ocular surface was proposed. In that method, the user must first locate four points P_1, P_2, P_3, and P_4, which correspond to the left, right, top, and bottom of the palpebral fissure [21]. Then four curves y_{13}, y_{32}, y_{42}, y_{14} are produced between points P_1P_3, P_3P_2, P_4P_2, P_1P_4, respectively to form a closed contour, with each curve y_{ij} defined as

$$y_{ij} = a - \frac{a}{b^2}x^2$$

where a and b denote the horizontal and vertical distance between point P_i and P_j, respectively [21]. Such a region-of-interest selection was claimed to enable straightforward localization, and also to avoid reading of eyelash temperature [21].

7.5 CONCLUSION

Many subtle details of ocular physiology and pathologies can be unraveled using infrared thermography. However, better and sophisticated methodology is required to facilitate deeper revelation on the relationships between the surface temperature and ocular diseases. There are two main directions for further improvement in the methodology: ocular/corneal localization and analytical techniques. With advances in these aspects, it will be possible to develop an automated ocular disease diagnosis algorithm based on ocular surface temperature.

REFERENCES

1. A. Holmberg, The temperature of the eye during application of hot packs and after milk injections, *Acta Ophthalmologica* (Copenhagen), 30 (1952) 347–364.
2. R. Mapstone, Ocular thermography, *British Journal of Ophthalmology*, 54 (1970) 751–754.
3. L. Wachtmeister, Thermography in the diagnosis of diseases of the eye and the appraisal of therapeutic effects: a preliminary report, *Acta Ophthalmologica*, 48 (1970) 945–958.
4. N. Efron, G. Young, N. Brennan, Ocular surface temperature, *Current Eye Research*, 8 (1989) 901–906.
5. L. Tan, Z.-Q. Cai, N.-S. Lai, Accuracy and sensitivity of the dynamic ocular thermography and inter-subjects ocular surface temperature (OST) in Chinese young adults, *Contact Lens & Anterior Eye*, 32 (2009) 78–83.
6. P. Cho, B. Brown, I. Chan, R. Conway, M. Yap, Reliability of the tear break-up time technique of assessing tear stability and the locations of the tear break-up in Hong Kong Chinese, *Optometry and Vision Science*, 69 (1992) 879–885.
7. P. Cho, B. Brown, Review of the TBUT technique and a closer look at the TBUT of HK-Chinese, *Optometry and Vision Science*, 70 (1993) 30–38.
8. P. Cho, M. Yap, Age, gender, and tear break-up time, *Optometry and Vision Science*, 70 (1993) 828–831.
9. S. Patel, S. Laidlaw, L. Mathewson, L. McCallum, C. Nicholson, Iris color and the influence of local anaesthetics on precorneal tear film stability, *Acta Ophthalmol* (Kbh), 69 (1991) 387–392.
10. C. Purslow, J.S. Wolffsohn, The relation between physical properties of the anterior eye and ocular surface temperature, *Optometry and Vision Science*, 84 (2007) 197–201.
11. P. Bourjat, M. Gautherie, Unilateral exophthalmos investigated by infrared thermography, *Modern Problems in Ophthalmology*, 14 (1975) 278–285.
12. T.-C. Chang, Y.-L. Hsiao, S.-L. Liao, Application of digital infrared thermal imaging in determining inflammatory state and follow-up effect of methylprednisolone pulse therapy in patients with Graves' ophthalmopathy, *Graefe's Archive for Clinical and Experimental Ophthalmology*, 246 (2008) 45–49.
13. P.B. Morgan, A.B. Tullo, N. Efron, Infrared thermography of the tear film in dry eye, *Eye*, 9 (1995) 615–618.
14. W.d. Mathers, G. Binarao, M. Petroll, Ocular water evaporation and the dry eye: a new measuring device, *Cornea*, 12 (1993) 335–340.
15. M. Rolando, M. Refojo, K. Kenyon, Increased tear evaporation in eyes with keratoconjunctivitis sicca, *Arch Ophthalmol*, 101 (1983) 557–558.

16. J.P. Craig, I. Singh, A. Tomlinson, et al., The role of tear physiology in ocular surface temperature, *Eye*, 14 (2000) 635–641.
17. A. Mori, Y. Oguchi, Y. Okusawa, M. Ono, H. Fujishima, K. Tsubota, Use of high-speed, high-resolution thermography to evaluate the tear film layer, *American Journal of Ophthalmology*, 124 (1997) 729–735.
18. H.K. Chiang, C.Y. Chen, H.Y. Cheng, K.-H. Chen, D.O. Chang, Development of infrared thermal imager for dry eye diagnosis, in: *Proceedings of SPIE—The International Society for Optical Engineering*, San Diego, CA, USA, 2006.
19. J. Nepp, K. Tsubota, E. Goto, J. Schauersberger, G. Schild, K. Jandrasits, C. Abela, A. Wedrich, The effect of acupuncture on the temperature of the ocular surface in conjunctivitis sicca measured by non-contact thermography: preliminary results, *Adv. Exp. Med. Biol.*, 506 (2002) 723–726.
20. T. Kamao, M. Yamaguchi, S. Kawasaki, S. Mizoue, A. Shiraishi, Y. Ohashi, Screening for dry eye with newly developed ocular surface thermographer, *American Journal of Ophthalmology*, 151 (2011) 782–791.e781.
21. T.Y. Su, C.K. Hwa, P.H. Liu, M.H. Wu, D.O. Chang, P.F. Su, S.W. Chang, H.K. Chiang, Noncontact detection of dry eye using a custom designed infrared thermal image system, *Journal of Biomedical Optics*, 16 (2011) doi: 10.1117/1.3562964.
22. M.J. Giraldez, S.A. Naroo, C.G. Resua, A preliminary investigation into the relationship between ocular surface temperature and lipid layer thickness, *Contact Lens & Anterior Eye: The Journal of the British Contact Lens Association*, 32 (2009) 177–180.
23. J.P. Guillon, M. Guillon, Tear film examination of the contact lens patient, *Optician*, 206 (1993) 21–29.
24. K. Gugleta, S. Orgül, J. Flammer, Is corneal temperature correlated with blood-flow velocity in the ophthalmic artery? *Current Eye Research*, 19 (1999) 496–501.
25. F. Galassi, B. Giambene, A. Corvi, G. Falaschi, Evaluation of ocular surface temperature and retrobulbar hemodynamics by infrared thermography and color Doppler imaging in patients with glaucoma, *British Journal of Ophthalmology*, 91 (2007) 878–881.
26. A.A. Sodi, B.A.D. Giambene, G.B. Falaschi, R.C. Caputo, B.B. Innocenti, A.B. Corvi, U.A. Menchini, Ocular surface temperature in central retinal vein occlusion: preliminary data, *European Journal of Ophthalmology*, 17 (2007) 755–759.
27. J.H. Tan, E.Y.K. Ng, U.R. Acharya, C. Chee, Infrared thermography on ocular surface temperature: a review, *Infrared Physics & Technology*, 52 (2009) 97–108.
28. U.R. Acharya, E.Y.K. Ng, C.Y. Gerk, J.H. Tan, Analysis of normal human eye with different age groups using infrared images, *Journal of Medical System*, 33 (2008) 207–213.
29. J.H. Tan, E.Y.K. Ng, A.U. Rajendra, Automated detection of eye and cornea on infrared thermogram using snake and target tracing function coupled with genetic algorithm, *Quantitative InfraRed Thermography International Journal*, 6 (2009) 21–36.
30. J.H. Tan, E.Y.K. Ng, U.R. Acharya, C. Chee, Automated study of ocular thermal images: comprehensive analysis of corneal health with different age group subjects and validation, *Digital Signal Processing*, 20 (2010) 1579–1591.
31. J.H. Tan, E.Y.K. Ng, U.R. Acharya, An efficient automated algorithm to detect ocular surface temperature on sequence of thermograms using snake and target tracing function, *Journal of Medical Systems*, (2010) DOI:10.1007/s10916-10010-19552-10916.
32. J.-H. Tan, E.Y.K. Ng, U. Rajendra Acharya, C. Chee, Study of normal ocular thermogram using textural parameters, *Infrared Physics & Technology*, 53 (2010) 120–126.
33. G. Schaefer, M. Závišek, T. Nakashima, Thermography based breast cancer analysis using statistical features and fuzzy classification, *Pattern Recognition*, 42 (2009) 1133–1137.
34. J.H. Tan, E.Y.K. Ng, U.R. Acharya, Evaluation of tear evaporation from ocular surface by functional infrared thermography, *Medical Engineering & Physics*, 37 (2010) 6022.

8 Computer Methods in the Estimation of Tear Evaporation by Thermography

Jen Hong Tan, E. Y. K. Ng, and U. Rajendra Acharya

CONTENTS

8.1 INTRODUCTION

Tear evaporation at the ocular surface is one of the major topics in tear dynamics. The primary motivation behind the intense interest in the topic was to deepen understanding of dry eye, an ocular disease that has affected numerous adults [1–6]. The Singapore National Eye Centre alone had 54,051 patients seeking treatment for dry eye in 2009, with medication costs totaling S\$181,354.17 [7]. This ocular disease has not only affected work productivity but also further added to the socioeconomic burden [8].

The diagnosis of this abnormality is performed mainly through tests such as tear breakup time, ocular surface staining, or Schirmer's test. These tests, however, have poor repeatability, and can be unreliable and invasive [9]. In most clinical investigations, symptomatic improvements are the primary outcome measures for dry eye treatment, and they are in fact poor and unreliable indicators in the determination of treatment effectiveness. With better, more straightforward, and consistent measurement of tear evaporation, it is possible to overcome the above difficulties.

The measurement of tear evaporation was first performed on rabbits. The workers fixed a chamber around the rabbits' corneas [10] and found a rate of 4.16×10^{-7}

$gcm^{-2}s^{-1}$. This work was later followed by two other similar studies [11,12], which gave values of 7.8×10^{-7} $gcm^{-2}s^{-1}$ [11] and 10.1×10^{-7} $gcm^{-2}s^{-1}$ [12], respectively. *In vivo* measurement for evaporation in the normal human eye, on the other hand, was first made by Hamano et al. [13], who reported an average value of 26.9×10^{-7} $gcm^{-2}s^{-1}$. This seminal work in the measurement of human tear evaporation was succeeded by Rolando and Refojo, who measured the evaporation rate by an instrument setup consisting of a tightly fitted goggle, with its chamber pumped with dry air [14,15]. They reported an average value of 4.07×10^{-7} $gcm^{-2}s^{-1}$ [14].

These were the initial measurements of tear evaporation, and they had shortcomings. For example, the tightly fitted goggle of Rolando and Refojo could not measure the rate of evaporation at any specific relative humidity and temperature [15]. Furthermore, petroleum jelly was required to reduce skin-contributed evaporation [14]. In the 1990s, however, a number of enhanced techniques were proposed to measure the evaporation, and the methodologies in general can be approximated in the following fashion. The rate of tear evaporation was recorded twice and its corresponding analysis had two portions: one while the eyes were open (blinking was allowed); another while the eyes were continuously shut. Such arrangements were considered because the workers wanted to eliminate the undesired portion of the skin-contributed evaporation in their recording values.

This idea was first carried out by Tsubota and Yamada, who reported a value of 16.2×10^{-7} in the unit gs^{-1} for normal subjects [16], and Tomlinson et al. employed a servomed evaporimeter, reporting values between $2.7 \times 10^{-7} \sim 19.4 \times 10^{-7} gcm^{-2}s^{-1}$ [17]. Mathers et al. performed the measurement in a slightly different fashion: they first measured water evaporation from the skin and eyelid (with the eye closed) for a 2-minute period, then the tear evaporation, with blinking allowed [18]. By subtracting the first measurement value from the second one, they obtained the final corrected tear evaporation and reported $14.7 \times 10^{-7} gcm^{-2}s^{-1}$ for normal evaporation.

More recently, an evaporimeter with greater responsivity was adopted to measure tear evaporation, based on the variations in frequency shift due to relative humidity change [19]. In this work, again one set of measurements was first made while the subject's eye was closed, followed by another while the eye was open with natural blinking allowed. The final rate was derived by the subtraction between the measurement values acquired while the eye was open and the other while the eye was closed.

Besides the above methodologies, there were also estimations of tear evaporation based on other measuring modalities, such as fluorophotometry (which measures the tear flow) and other devices. These investigations provided an estimated rate of evaporation in the range of $10 \times 10^{-7} \sim 40 \times 10$ $gcm^{-2}s^{-1}$ [15], around 10% of the tear produced [18]. There was also a study that determined the rate to be 14.7×10^{-7} $mg cm^{-2}h^{-1}$ [20], or equivalently 100 Wm^{-2} (the power loss per area) [21].

In summary, the rate of tear evaporation generally was deemed higher in patients suffering from dry eye disease, although the findings of the literature in regard to this were inconsistent [15]. Such disagreement may be due to the selection of subjects rather than the dissimilar physiology, measurement techniques, or instrumentation [15]. In addition, the reported rates of tear evaporation on both normal and dry eye subjects were found inconsistent in the studies.

In this chapter we develop a technique to measure the rate of tear evaporation based on dynamic/functional infrared (IR) thermography instead of relative humidity. Infrared thermography is commonly used in the medical field currently, with applications in areas such as tumor localization, diagnosis of fever, open heart surgery, and so on [9,22,23]. This imaging modality is noninvasive, noncontact, and capable of real-time thermal recording, especially the distribution of surface temperature. It has become the main tool in ophthalmology to access human ocular surface temperature (OST), due to its noninvasiveness and nonalteration to ocular surface temperature. A number of investigations have been performed using this technology, on glaucoma, human lacrimal drainage system, cataract, Graves' ophthalmopathy, and dry eye [9].

However, ocular thermography (both thermal image and thermographic recording/sequence) has so far not been used to estimate the rate of tear evaporation. Instead, comparisons have been made between normal and dry eye subjects, on the temperature at the ocular surface, and its corresponding temporal and topographical variation. For example, Craig et al. [24] have observed a higher temperature variation factor in dry eye subjects. Central corneal temperature was determined to be inversely correlated to temperature variation factor. Also, some attempts were made to model the variation in corneal surface temperature during the inter-blink period, in the form of $T(t) = (T_0 - T_\infty)e^{-kt} + T_\infty$, and use it to diagnose dry eye. However, it is important to note that in the literature so far there is no firm conclusion on whether the dry eye subject has a warmer ocular surface.

We estimated the rate of tear evaporation by the first law of thermodynamics, based on the ocular surface temperature at each moment. The heat exchange at the ocular surface can be watered down into five components: the heat loss due to convection, radiation, and tear evaporation, the heat produced/absorbed at the thin layer on the ocular surface (the control volume), and the inflow of heat into the eyeball. By estimation, it is possible to determine the heat loss due to convection, radiation, and the heat exchange at the control volume. Furthermore, the inflow of heat into the eyeball is conceivably approximated based on a three-dimensional finite element model, which was developed earlier to study the heat transfer within the human eye [25]. By solving these unknowns, the rate of tear evaporation can be determined. This measuring modality also allows observation on variation in the rate with respect to time.

8.2   THE THEORY

Consider a small-piece element on the corneal or conjunctival epithelium with an area of dA. The element has a thickness of $d = d_2 - d_1$ such that both of the following conditions are satisfied (see Figure 8.1):

$$T(x, y, t, d_2) \approx T(x, y, t, d_1) \approx T(x, y, t)$$

$$mC_p(T_2 - T_1) \approx 0 \quad or \quad mC_p(T_2 - T_1) \text{ is negligible in calculation}$$

$$(8.1)$$

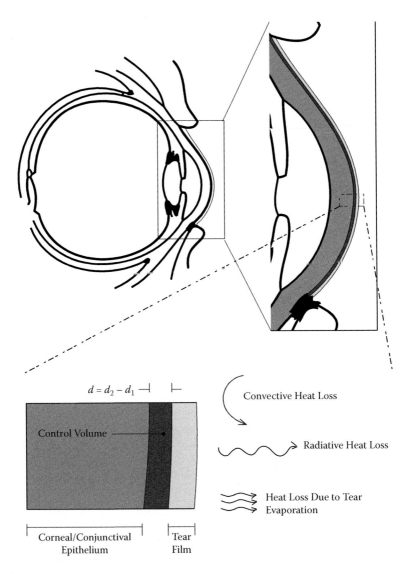

FIGURE 8.1 Tear film layer, the control volume of interest and the heat loss. (Please see color insert.)

Assume the temperature within the element is homogeneous; then, T_2, T_1 are the element temperatures at times t_2, t_1, respectively. The above-stated conditions (as in equation 8.1) suggest the element of interest needs to be very thin such that the difference $T_2 - T_1$ is small and the net heat exchange $mC_p(T_2 - T_1)$ within the element can be considered negligible. If the thickness d is set to be about the thickness of the lipid layer, it has been illustrated that the above conditions can be comfortably satisfied. (For more details see [26]). Moreover, except for moments before and after a blink, the ocular surface temperature in general fluctuates narrowly.

Therefore it is justified to argue that within a short time period Δt the net change in the element's internal energy is in fact insignificant and hence negligible. Then when an eye opens immediately after a blink, from the first law of thermodynamics, in a short period of time $\Delta t = t_2 - t_1$ the heat exchange at the ocular surface can be described by

$$(Q_{in} + W_{in} + \Sigma m_i h_i) - (Q_{out} + W_{out} + \Sigma m_e h_e) = mC_p(T_2 - T_1) \tag{8.2}$$

For our case, the above can be simplified to

$$Q_{in} - Q_{out} = mC_p(T_2 - T_1) \tag{8.3}$$

The heat inflow to the control volume is

$$Q_{in} = \int_{t_1}^{t_2} \ddot{q}(x,y,t)\,dAdt \tag{8.4}$$

where $\ddot{q}(x,y,t)$ is heat flux, and the outflow of heat from the element can be obtained by

$$Q_{out} = \int_{t_1}^{t_2} \left\{ h_{amb} \left[[T(x,y,t) - T_{amb}] \right] dA + \sigma \varepsilon [T(x,y,t)^4 - T_{amb}^4] dA \right\} dt$$
$$+ \int_{t_1}^{t_2} E(x,y,t) dA dt \tag{8.5}$$

The right-hand side of equation (8.5) consists of three components, which correspond to the three types of heat losses occurring on the small-piece control volume within the inter-blink period: tear evaporation, convective and radiative heat transfer. h_{amb} is the convection coefficient in ambient environment, and its value is 10 $Wm^{-2}k^{-1}$ [27]. ε is emissivity, 0.975 for cornea [25]; σ is the Stefan-Boltzmann constant 5.67×10^{-8} $Wm^{-2}k^{-4}$. $T(x, y, t)$ is the ocular surface temperature at the location of (x, y) (the coordinates definition is in line with Figure 8.5a) and T_{amb} is the ambient room temperature, which in our case we assume to be constant. $E(x, y, t)$ is the rate of tear evaporation in energy form. Substitute (8.4), (8.5) into (8.2) and we get

$$\int_{t_1}^{t_2} \ddot{q}(x,y,t) dA dt - \int_{t_1}^{t_2} h_{amb}[T(x,y,t) - T_{amb}] dA dt$$
$$- \int_{t_1}^{t_2} \sigma \varepsilon [T(x,y,t)^4 - T_{amb}^4] dA dt - \int_{t_1}^{t_2} E(x,y,t) dA dt = 0 \tag{8.6}$$

From the above we obtain the total heat transfer at the entire ocular surface by

$$\int_{t_1}^{t_2} \int_S \ddot{q}(x,y,t) dA\, dt - \int_{t_1}^{t_2} \left\{ h_{amb} \int_S [T(x,y,t) - T_{amb}] dA \right.$$
$$\left. + \sigma \varepsilon \int_S [T(x,y,t)^4 - T_{amb}^4] dA \right\} dt - \int_{t_1}^{t_2} \int_S E(x,y,t) dA\, dt = 0 \tag{8.7}$$

where S is the total ocular surface area. Rearrange,

$$\int_{t_1}^{t_2} \int_S E(x,y,t)dA\,dt = \int_{t_1}^{t_2} \int_S \ddot{q}(x,y,t)dA\,dt - \int_{t_1}^{t_2} \left\{ h_{amb} \int_S [T(x,y,t) - T_{amb}]dA \right.$$
$$\left. + \sigma\varepsilon \int_S [T(x,y,t)^4 - T_{amb}^4]dA \right\} dt \tag{8.8}$$

Divide the above equation by $S\Delta t$ and let

$$E_{t_1 t_2} = \int_{t_1}^{t_2} \int_S E(x,y,t)dA\,dt \Big/ S\Delta t$$

$$L_{t_1 t_2} = \int_{t_1}^{t_2} \left\{ h_{amb} \int_S [T(x,y,t) - T_{amb}]dA + \sigma\varepsilon \int_S [T(x,y,t)^4 - T_{amb}^4]dA \right\} dt \Big/ S\Delta t$$

$$Q_{t_1 t_2} - \int_{t_1}^{t_2} \int_S \ddot{q}(x,y,t)\,dA\,dt \Big/ S\Delta t$$

Then we have

$$E_{t_1 t_2} = Q_{t_1 t_2} - L_{t_1 t_2} \tag{8.9}$$

where $E_{t_1 t_2}$, $Q_{t_1 t_2}$, $L_{t_1 t_2}$ are the mean tear evaporation rate, mean heat flux (into an element), and mean heat loss (due to convection and radiation) across the anterior ocular surface during the time period $\Delta t = t_2 - t_1$. Hence for a short period $\Delta t = t_{k+1} - t_k$, we have

$$E_{t_k t_{k+1}} = Q_{t_k t_{k+1}} - L_{t_k t_{k+1}} \tag{8.10}$$

Finally, we get the average tear evaporation rate by

$$E_{avg} = \frac{1}{n_t} \sum_{k=1}^{n_t} E_{t_k t_{k+1}} \tag{8.11}$$

Due to homeostatic regulation, humans generate heat to preserve the level of body temperature, especially when the external environment is much cooler than the core body temperature. The varying level of heat in the human body is produced in response to ambient temperature, and hence is generally a function of the external temperature.

In the case of the human eye, the ocular globe is warm due to ocular blood flow; metabolism of several ocular tissues also contributes some of the heat to the globe. As long as no major variations occur in both the internal and the external environment, and in the absence of stimulants, the amount of heat delivered to the ocular globe by blood flow and metabolism is likely to remain constant. Under this argument, the heat is considered as flowing uniformly across the ocular globe, and the total heat inflow into the control volume over a period of time can be assumed to be constant, that is,

$$Q = Q_{t_1 t_2} = Q_{t_2 t_3} = Q_{t_3 t_4} = \cdots = constant \tag{8.12}$$

Inflow heat to the entire anterior surface can be given by

$$Q \cdot S = \int_{\Delta t} \int_S \ddot{q}(x,y,t) dA dt \Big/ \Delta t = \frac{1}{\overline{R}} \{T_b - T_{amb}\} \tag{8.13}$$

where T_b is the body temperature and $\overline{R}$ is the total mean thermal resistance, which denotes the total resistance of all the conceivable heat transfer in the ocular globe. Furthermore, since

$$R \cdot A_r = \frac{L}{KA_r} \cdot A_r = \frac{1}{U} \tag{8.14}$$

where L, A_r, K, are the length, heat transfer area, and thermal conductivities of an object of interest, respectively, and U is the overall heat transfer coefficient (detailed explanation can be located in [28]), we can determine the inflow heat flux by

$$Q = \frac{T_b - T_{amb}}{\overline{R} \cdot S} = \overline{h}(T_b - T_{amb}) \tag{8.15}$$

where $\overline{h}$ is the mean heat transfer coefficient.

8.3 DISCRETE APPROXIMATION

In practice, the absence of continuous function $T(x, y, t)$ makes the calculation in equations (8.9), (8.10), (8.11) not possible. For ocular thermal images, we have only finite numbers of temperature data points pertinent to the anterior surface; hence, by considering each temperature data point as a small-piece element, we can discretize the formulation derived earlier. Denote $T(i, j, t)$ a temperature data point in a thermal image, and substitute $T(x, y, t)$ with $T(i, j, t)$ in the above-mentioned equations. We have, for example,

$$\left\{ h_{amb} \int_S [T(x,y,t) - T_{amb}] dA \right\} \Big/ S \approx \frac{h_{amb}}{n_p dA} \Sigma_i \Sigma_j [T(i,j,t) - T_{amb}] dA$$

$$\approx \frac{h_{amb}}{n_p} \Sigma_i \Sigma_j [T(i,j,t) - T_{amb}] \tag{8.16}$$

and

$$\left\{ \sigma\varepsilon \int_S [T(x,y,t)^4 - T_{amb}^4] dA \right\} \Big/ S \approx \frac{\sigma\varepsilon}{n_p dA} \Sigma_i \Sigma_j [T(i,j,t)^4 - T_{amb}^4] dA$$

$$\approx \frac{\sigma\varepsilon}{n_p} \Sigma_i \Sigma_j [T(i,j,t)^4 - T_{amb}^4] \tag{8.17}$$

where n_p is the number of points pertained to anterior ocular surface. By trapezoidal rule, we get the discretized $L_{t_k t_{k+1}}$ by substituting (8.16), (8.17) and obtain

$$L_{t_k t_{k+1}} = \int_{t_{k+1}}^{t_k} \{h_{amb} \int_S [T(x,y,t) - T_{amb}] dA + \sigma\varepsilon \int_S [T(x,y,t)^4 - T_{amb}^4] dA\} dt / S\Delta t$$

$$\approx \frac{1}{\Delta t \cdot n_p} \cdot$$

$$\frac{1}{2} \Big[\Big\{ h_{amb} \sum_i \sum_j [T(i,j,t_k) - T_{amb}] + \sigma\varepsilon \sum_i \sum_j [T(i,j,t_k)^4 - T_{amb}^4] \Big\}$$

$$+ \Big\{ h_{amb} \sum_i \sum_j [T(i,j,t_{k+1}) - T_{amb}] + \sigma\varepsilon \sum_i \sum_j [T(i,j,t_{k+1})^4 - T_{amb}^4] \Big\} \Big] \Delta t$$

$$\quad (8.18)$$

$$\approx \frac{1}{2n_p} \Big[\Big\{ h_{amb} \sum_i \sum_j [T(i,j,t_k) - T_{amb}] + \sigma\varepsilon \sum_i \sum_j [T(i,j,t_k)^4 - T_{amb}^4] \Big\}$$

$$+ \Big\{ h_{amb} \sum_i \sum_j [T(i,j,t_{k+1}) - T_{amb}] + \sigma\varepsilon \sum_i \sum_j [T(i,j,t_{k+1})^4 - T_{amb}^4] \Big\} \Big]$$

8.4   DETERMINATION OF THE MEAN HEAT TRANSFER COEFFICIENT

In equation (8.15), the mean heat transfer coefficient so far is yet to be known. In our case, we assume that this coefficient does not vary significantly among subjects. Although it is possible to derive the mean heat transfer coefficient based on reported values on the rate of tear evaporation, which falls between 9 Wm^{-2} and 100 Wm^{-2}, none of the investigations reported ocular surface temperature. Hence those values were not eligible for the determination of the coefficient value. This was overcome by looking into a finite element model on the ocular globe, on which several bioheat analyses were carried out previously [25].

The finite element model is basically a three-dimensional ocular globe, and the investigation looked into the steady-state heat transfer across the globe. By the first law of thermodynamics, for steady state we have

$$Q_{in} = Q_{out}$$

Then equation (8.7) is reduced to

$$\int_S \ddot{q}(x,y) dA - h_{amb} \int_S [T(x,y) - T_{amb}] dA$$

$$\quad (8.19)$$

$$- \sigma\varepsilon \int_S [T(x,y)^4 - T_{amb}^4] dA - \int_S E(x,y) dA = 0$$

Divide the above equation by S

$$\left[\int_S \ddot{q}(x,y)dA\right]/S - \left\{h_{amb}\int_S[T(x,y)-T_{amb}]dA\right\}/S$$

$$-\left\{\sigma\epsilon\int_S[T(x,y)^4 - T_{amb}^4]dA\right\}/S - \left[\int_S E(x,y)dA\right]/S = 0 \tag{8.20}$$

And since

$$\left[\int_S \ddot{q}(x,y)dA\right]/S = \frac{T_b - T_{amb}}{R\cdot S} \approx \overline{h}(T_b - T_{amb}) \tag{8.21}$$

$$\left\{h_{amb}\int_S[T(x,y)-T_{amb}]dA\right\}/S \approx \left\{h_{amb}\,\Sigma_i\,\Sigma_j[T(i,j)-T_{amb}]dA\right\}/n_p dA$$

$$\approx \frac{h_{amb}}{n_p}\,\Sigma_i\,\Sigma_j[T(i,j)-T_{amb}] \tag{8.22}$$

$$\left\{\sigma\epsilon\int_S[T(x,y)^4 - T_{amb}^4]dA\right\}/S \approx \left\{\sigma\epsilon\,\Sigma_i\,\Sigma_j[T(i,j)^4 - T_{amb}^4]dA\right\}/n_p dA$$

$$\approx \frac{\sigma\epsilon}{n_p}\,\Sigma_i\,\Sigma_j[T(i,j)^4 - T_{amb}^4] \tag{8.23}$$

$$\left[\int_S E(x,y)dA\right]/S \approx \left\{\Sigma_i\,\Sigma_j[E(i,j)dA]\right\}/n_p dA \approx \frac{1}{n_p}\Sigma_i\,\Sigma_j E(i,j) \tag{8.24}$$

Substitute (8.21)–(8.24) into (8.20) and we get

$$\overline{h}(T_b - T_{amb}) = \frac{h_{amb}}{n_p}\,\Sigma_i\,\Sigma_j[T(i,j)-T_{amb}]$$

$$+\frac{\sigma\epsilon}{n_p}\,\Sigma_i\,\Sigma_j[T(i,j)^4 - T_{amb}^4] + \frac{1}{n_p}\Sigma_i\,\Sigma_j E(i,j) \tag{8.25}$$

Rearrange,

$$\overline{h} = \frac{1}{T_b - T_{amb}}\cdot\left\{h_{amb}\left[\frac{\Sigma_i\,\Sigma_j\,T(i,j)}{n_p} - T_{amb}\right]\right.$$

$$\left. +\sigma\epsilon\left[\frac{\Sigma_i\,\Sigma_j\,T(i,j)^4}{n_p} - T^4_{amb}\right] + \frac{1}{n_p}\Sigma_i\,\Sigma_j E(i,j)\right\} \tag{8.26}$$

To determine $\overline{h}$, we need $T(i,j)$ of the ocular surface; however, this was not provided in the investigation. It was found that the central corneal temperature was 34.48°C [25] and limbus (which is 6.44 mm from the geometric centre of cornea) was 1.07°C lower than central corneal temperature. Furthermore it was observed that the temperature difference between a point on the ocular surface and the corneal center forms a paraboloid of revolution, which can be approximated by

$$z(x,y) = \frac{x^2}{a^2} + \frac{y^2}{b^2} \qquad (8.27)$$

and $a = b$ for the paraboloid of revolution; then,

$$z(x,y) = \frac{x^2 + y^2}{a^2} \qquad (8.28)$$

where $z(x, y)$ denotes the temperature difference in between a point (x, y) and the corneal center (the coordinates defined on x- and y-axis in the above are in line with the coordinates defined in Figure 8.5); a and b are the semi-major and semi-minor axis, respectively. Then the ocular surface temperature of the model can be approximated by

$$T(x,y) = \frac{x^2 + y^2}{a^2} + 34.38 \qquad (8.29)$$

In the model, on limbus region where $x^2 + y^2 = 0.00644^2$ (m^2), it has $z(x, y) = 1.07$ (°C); besides, it is possible to interpolate further values pair $(x^2 + y^2, z)$ from the paper's reported results, as tabulated in Table 8.1. Then we can approximate these values pair using least square and get

$$T(x, y) = 20992\ (x^2 + y^2) + 34.38 \qquad (8.30)$$

Based on the above, we produce Figure 8.2 and obtain the mean ocular surface temperature

TABLE 8.1
Interpolated Values Pair for $x^2 + y^2$ and $z(x, y)$

$x^2 + y^2$	$z(x, y)$
0.001^2	0.01
0.00125^2	0.02
0.002^2	0.055
0.0025^2	0.09
0.003^2	0.14
0.0035^2	0.19
0.004^2	0.25
0.0045^2	0.34
0.005^2	0.445
0.0055^2	0.58
0.006^2	0.76
0.00644^2	1.07

Source: E.Y.K. Ng, E.H. Ooi, Ocular surface temperature: A 3D FEM prediction using bioheat equation, Computers in Biology and Medicine, 37 (2007) 829–835.

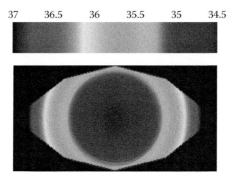

37   36.5   36   35.5   35   34.5

FIGURE 8.2   OST stimulated according to a 3D ocular model. (Please see color insert.)

$$[\Sigma_i \Sigma_j T(i,j)]/n_p = 35.31°C \tag{8.31}$$

Besides, the finite element analysis adopted a tear evaporation rate of 40 Wm^{-2} in their simulation, so we know

$$[\Sigma_i \Sigma_j T(i,j)]/n_p = 35.31°C \tag{8.32}$$

By calculation

$$h_{amb}\left[\frac{\Sigma_i \Sigma_j T(i,j)}{n_p} - T_{amb}\right] = 103.1$$

$$\sigma\varepsilon\left[\frac{\Sigma_i \Sigma_j T(i,j)^4}{n_p} - T_{amb}^4\right] = 63.57$$

From (8.26),

$$\bar{h} = \frac{103.1 + 63.5 + 40}{37 - 25}$$

$$\bar{h} = 17.22 \ (K^{-1}Wm^{-2}) \tag{8.33}$$

Together with (8.10), (8.18) and (8.33), we have

$$E_{t_1t_2} = 17.22 \ (T_b - T_{amb}) - L_{t_1t_2}$$

where

$$L_{t_kt_{k+1}} = \frac{1}{2n_p}\left[\left\{h_{amb}\Sigma_i\Sigma_j[T(i,j,t_k) - T_{amb}] + \sigma\varepsilon\Sigma_i\Sigma_j[T(i,j,t_k)^4 - T_{amb}^4]\right\}\right.$$

$$\left. + \left\{h_{amb}\Sigma_i\Sigma_j[T(i,j,t_{k+1}) - T_{amb}] + \sigma\varepsilon\Sigma_i\Sigma_j[T(i,j,t_{k+1})^4 - T_{amb}^4]\right\}\right] \tag{8.34}$$

It is also possible to calculate the tear evaporation rate on cornea and sclera:

$$_{cor}E_{t_k t_{k+1}} = {}_{cor}Q_{t_k t_{k+1}} - {}_{cor}L_{t_k t_{k+1}} \tag{8.35}$$

$$_{scl}E_{t_k t_{k+1}} = {}_{scl}Q_{t_k t_{k+1}} - {}_{scl}L_{t_k t_{k+1}} \tag{8.36}$$

Since we consider the total inflow heat to the anterior surface to be constant, as the heat is assumed to flow uniformly across the ocular globe, then

$$_{cor}Q_{t_k t_{k+1}} = {}_{scl}Q_{t_k t_{k+1}} = Q_{t_k t_{k+1}} = \bar{h}(T_b - T_{amb}) \tag{8.37}$$

In regard to the mean heat loss for corneal and scleral regions, for each of them it can be obtained by summing the heat loss across the respective region over time Δt, and divided by the product of region's area and time period Δt:

$$_{cor}L_{t_k t_{k+1}} = \frac{1}{2n_{cor}} \Big[\{ h_{amb} \Sigma_i \Sigma_j [T(i,j,t_k) - T_{amb}]$$
$$- \sigma \varepsilon \Sigma_i \Sigma_j [T(i,j,t_k)^4 - T_{amb}^4] \}_{cor}$$
$$+ \{ h_{amb} \Sigma_i \Sigma_j [T(i,j,t_{k+1}) - T_{amb}]$$
$$+ \sigma \varepsilon \Sigma_i \Sigma_j [T(i,j,t_{k+1})^4 - T_{amb}^4] \}_{cor} \Big] \tag{8.38}$$

$$_{scl}L_{t_k t_{k+1}} = \frac{1}{2n_{scl}} \Big[\{ h_{amb} \Sigma_i \Sigma_j [T(i,j,t_k) - T_{amb}]$$
$$+ \sigma \varepsilon \Sigma_i \Sigma_j [T(i,j,t_k)^4 - T_{amb}^4] \}_{scl}$$
$$+ \{ h_{amb} \Sigma_i \Sigma_j [T(i,j,t_{k+1}) - T_{amb}]$$
$$+ \sigma \varepsilon \Sigma_i \Sigma_j [T(i,j,t_{k+1})^4 - T_{amb}^4] \}_{scl} \Big] \tag{8.39}$$

Furthermore, from (8.8) we divide the equation by dA and Δt,

$$\frac{1}{dA \cdot \Delta t} \int_{t_1}^{t_2} E(x,y,t)dAdt = \frac{1}{dA \cdot \Delta t} \int_{t_1}^{t_2} \ddot{q}(x,y,t)dAdt$$
$$- \frac{1}{dA \cdot \Delta t} \int_{t_1}^{t_2} h_{amb}[T(x,y,t) - T_{amb}]dAdt \tag{8.40}$$
$$- \frac{1}{dA \cdot \Delta t} \int_{t_1}^{t_2} \sigma \varepsilon[T(x,y,t)^4 - T_{amb}^4]dAdt$$

Let

$$_eE = \frac{1}{dA \cdot \Delta t} \int_{t_1}^{t_2} E(x, y, t) dAdt \tag{8.41}$$

$$_eQ = \frac{1}{dA \cdot \Delta t} \int_{t_1}^{t_2} \ddot{q}(x, y, t) dAdt \tag{8.42}$$

$$_eL = \frac{1}{dA \cdot \Delta t} \int_{t_1}^{t_2} h_{amb}[T(x, y, t) - T_{amb}] dAdt$$

$$+ \frac{1}{dA \cdot \Delta t} \int_{t_1}^{t_2} \sigma\varepsilon[T(x, y, t)^4 - T_{amb}^4] dAdt \tag{8.43}$$

Substitute (8.41)–(8.43) into (8.40), and we have

$$_eE = {}_eQ - {}_eL \tag{8.44}$$

where $_eE$ refers to the mean tear evaporation of a small-piece element during Δt. From (8.44), we equate $_eQ$ to (8.15) and get the relative mean tear evaporation of that element:

$$_e^rE = 17.22(T_b - T_{amb}) - {}_eL \tag{8.45}$$

8.5   THERMOGRAPHIC ESTIMATION

In ocular thermography, it has been concluded that the temperature data captured by the thermal images was pertinent to the thin tear film [9], which generally consists of three layers: an outer lipid layer, a middle aqueous layer, and a mucous layer. The thin film has a thickness of around 3 to 10 μm, in which the aqueous layer accounts for 90% thickness [29]; the lipid layer, on the other hand, is approximately 100 nm thick [30]. Despite this, in the literature it is still a common practice to regard the temperature captured by the ocular thermography as the temperature of the corneal and conjunctival surfaces. Hence this temperature data serves as the basis for $T(i, j)$ in the calculation of (8.34)–(8.36).

To realize the estimation of the rate of tear evaporation as laid out above, we need thermal recordings on the region of the ocular surface, with a reasonable frame rate so that Δt can be considerably small. After that, in the recording we need to efficiently segment the anterior surface from the other facial regions and warp the thermal images into a standardized form. Only then can we perform an estimation of evaporation rate based on (8.34)–(8.36).

8.5.1   IMAGE WARPING

It is well known that the cornea–sclera boundary is indiscernible in ocular thermal images, and this makes the discrimination between the cornea and sclera regions a daunting task. Hence, we need a good scheme to efficiently resolve this issue.

In this case we use an image warping/metamorphosis technique. This methodology is proposed to solve the two issues—localization of the ocular surface and segmentation of the cornea—at once. In warping, the thermal data at the anterior surface is transformed into a standard form, in which the corneal region is well defined. The following explanation covers the basic idea behind the methodology, and then actual procedures are explained.

Two approaches are available for image warping: forward mapping and reverse mapping [31]. The former methodology goes through each of the pixels in the source image pixel by pixel and puts them into appropriate locations on the destination image. For the latter, the algorithm runs through the destination image pixel by pixel and samples the relevant pixels in the source image [32]. In this application, we adopted a sort of reverse mapping, proposed by Beier and Neely [32]. Starting with a number of pairs of lines defined on a source image and its corresponding destination image, for each line $Q_{q_i}Q_{q_{i+1}}$, the algorithm calculates

$$u = \frac{(D - Q_{q_i}) \cdot (Q_{q_{i+1}} - Q_{q_i})}{\left\| Q_{q_{i+1}} - Q_{q_i} \right\|^2} \qquad (8.46)$$

$$v = \frac{(D - Q_{q_i}) \cdot perpendicular\, (Q_{q_{i+1}} - Q_{q_i})}{\left\| Q_{q_{i+1}} - Q_{q_i} \right\|^2} \qquad (8.47)$$

$$D' = Q'_{q_i} + u \cdot (Q'_{q_{i+1}} - Q'_{q_i}) + \frac{v \cdot perpendicular\, (Q'_{q_{i+1}} - Q'_{q_i})}{\left\| Q'_{q_{i+1}} - Q'_{q_i} \right\|^2} \qquad (8.48)$$

where D and D' are coordinates of destination image pixel and source image pixel, respectively, as illustrated in Figure 8.3; function *perpendicular* () returns the vector perpendicular to and equal to the input vector. Then, for the case of multiline, the algorithm does the following:

For each pixel D in destination image

```
DSUM = 0
weightsum = 0
For each line Q_{q_i}Q_{q_{i+1}}
      Get u, v determined on Q_{q_i}Q_{q_{i+1}}
      Get D'_{q_i}
      Calculate Ds_{q_i} = D'_{q_i} - D
      dist = shortest distance from D to Q_{q_i}Q_{q_{i+1}}
      weight = ( ‖Q_{q_i}Q_{q_{i+1}}‖^{c_1} / (c_2 + dist) )^{c_3}
      DSUM += Ds_{q_i} · weight
      weightsum += weight
D' = D + DSUM/weightsum
destinationImage(D) = sourceImage(D')
```

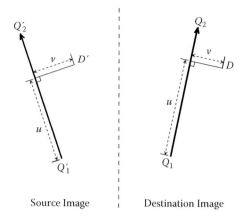

Source Image   Destination Image

FIGURE 8.3   Single line pair between source image and destination image.

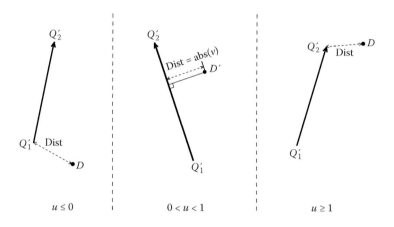

FIGURE 8.4   The defined shortest distances from D to $Q_{q_i}Q_{q_{i+1}}$.

The shortest distance from D to $Q_{q_i} Q_{q_{i+1}}$ is $abs(v)$ if $0 < u < 1$; if $u \leq 0$, that value equals the straight-line distance between D and Q_{q_i}; if $u \geq 1$, it equals the straight-line distance between D and $Q_{q_{i+1}}$ (see Figure 8.4).

In the actual application, on the first thermal image of any length of sequence, we pick up eight points around the palpebral fissure, on which the algorithm will in turn form eight lines that approximately enclose the entire eye, as shown in Figure 8.5. The selection of the eight points needs to proceed in this fashion: four points $Q_1', Q_3', Q_5',$ and Q_7' are first determined, as seen in Figure 8.5(a); these points correspond to medial canthus, middle upper edge, lateral canthus, and middle lower edge of a left eye (similarly, these points correspond to the lateral canthus, middle upper edge, medial canthus, and middle lower edge of a right eye), followed by the

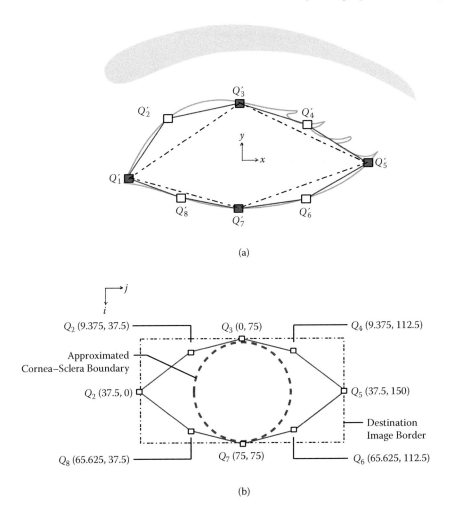

(a)

(b)

FIGURE 8.5 Points and lines defined in the source and the destination images in the warping of ocular thermal images. (Please see color insert.)

points $Q_2', Q_4', Q_6',$ and Q_8'. Q_2' falls somewhere between Q_1' and Q_3' along the edge of an eye; similarly Q_4' falls somewhere between Q_3' and Q_5' along the edge of the eye. Q_6' and Q_8' are also selected by the same principle (Figure 8.5(a)). The details on the corresponding points and lines in the destination image (which has a size of 75×150 pixels) are illustrated in Figure 8.5(b).

After the above point determination, the entire thermographic sequence is warped accordingly. This is possible because the movement and variation in the shape of the palpebral fissure are insignificant. Therefore a single round of point selection is sufficient for the warping of the whole sequence. Figure 8.6 illustrates the estimation of the rate of tear evaporation on both eyes of a normal subject.

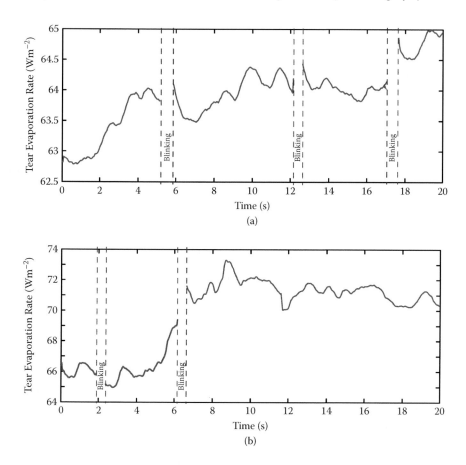

FIGURE 8.6   Tear evaporation rate of a normal subject: (a) left eye; (b) right eye. (Please see color insert.)

8.6   CONCLUSION

Previously, the rate of tear evaporation was measured mostly by relative humidity. A closed chamber was fixed around the subject's eye to collect data on the change in relative humidity and derive the rate value. In some investigations, the air was consistently trapped within the chamber. In the absence of constant airflow in and out of the chamber, the rise in humidity within the chamber in practice retards the ongoing tear evaporation at the ocular surface. The observed value in the rate may not be the actual evaporation of tear under a usual ambient environment. Furthermore, it is unclear if the application of a closed chamber around the eye has an effect on the measurement outcome.

In this chapter, we have illustrated possible ways to measure the rate of evaporation on thermographic sequence. The developed idea does not need any contact with the facial and ocular region. It is possible to perform repeated measurement by this method on the rate, as it does not interfere with any part of the anterior ocular surface. The data can be captured with ease and the procedure is simple. During the eye blinks, the corresponding thermal data can be easily removed and avoided in analysis. By warping, users have full control over the evaluation of the rate; for regions other than the ocular surface it can be easily excluded. The application of petroleum jelly around the eye is not required. The recording can be achieved in a single shot and does not need two observations, and there is no ambiguous subtraction in values. This method can be used by physicians and ophthalmologists in the diagnosis of dry eye.

REFERENCES

1. K.B. Bjerrum, Keratoconjunctivitis sicca and primary Sjögren's syndrome in a Danish population aged 30–60 years, *Acta Ophthalmologica Scandinavica*, 75 (1997) 281–286.
2. B.E. Caffery, D. Richter, T. Simpson, D. Fonn, M. Doughty, K. Gordon, CANDEES. The Canadian Dry Eye Epidemiology Study, *Adv Exp Med Biol*, 438 (1998) 805–806.
3. W.D. Mathers, A.M. Dolney, D. Kraemer, The effect of hormone replacement therapy on the symptoms and physiologic parameters of dry eye, *Adv Exp Med Biol*, 506 (2002) 1017–1022.
4. C.A. McCarty, A.K. Bansal, P.M. Livingston, Y.L. Stanislavsky, H.R. Taylor, The epidemiology of dry eye in Melbourne, Australia, *Ophthalmology*, 105 (1998) 1114–1119.
5. C.W. McMonnies, A. Ho, Responses to a dry eye questionnaire from a normal population, *J Am Optom Assoc*, 58 (1987) 588–591.
6. O.D. Schein, B. Munoz, J.M. Tielsch, Prevalence of dry eye among the elderly, *Am J Ophthalmol*, 124 (1997) 723–728.
7. S.H. Waduthantri, H.L. A., C.H. Tan, L. Tong, Annual medical expenditure of dry eye syndrome in Singapore, in 2011.
8. J. Yu, C.V. Asche, C.J. Fairchild, The economic burden of dry eye disease in the United States: A decision tree analysis, *Cornea*, 30 (2011) 379–387 310.1097/ICO. 1090b1013e3181f1097f1363.
9. J.H. Tan, E.Y.K. Ng, U.R. Acharya, C. Chee, Infrared thermography on ocular surface temperature: A review, *Infrared Physics Technology*, (2009).
10. G. Von Bahr, Könnte die Flussigkeitsabgang durch die Cornea von physiologischer Bedeutung sein, *Acta Opthalmol (Copenh)*, 19 (1941) 125–134.
11. S. Mishima, D.M. Maurice, The oily layer of the tear film and evaporation from the corneal surface, *Exp Eye Res*, 1 (1961) 39–45.
12. S. Iwata, M.A. Lemp, F.J. Holly, C.H. Dohlman, Evaporation rate of water from the precorneal tear film and cornea in the rabbit, *Invest Ophthalmol*, 8 (1969) 613–619.
13. H. Hamano, M. Hori, H. Kawabe, S. Mitsunaga, Y. Ohnishi, I. Koma, Modification of the superficial layer of the tear film by the secretion of the meibomian glands, *Folia Ophthalmol Japonica*, 31 (1980) 353–360.
14. M. Rolando, M.F. Refojo, Tear evaporimeter for measuring water evaporation rate from the tear film under controlled conditions in humans, *Exp Eye Res*, 36 (1983) 25–33.
15. W. Mathers, Evaporation from the ocular surface, *Exp Eye Res*, 78 (2004) 389–394.
16. K. Tsubota, M. Yamada, Tear evaporation from the ocular surface, *Invest Ophthalmol Vis Sci*, 33 (1992) 2942–2950.
17. A. Tomlinson, G.R. Trees, J.R. Occhipinti, Tear production and evaporation in the normal eye, *Ophthalmic Physiol Opt*, 11 (1991) 44–47.

18. W.D. Mathers, G. Binarao, M. Petroll, Ocular water evaporation and the dry eye. A new measuring device, *Cornea*, 12 (1993) 335–340.
19. E. Goto, K. Endo, A. Suzuki, Y. Fujikura, Y. Matsumoto, K. Tsubota, Tear evaporation dynamics in normal subjects and subjects with obstructive meibomian gland dysfunction, *Invest Ophthalmol Vis Sci*, 44 (2003) 533–539.
20. F.H. Adler, R.A. Moses, *Adler's physiology of the eye: Clinical application*, 5th ed., Mosby, Saint Louis, 1970.
21. J.A. Scott, A finite element model of heat transport in the human eye, *Phys Med Biol*, 33 (1988) 227–241.
22. S.J. Erickson, A. Godavarty, Hand-held based near-infrared optical imaging devices: A review, *Med Eng Physics*, 31 (2009) 495–509.
23. V.S. Cheng, J. Bai, Y. Chen, A high-resolution three-dimensional far-infrared thermal and true-color imaging system for medical applications, *Med Eng Physics*, 31 (2009) 1173–1181.
24. J.P. Craig, I. Singh, A. Tomlinson, et al., The role of tear physiology in ocular surface temperature, *Eye*, 14 (2000) 635–641.
25. E.Y.K. Ng, E.H. Ooi, Ocular surface temperature: A 3D FEM prediction using bioheat equation, *Computers Biol Med*, 37 (2007) 829–835.
26. J.-H. Tan, E.Y.K. Ng, U.R. Acharya, Evaluation of tear evaporation from ocular surface by functional infrared thermography, *Med Physics*, 37 (2010) 6022–6034.
27. A.F. Emery, P.O. Kramar, A.W. Guy, J.C. Lin, Microwave induced temperature rises in rabbit eyes in cataract research, *J Heat Transfer*, C97 (1975) 123–128.
28. Y.A. Cengel, *Introduction to thermodynamics and heat transfer*, McGraw-Hill, 1996.
29. L. Remington, *Clinical anatomy of the visual system*, 2nd ed., Butterworth-Heinemann, 2004.
30. J.P. Craig, A. Tomlinson, Importance of the lipid layer in human tear film stability and evaporation, *Optometry Vision Sci*, 74 (1997) 8–13.
31. G. Wolberg, *Digital image warping*, IEEE Computer Society Press, 1990.
32. T. Beier, S. Neely, Feature-based image metamorphosis, *Computer Graphics*, 26 (1992) 35–42.

9 Tear Film Thermal Image Characteristics Analysis in Temporal and Spatial Aspects

Huihua Kenny Chiang, Tai Yuan Su, Shu Wen Chang, Joe Chang, and David O. Chang

CONTENTS

9.1 INTRODUCTION

Dry eye syndrome (keratoconjunctivitis sicca) is one of the most common eye diseases in developed countries. The syndrome is caused by various types of etiology and is a result of loss in tear film quality. Clinical assessments of tear film conditions include stability of the tear film, the amount of tear, osmolality of the tear, superficial punctate keratopathy, and meibomian gland dysfunction.

Current clinical diagnostic methods for dry eye syndrome are contact procedures, which are uncomfortable for patients. In recent years, the development of noncontact or noninvasive dry eye diagnostic methods has received significant attention among researchers. One promising method uses infrared thermal imaging to examine the quality of the tear film, playing a critical role in noncontact dry eye diagnoses.

This chapter presents a study of the characteristics of infrared thermal images of normal and dry eye patients. These characteristics relate to the quality of the tear film, which we investigated in the spatial and temporal aspect.

9.2   DRY EYE SYNDROME AND TEAR FILM

9.2.1   DRY EYE SYNDROME

Dry eye syndrome is characterized by symptoms of ocular discomfort and represents a wide variety of conditions associated with decreased tear production and/or abnormally rapid tear-film evaporation. In developed countries, more than 15% of the population suffers from the syndrome, and the number is increasing. The prevalence of dry eye syndrome relates to the wide use of computers, contact lense wear, air conditioning, and air pollution problems. The eyes become dry because (1) not enough tear is produced and (2) the rate of the evaporation of tear is abnormally high.

Common symptoms of dry eye syndrome include feelings of sandy-gritty irritation, dryness, blurred vision, excessive tearing, burning, or increased awareness of the eyes. Dry eye syndrome may worsen with time and eventually damage the surface of the cornea.

9.2.2   TEAR FILM STRUCTURE

The tear film is a thin liquid film that covers the cornea. The tear film provides moisture and lubrication to maintain eye function. If any unbalance occurs to the tear film, a person may experience dry eye syndrome.

The tear film comprises three main layers: the mucin layer, the aqueous layer, and the lipid layer.[1] There is no distinct barrier between the layers. Instead, each layer gradiently transitions into another.

The inner layer of the tear film is the mucin layer, which creates a hydrophilic surface that allows the aqueous layer to spread smoothly and evenly over the ocular surface. The aqueous layer, which is composed primarily of water, is located between the mucin layer and the lipid layer. The aqueous layer is produced by lacrimal glands to create a proper environment for epithelial cells of the eyes. The aqueous layer also provides oxygen to the cornea and enables epithelial cells to move on the ocular surfaces. The water remains mainly in this layer; a lack of water may cause aqueous deficiency in the tear film. Uneven distribution of the aqueous layer increases the risk of excessive evaporation, which may result in dry eye syndrome. The outer layer of the tear film is the lipid layer, which is secreted from the meibomian glands. The main function of the lipid layer is to prevent evaporation of the aqueous layer.

The blink reflex of the eyes releases the oily product from the meibomian glands to the tear film, increasing the thickness of the lipid layer. A lack of lipid secretion may result in excessive evaporation of the aqueous layer.

The tear film is restored with the blink reflex. A person may increase the frequency of blinking when experiencing dryness of the eyes, indicating a minor or early stage of dry eye syndrome.

9.2.3   DRY EYE DIAGNOSIS METHODS

Numerous studies have presented clinical diagnostic methods to evaluate dry eye syndrome, which are based chiefly on measuring the quality of the tear film, and are listed as follows:

1. Schirmer's test: This test is performed by placing a filter paper inside the lower lid of the eye and waiting for the filter paper to absorb tears for 5 min. The length of the wet filter paper is used to evaluate the amount of tear production. If the length is longer than 10 mm, the amount of tear production is normal. The major drawbacks of the test are its invasiveness and low repeatability.

2. Tear film breakup time (TBUT): TBUT is performed by applying fluorescent sodium drops on the ocular surface and measuring the time of tear film breakage. If tear film breakage does not occur within 10 seconds, tear film stability is normal. The drawbacks of TBUT are its invasiveness, subjectivity, and low chances for repeatability.

3. Tear osmolality: Tear osmolality is performed by extracting tears and measuring the osmolality of the tears. For dry eye patients, continuous evaporation of tears results in a lack of water in the tear film, and increases tear osmolality. When tear osmolality is greater than 315 mOsmol/L, the patient likely has dry eye disease.[2]

4. Superficial punctate keratopathy (SPK): Superficial punctate keratitis, or corneal erosion, is the death of small cell groups on the surface of the cornea. The most readily available and commonly used diagnostic tool for SPK is the slit lamp or an ophthalmoscope examination of the cornea, which can reveal a characteristic hazy appearance with multiple punctate speckles that stain with fluorescein. Rose bengal staining is another method for evaluating patients with dry eye syndrome. Rose bengal is a water-soluble dye that is applied to the ocular surface and absorbed by devitalized (sick) epithelial cells and mucin. Positive staining of the conjunctiva with rose bengal is consistent with a diagnosis of dry eye syndrome. Dry eye-related fluorescein/rose bengal staining first appears at the interpalpebral (exposure) area of both the cornea and conjunctiva in early cases, while staining could extend to non-exposure areas in severe cases. Fluorophotometry is useful for assessing the severity of dry eyes from the aspect of the corneal epithelial barrier function and measuring the tear turnover rate.

5. Meibomian gland dysfunction (MGD): Both videomeibography and meibometry are useful for screening meibomian gland dysfunctions. Meibography

assesses the structure of the meibomian gland by transilluminating the lid from the skin while turning over the lid.[3-8] Meibometry is the blotting of lipid onto a loop of translucent plastic tape from the central region of the lower lid. The process is a simple test to quantify the amount of lipids at the lid margin. Standard meibometry uses the clinical Meibometer (MB 550; Courage & Khazaka Electronic GmbH, Cologne, Germany). After modification from standard meibometry, direct meibometry modifies the Goldman applanation tonometer probe (Keeler, Windsor, England), which is mounted on a slit-lamp biomicroscope.[3] This permits controlled placement of the probe on the lid margin under direct vision. Integrated meibometry provides a cohesive analysis of densities over the entire area of the imprint.[3]

6. Ocular surface disease index (OSDI): OSDI is a questionnaire-based dry eye syndrome diagnostic method, which contains twelve questions to be graded on a scale from 0 to 4 for each question. The total scores are added to identify the degree of dry eyes.[9]

7. Infrared thermal imaging method: Several researchers have proposed using infrared thermal cameras to measure the quality of tear film. The camera records the temperature distribution on the ocular surface, which indicates the amount of tear evaporation. Evaporation shows a strong correlation to the quality of the tear film.[10]

9.2.4 DRY EYE CLASSIFICATION

The diagnostic classification of dry eye syndrome has been complicated in the past by the lack of accepted diagnostic criteria and standardized specific diagnostic tests. A commonly used subclassification in this regard separates dry eye patients into those with decreased aqueous tear production (aqueous tear deficiency, ATD) and those with excessive tear evaporation (evaporative tear dysfunction, ETD). These two conditions often coexist.

9.2.4.1 Aqueous Tear Deficiency (ATD)

Particular signs of ATD include decreased aqueous tear production measured via Schirmer testing, exposure pattern of conjunctival and/or corneal staining with rose bengal and/or fluorescein, and filamentary keratopathy. Patients displaying signs and symptoms of ATD can be subdivided into those who have Sjögren syndrome and those who do not (non-Sjögren syndrome), as shown in Figure 9.1.

9.2.4.2 Evaporative Tear Dysfunction (ETD)

Increased tear film evaporation is most commonly caused by meibomian gland dysfunction. Meibomian gland diseases, poor eyelid apposition to the ocular surface, increased palpebral aperture, and contact lens wear could also lead to ETD. Symptoms include burning, foreign-body sensations, redness of the eyelids and conjunctiva, filmy vision, and recurrent chalazia. Signs of ETD include decreased tear breakup time, meibomian gland dysfunction, abnormal aqueous tear production, and a characteristic linear pattern of rose bengal/fluorescein staining of the inferior conjunctiva, the cornea, and the eyelid margin.

Aqueous tear deficiency (ATD)
Sjögren syndrome
        Primary
        Secondary

Non-Sjögren syndrome
        Lacrimal disease (primary or secondary)
        Lacrimal obstructive disease
        Reflex hyopsecretion
        Other (e.g., multiple neuromatosis)

Evaporative tear dysfunction (ETD)
Evaporative tear dysfunction
        Meibomian gland disease or dysfunction
        Increased palpebral aperture
        Poor eyelid/lobe congruity
        Contact lens wear

FIGURE 9.1 Classification of dry eye syndrome. ATD and ETD are commonly used subclassifications.

9.3 TEAR FILM SURFACE TEMPERATURE AND THERMAL IMAGE

Many clinical utility imaging tools are available for the assessment of ocular surface disease; the advantages and disadvantages of the imaging modality are listed in Table 9.1.

Since 1990, researchers have used infrared thermal imaging systems to observe the ocular surface temperature (OST) and tear film stability noninvasively.[10–14] The evaporation of tear film reduces the ocular surface temperature. The ocular surface temperature reveals the tear film stability.[12,13] The tear film stability is related to the thickness of the lipid layer, which is associated with dry eye syndrome.[15]

The lipid layer covers the aqueous layer to prevent water evaporation. The lipid layer thins continuously while the eyes are open. The lipid layer eventually breaks; the time period over which this occurs is the TBUT. The longer the tear breakup time, the more stable the tear film, which subsequently signifies less evaporation.

An IR camera can measure tear film evaporation by monitoring the temperature change across the ocular surface during the open-eye period. Researchers have found that temperature characteristics on the ocular surface are related to dry eye syndrome. A series of thermal images of a dry eye (Figure 9.2) shows the temperature distribution on the ocular surface. The darker area represents a relatively lower temperature, and the lighter area represents a relatively warmer area. The darker area also represents a larger amount of tear film evaporation occurrence. The distribution of the darker area signifies the irregularity of the tear film.

TABLE 9.1

Clinical Use and Limitations of Imaging Modalities

Imaging Modality	Clinical Use	Advantages	Limitations
Topography-based imaging	Evaluation of corneal radius and thickness Screening and diagnosis of keratoconus Assessment of tear film quality	Noninvasive, objective measurement Highly accurate for tear breakup time	Costly equipment
Angiography	Observation of blood flow in ocular surface	Visualization and differentiation of blood flow Indocyanine-green angiography No leakage from normal blood vessels, which enables thorough examination Fluorescein angiography Quick visualization of changes in blood perfusion	Invasiveness due to intravenous administration of dyes with discomfort for patients Possible allergic reaction Indocyanine-green angiography Possible allergic reaction to iodine Fluorescein angiography Fast leakage from normal blood vessels, which reduces necessary examination times
Confocal microscopy (CM)	*In vivo* clinical imaging of ocular surface structures and optical sectioning of human eye	*In vivo* usage High magnification and resolution Detailed visualization of cornea, conjunctiva, and meibomian glands	Possible discomfort to patients Costly equipment
Meibomian gland imaging	Visualization of meibomian gland embedded in the eyelids Diagnosis of MGD	Meibography Mounting onto slit-lamp biomicroscope Affordable equipment CM meibography High magnification Detailed imaging of glandular ducts and acinar cells	Meibography Decreased image quality due to overexposure or reflection Eversion of eyelid with discomfort to patients CM meibography Invasive as objective touches the eyelid with possible discomfort to patients Costly equipment
Tear interferometry	Diagnosis of abnormal tear film	Noninvasive Fast measurement Detailed assessment of tear film quality	Constant temperature and humidity required Costly equipment

TABLE 9.1 (CONTINUED)
Clinical Use and Limitations of Imaging Modalities

Imaging Modality	Clinical Use	Advantages	Limitations
Anterior segment optical coherence tomography	Diagnosis of abnormalities in cornea and tear film	Noninvasive	Constant temperature and humidity required for tear film evaluation External analysis tools Costly equipment
Ocular thermography	Measurement of ocular surface temperature Diagnosis of tear abnormalities using tear evaporation	Noninvasive Fast measurement Calculation of tear evaporation	External analysis tools Costly equipment

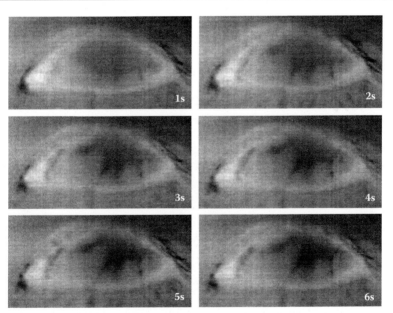

FIGURE 9.2 A series of 6-second thermal images of an abnormal tear film during an open-eye period.

9.3.1 TEAR FILM THERMAL IMAGING SYSTEM

An IR camera system is custom designed for tear film temperature measurement, as shown in Figure 9.3. This system records the thermal image of the tear film at a rate of 30 films per second, with a spatial resolution of 320×240 pixels. The IR camera can be moved with a joystick for adjusting the camera to align with the eye. The camera and eye are maintained at the same distance during the measurement.

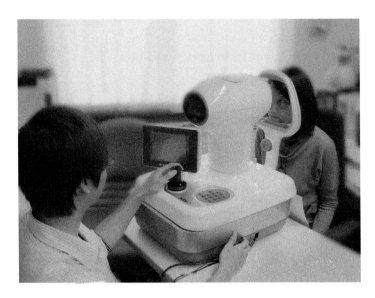

FIGURE 9.3   The tear film thermal image measurement system. (Please see color insert.)

An infrared radiation detector module, a microbolometer sensor (BOEING U3000A, DRS Sensors & Targeting Systems, Parsippany, NJ), is operated at uncooled room temperature. This module is sensitive to infrared radiation between 8 to 12 μm. The size of the sensor is 51×51 (μm^2). The noise equivalent temperature difference (NETD) of the image system is 0.07°C, and the measurement accuracy is 0.1°C. For considering background radiation, a black body plate is inserted to adjust the sensor before the measurement. The IR camera has a Germanium lens with a 120-mm working distance. With this working distance, the camera acquires and records the thermography of the tear film without causing uncomfortable sensation for patients.

9.3.2   Region of Interest Selection Method

The region of interest (ROI) selection method selects the region on the ocular surface for analysis. Four apex points, P1–P4, define the entire ROI, as shown in Figure 9.4. This selection method is based on the equations of the eye template method.[16] The four apex points are set by the operator manually to exclude the influence from the eyelashes. The points P3 and P4 are located on the top and bottom of the eye, above and below the eyelashes, respectively. The points P1 and P2 are located on the left and right corner of the eye, respectively, to avoid line y_{ij} contacting the eyelashes.

9.3.3   Temperature versus Gray Level Mapping Method

The infrared radiation detector module acquires the temperature value with 12-bit resolution. For operation convenience and visualization purposes, the ocular surface temperature is presented in a 256 gray level. The averaging temperature is set at a gray level of 127. The temperature ±1.8°C above or below the average temperature

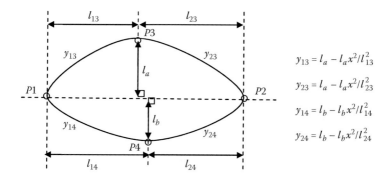

$$y_{13} = l_a - l_a x^2 / l_{13}^2$$

$$y_{23} = l_a - l_a x^2 / l_{23}^2$$

$$y_{14} = l_b - l_b x^2 / l_{14}^2$$

$$y_{24} = l_b - l_b x^2 / l_{24}^2$$

FIGURE 9.4   The ROI is connected by four curves: y_{13}, y_{32}, y_{42}, and y_{14}.

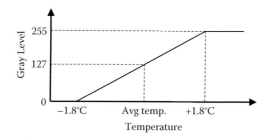

FIGURE 9.5   The mapping relationship between the ocular surface temperature and the [0, 255] gray level.

of the ROI is set at a gray level of 255 and 0, as shown in Figure 9.5. This range also provides an adequate temperature resolution, $3.6/256 = 0.014$ (°C/gray level), for image recording and further processing purposes.

9.3.4   MEASUREMENT CONDITIONS

Ocular surface temperature was recorded in an examination room, which was controlled at a stable temperature and humidity. The forehead and the chin of participants were placed against a measuring bracket to stabilize the position of the eye during the measurement. The geometric center of the cornea was aligned with the camera lens by controlling the joystick on the control panel. During the measurement, participants were asked to close their eyes for 2 s before opening them for 6 s. The ocular surface IR image was recorded and displayed in real time.

9.4   THERMAL IMAGE CHARACTERISTICS

The temperature characteristics of the tear film are presented in temporal and spatial aspects. The temporal features illustrate the changes in ocular surface temperature due to tear film evaporation once the eyes are open. The spatial features illustrate the distribution changes in ocular surface temperature during the evaporation process.

9.4.1 TEMPORAL CHARACTERISTICS

The temporal characteristic is the evaluation of the averaged temperature change of the ocular surface. The ocular surface temperature is an indicator for identifying the tear film quality. Several groups have reported that the abnormal eye group had a greater degree of temperature decrease compared to the control group.[11,17] The phenomenon may be due to faster tear film evaporation and faster temperature decrease in the abnormal eye group.

To demonstrate this phenomenon, a gold standard of normal and abnormal eye groups was required, which was provided in the clinical test. The participants were classified as normal and abnormal eye groups via Schirmer's test and the TBUT test. After the clinical tests, the IR images were recorded and analyzed.

The abnormal and normal eyes were first classified according to Schirmer's test and the TBUT test. Fourteen eyes had low Schirmer's test scores (<5 mm/5 min), and the TBUT (<10 s) results indicate abnormal tear film conditions; twelve eyes achieved high Schirmer's test scores (>5 mm/5 min), and TBUT (>10 s) indicated normal tear film conditions. The two groups were subsequently measured via the IR thermal imaging system to obtain the ocular surface temperature.

The ocular surface temperature was obtained in each IR image. The image first selected the region of interest before the pixel value was averaged within the area to acquire the average temperature. All the eyes were measured with the IR thermal imaging system 6 s upon opening the eye. All the participants were asked to close their eyes for 2 s before opening them for 6 s. The eyes are open normally during the measurement to avoid reflex tearing. The participants were recommended to take deep breaths during the measurement; this stabilizes body movement to ensure that the eye stays on the correct focusing region.

The results of the temporal change in the ocular surface temperature with time are shown in Figure 9.6.

The average temperature of the abnormal eye group is lower than that of the normal eye group, indicating the existence of fast evaporation in the tear film of the abnormal eye group. The standard deviation rises as the eye stays open longer; this phenomenon indicates the inhomogeneity in the ocular surface temperature during the open-eye period.

Though using the temporal characteristic to classify tear film conditions is statistically significant, the error bar reveals that standard deviation increases with time, even when environmental conditions are carefully controlled. The temperature measurement is sensitive to environmental conditions, such as the temperature, moisture, and wind around the eye.

9.4.2 SPATIAL CHARACTERISTICS

Recent studies showed that temperature distributions on the ocular surface of normal eyes were smooth, with homogeneity curves.[18,19] Thermal image patterns of the dry eye group appeared more irregular and unstable compared to those of the normal eye group.[20–23]

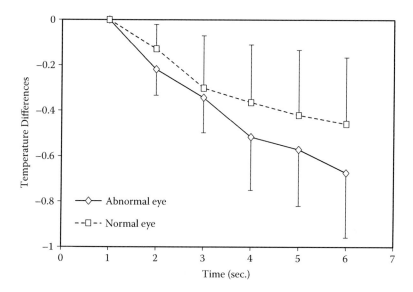

FIGURE 9.6   The temporal characteristics of the ocular surface temperature during the open-eye period. The error bar is the standard deviation. The abnormal eye group experienced a larger temperature drop in ocular surface temperature.

Tear film evaporates before cooling down the ocular surface. The IR imaging system captures the temperature distribution during the eye-opening period. The degree of temperature variation of the tear film can subsequently be quantified by measuring the compactness value of the thermal image of the tear film.

The compactness value is defined as the square root of a perimeter divided by its region. The perimeter and the region of the compactness value are defined by a relatively lower temperature area of the IR image. The temperature of this area is colder compared to other regions on the ocular surface.

The IR images were first selected according to the region of interest before processing the areas within. The contrast stretching method was used to enhance the region, and the power-law transformation method revealed the relatively lower temperature area. The area was consequently filtered with a medium filter to remove the noise before sharpening with a Laplacian operator. The image was converted to a binary image with a threshold of 100, and the dilation and erosion algorithm was subsequently used to reconnect the relatively lower temperature area. We recorded the control of this area before superimposing it to the original images, as shown in Figure 9.7 and Figure 9.8.

A series of IR thermal images of a normal condition in the tear film is also shown in Figure 9.7. A thirty-three-year-old participant with an IR image that scored 10 mm/5 min in Schirmer's test and 9 s in the TBUT showed a stable tear film condition and adequate tear production. In this participant, the tear film evaporation started at the center of the eye before evenly spreading from the center. This revealed that the spatial variation of the temperature was smooth and roundish. This result is in agreement with the lipid layer of the tear film normally thinning from the center of the eye.[24]

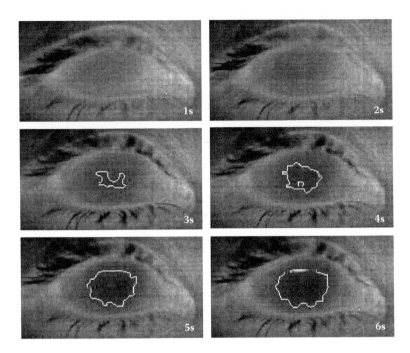

FIGURE 9.7   The contour of relatively lower temperature areas of a normal tear film condition. The final compactness value is 14 after a 6-second open-eye period.

The abnormal tear film is displayed in Figure 9.8, which is a series of IR images of a fifty-four-year-old participant, with a Schirmer's test score of 4 mm/5 min and a TBUT of 3 s. Both tests showed that the eye had a shortage of tear production and tear film instability. The unstable tear film caused uneven tear evaporation across the surface of the eye. The area with extra evaporation was a relatively lower temperature area where the structure of tear film collapsed. Tear film breakage affects the uniformity of the spatial variation of the temperature.

The compactness values of the normal and abnormal tear film are plotted versus the open-eye period in Figure 9.9. In the first 2 s, the compactness values are 0 because the image enhancement method is unable to detect the relatively lower temperature area. With time, the evaporation continued before the relatively lower temperature area appeared; the first appearance of this area was small, and the compactness value was unstable. After a few seconds, the compactness value grew stable. The compactness value of the dry eye is larger than that of the normal eye, demonstrating that a greater compactness value signifies a less stable tear film.

9.5   CONCLUSIONS

Dry eye syndrome is one of the most common eye diseases in developed countries. However, clinical diagnostic methods for dry eye syndrome are invasive methods that are uncomfortable for patients. This chapter presents the use of infrared thermal image to examine the quality of the normal and abnormal tear films, as well as

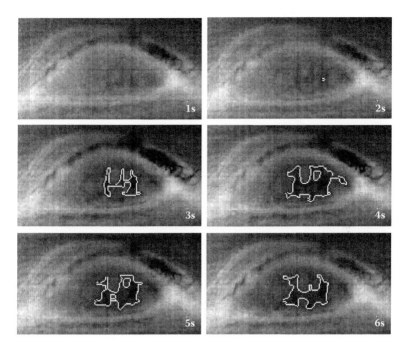

FIGURE 9.8 The contour of relatively lower temperature areas of an abnormal tear film condition. The final compactness value is 60. The irregular pattern indicates the unstable tear film condition.

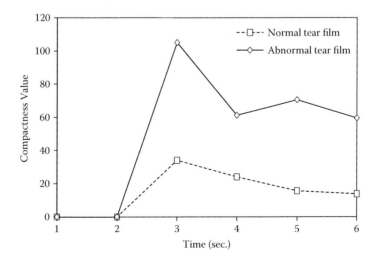

FIGURE 9.9 The compactness value of a normal and abnormal tear film versus the open-eye period.

the temporal and spatial characteristics. The results may lead to the implementation of infrared thermal imaging systems to facilitate noncontact diagnosis of dry eye syndrome.

REFERENCES

1. M. Rolando and M. Zierhut, The ocular surface and tear film and their dysfunction in dry eye disease. *Survey of Ophthalmology* 45, S203–S210 (2001).
2. A. Tomlinson, S. Khanal, K. Ramaesh, C. Diaper and A. McFadyen, Tear film osmolarity: determination of a referent for dry eye diagnosis. *Investigative Ophthalmology & Visual Science* 47 (10), 4309 (2006).
3. N. Yokoi, F. Mossa, J. M. Tiffany, and A. J. Bron, Assessment of meibomian gland function in dry eye using meibometry. *Archives Ophthalmology* 117 (6), 723–729 (1999).
4. J. B. Robin, J. V. Jester, J. Nobe, N. Nicolaides and R. E. Smith, In vivo transillumination biomicroscopy and photography of meibomian gland dysfunction. *Ophthalmology* 92 (10), 1423–1426 (1985).
5. W. D. Mathers, W. J. Shields, M. S. Sachdev, W. M. Petroll and J. V. Jester, Meibomian gland dysfunction in chronic blepharitis. *Cornea* 10 (4), 277–285 (1991).
6. N. Yokoi, A. Komuro, H. Yamada, K. Maruyama and S. Kinoshita, Newly developed video-meibography system featuring a newly designed probe. *Jpn J Ophthalmol* 51 (1), 53–56 (2007).
7. Mathers WD, Daley T and V. R., Video imaging of the meibomian gland. *Arch Ophthalmol* 112 (4), 448–449 (1994).
8. Yokoi N and K. A., Non-invasive methods of assessing the tear film. *Exp Eye Res* 78 (3), 399–407 (2004).
9. C. G. Begley, B. Caffery, R. L. Chalmers, G. L. Mitchell and Dry Eye Investigation (DREI) Study Group. Use of the dry eye questionnaire to measure symptoms of ocular irritation in patients with aqueous tear deficient dry eye. *Cornea* 21 (7), 664 (2002).
10. J. H. Tan, E. Y. K. Ng, U. R. Acharya and C. Chee, Infrared thermography on ocular surface temperature: A review. *Infrared Physics & Technology* 52 (4), 97–108 (2009).
11. P. B. Morgan, A. B. Tullo and N. Efron, Ocular surface cooling in dry eye–A pilot study. *Journal of the British Contact Lens Association* 19 (1), 7–10 (1996).
12. C. Purslow and J. Wolffsohn, The relation between physical properties of the anterior eye and ocular surface temperature. *Optometry & Vision Science* 84 (3), 197–201 (2007).
13. J. H. Tan, E. Y. K. Ng and U. R. Acharya, Evaluation of tear evaporation from ocular surface by functional infrared thermography. *Medical Physics* 37 (11), 6022 (2010).
14. J. H. Tan, E. Y. K. Ng and U. R. Acharya, Automated study of ocular thermal images: Comprehensive analysis of corneal health with different age group subjects and validation. *Digital Signal Processing* 20 (6), 1579–1591 (2010).
15. E. Hosaka, T. Kawamorita, Y. Ogasawara, N. Nakayama, H. Uozato, K. Shimizu, M. Dogru, K. Tsubota and E. Goto, Interferometry in the evaluation of precorneal tear film thickness in dry eye. *American Journal of Ophthalmology* 151 (1), 18–23 (2010).
16. A. L. Yuille, P. W. Hallinan and D. S. Cohen, Feature extraction from faces using deformable templates. *International Journal of Computer Vision* 8 (2), 99–111 (1992).
17. H. K. Chiang, C. Y. Chen, H. Y. Cheng, K. H. Chen and D. O. Chang, Development of infrared thermal imager for dry eye diagnosis, in *Infrared and Photoelectronic Imagers and Detector Devices II* (R. E. Longshore, A. Sood, eds.) (*Proc. SPIE* 6294, 629406 2006).
18. U. R. Acharya, E. Y. K. Ng, G. C. Yee, T. J. Hua and M. Kagathi, Analysis of normal human eye with different age groups using infrared images. *Journal of Medical Systems* 33 (3), 207 (2009).

19. J. H. Tan, E. Y. K. Ng, U. R. Acharya and C. Chee, Study of normal ocular thermogram using textural parameters. *Infrared Physics & Technology* 53 (2), 120–126 (2010).
20. P. B. Morgan, A. B. Tullo and N. Efron, Infrared thermography of the tear film in dry eye. *Eye* 9 (5), 615–618 (1995).
21. J. H. Tan, E. Y. K. Ng and U. R. Acharya, An efficient automated algorithm to detect ocular surface temperature on sequence of thermograms using snake and target tracing function. *Journal of Medical Systems*, 1–10 (2010).
22. W. Mathers, Evaporation from the ocular surface. *Experimental Eye Research* 78 (3), 389–394 (2004).
23. J. P. Craig, I. Singh, A. Tomlinson, P. B. Morgan and N. Efron, The role of tear physiology in ocular surface temperature. *Eye* 14 (4), 635–641 (2000).
24. J. J. Nichols, G. L. Mitchell and P. E. King-Smith, Thinning rate of the precorneal and prelens tear films. *Investigative Ophthalmology & Visual Science* 46 (7), 2353 (2005).

Section II

10 Biomechanical Modeling of the Human Eye with a Focus on the Cornea

David Varssano, Roy Asher, and Amit Gefen

CONTENTS

10.1 ANATOMY AND PHYSIOLOGY OF THE CORNEA

The human eyeball is an imperfect globe, with the cornea having a smaller radius of curvature than the remaining portions of the eyeball. The visible white opaque portion of the eyeball is called the sclera. The cornea forms the transparent outer covering of the visible colored portion of the eyeball, the color being due to the underlying iris. The interface between air and the cornea forms most of the optical power of the eye. The curvature of the cornea is responsible for roughly two-thirds of the refraction of light in the eye and the slightest imperfection in its shape results

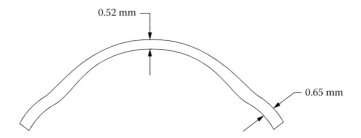

0.52 mm

0.65 mm

FIGURE 10.1 The corneal thickness in the central region is 0.52 mm. The cornea thickens toward its periphery where its value is about 0.65 mm.

in astigmatism and refractive error. The corneal thickness in the central region is 0.52 mm with a standard deviation of 0.04 mm. The cornea thickens toward its periphery, where its value is about 0.65 mm (Figure 10.1) (Pinsky and Dayte, 1991).

The cornea performs three major functions:

1. Protects the inner contents of the eye
2. Maintains the shape of the eye
3. Refracts light

Disease and injury can alter the shape, transparency, and thickness of the cornea, leading to serious changes in the visual performance of the eye. For this reason, understanding the biomechanical response of the cornea, particularly when a disease is present, is of great importance. This task is made difficult by the layered structure of the cornea and its lack of homogeneity (Anderson and Newson, 2004). Both factors mean that losing corneal tissue due to disease affects the cornea's tissue mechanical properties and makes predicting the effects of pathological factors more difficult.

10.2 MORPHOLOGY OF THE NORMAL CORNEA

The human cornea is divided into five layers lying parallel to its surface. The layers from outside to inside are the epithelium, Bowman's layer, the stroma, Descemet's membrane, and the endothelium (Maurice, 1984). The stroma makes up about 90% of the thickness of the cornea and gives it its strength and shape; the stroma is divided into 300–500 sheets of collagenous material—the stromal lamella—lying parallel to the corneal surface. Each lamella is composed of long collagen fibrils embedded in a ground substance. In each lamella the collagen fibrils lie parallel to each other and run continuous along the length of the lamella.

The central cornea contains between 200 and 400 lamellae, and it is implicit that lamellar organization and distribution must control corneal shape and curvature. In accordance with this microstructure, the mechanical properties of a lamella are orthotropic.

The transparency of the cornea requires a regular distribution of the collagen fibrils in addition to their being of equal diameter (Gallagher and Maurice, 1977;

Maurice, 1987a). The collagen fibrils are 20 times smaller than the average wavelength of visible light and make the cornea transparent. It would be opaque if the collagen fibrils were not uniformly arranged and of equal diameter.

Fibril arrangement in the corneal stroma was analyzed using synchrotron x-ray diffraction instrumentation to acquire diffraction patterns from the cornea and limbus under near physiological conditions (Daxer and Fratzl, 1997; Newton and Meek, 1998; Meek and Quantock, 2001). By analyzing the primary reflection derived from the lateral spacing of the collagen molecules within the individual fibrils, the overall preferred orientation of the collagen fibers throughout the entire cornea and limbus was determined. It reveals a highly complex arrangement of collagen and lamellae in the cornea and limbus. In the aforementioned studies, it was reported that there is a preferred orientation of collagen fibrils in the horizontal and vertical directions within the central region of the cornea; this central (optical) region of the cornea has a relatively uniform distribution of preferentially aligned collagen fibrils. Surrounding the central region in a diamond-like arrangement, a set of curved anchoring lamella is apparent to the researchers, but perhaps most interesting of all is the observation that an annulus of collagen fibers encircles the limbus. Meek and colleagues (Newton and Meek, 1998; Aghamohammadzadeh, Newton, and Meek, 2004) suggested that the change in orientation of the fibrils as they move toward the limbus accounts for the flattening of curvature of the cornea in this region, and their finding of the circumferential ring of fibrils at the limbus also provides a very elegant explanation as to how the transition in curvature between the cornea and sclera is achieved. The majority of corneal diseases result from disruption to the fibril arrangement in the corneal stroma.

Smolek (1993) showed regional differences in the interlamellar strength in different parts of the cornea, this strength being lowest in the inferior position. The results support the idea that there is a significant anisotropy in the cornea's physical properties, depending on direction. Indeed, by measuring elastic moduli of the cornea, Hjortdal (1996) showed that in the meridional direction, the highest stiffness was at the central and paracentral corneal regions, whereas the highest circumferential stiffness was found at the limbus. This suggests a meridionally oriented reinforcement of the paracentral parts of the human cornea and supports the notation of circumferentially oriented reinforcing structures in human limbal tissue.

The direction of collagen in different parts of the tissue also has implications for tissue shape. The cornea is approximately spherical in the central 4 mm or so, but then flattens. One benefit of the peripheral flattening is reduction of spherical aberrations. Moreover, the cornea is more curved than the rest of the eyeball, so flattening allows a smoother transition at the limbus. This change of curvature moving radially outward across the limbus has its own mechanical implications.

10.3   KERATOCONUS

Keratoconus is characterized by deterioration of the structure of the cornea mainly in the form of localized loss of up to 75% of the corneal tissue (Bron, 1988). As a result, the cornea changes shape under intraocular pressure (IOP), with serious implications on its refractive power (Andreassen, 1980; Edmund, 1989).

Corneal topography is characteristically altered in keratoconus; Mandell and Polse (1969) stated that compared to normal corneas, many keratoconic corneas become more hyperbolic in shape and furthermore that most keratoconic corneas have characteristically large differences between their central and peripheral thickness. Keratoconus may develop from a presumably normal cornea by an increased distensibility of keratoconic tissue. Thus the progressive alteration of the keratoconic corneal shape may be based on elastic deformation. Theoretically prolonged increased intraocular pressure, bursts of intense force as in eye rubbing, decreased corneal tissue strength, decreased corneal tissue mass, or a combination, may be pathogenetic factors.

In the literature, topics concerning tissue mass and strength have attracted the most attention. The magnitude of the corneal tissue mass depends on the corneal thickness. In general keratoconus is characterized as a corneal thinning disorder (Krachmer et al., 1984). The variability of the corneal thinning has been shown in different *in vivo* studies comparing normal and keratoconic eyes. In 18 eyes from 12 keratoconic patients a mean decrease of 25% in the central corneal thickness was demonstrated (Mandell and Polse, 1969). In 84 eyes from 55 keratoconic patients, no thinning in 42 eyes, a 10–60% thinning in 39 eyes, and >60% thinning in three eyes were shown (Foster and Yamamoto, 1978). In 27 eyes from 27 keratoconic patients, a 7% decrease in the mean central corneal thickness was demonstrated (Edmund, 1987b). By histopathological studies Poulquen (Poulquen et al., 1970) found normal-sized collagen fibers with a decrease in the number of collagen lamella.

Biomechanical studies have demonstrated a decreased amount of normal stromal collagen in keratoconus. In accordance with Polack (1976), collagen lamellas are released from their attachment to other lamella or to Bowman's layer and slide, resulting in a thinning of the cornea without actual collagenolysis. Thus, a thinning of the keratoconic cornea does not necessarily imply a decrease in the total corneal tissue mass (Edmund, 1988).

Rabinowitz (1998) lists the following clinical signs that may be present individually, or in combination, in moderate to advanced keratoconus: stromal thinning (centrally or paracentrally, most commonly inferiorly or inferotemporally); conical protrusion; an iron deposit line partially or completely surrounding the cone (Fleischer's ring); and fine vertical lines in the deep stroma and Descemet's membrane (Vogt's striae). Other accompanying signs might include epithelial nebulae, anterior stromal scars, enlarged corneal nerves, and increased intensity of the corneal endothelial reflex and subepithelial fibrillary lines.

Auffarth (Auffarth et al., 1999) used the Orbscan Topography System to evaluate corneal topography in a series of 38 keratoconus patients. The Orbscan is a three-dimensional (3D) slit-scan topography system designed for analysis of the corneal and anterior chamber surfaces. It uses a calibrated video and scanning slit-beam system to independently measure the x, y, and z locations of several thousand points on each surface of the cornea and anterior chamber. These points are used to construct topographic maps (Yaylali et al., 1977). The Orbscan Topography System was used to evaluate a series of keratoconus patients and analyze their topographic maps. Analysis of the Orbscan color maps was focused on quantitative topographic parameters at three points: the central point of the cornea; the apex, the point with maximum reading on the anterior elevation best-fit sphere map (anterior elevation BFS); and the thinnest point, the spot with minimum value on the pachymetry map. Thirty-three patients (86.8%) had bilateral keratoconus and five (13.2%) had unilateral keratoconus. On the anterior elevation BFS map, 68 cone apexes were located in the inferior temporal quadrant; three cone apexes were located above the horizontal meridian. The mean radius of the apex was 1.0 ± 0.5 mm. The mean elevation of the apex was 0.117 ± 0.076 mm. The mean tangential and composite curvatures were identical, 56.2 ± 8.5 diopters (D). The mean pachymetry of the thinnest point was 0.457 ± 0.094 mm (range 0.237 to 0.593 mm). The mean distance between the apex and the thinnest point was 0.917 ± 0.729 mm (range 3.364 to 0.068 mm) ($P < 0.001$). The correlations between apex elevation and apex composite curvature was high ($r = 0.938$; $P < 0.0001$).

10.4   INDICATION FOR THE SEVERITY OF KERATOCONUS

The diagnosis of keratoconus is based on observations of the refractive properties of the keratoconic cornea. Based on the inclination of the horizontal axis, Amsler (1937, 1938) classified keratoconus into four stages as follows:

1. A 1 to 3 degree of inclination angle
2. A 4 to 8 degree of inclination angle
3. An inclination angle > 8 degrees
4. Distortion with interminable inclination angle

Stages 1 and 2 are named *keratocone fruste* and stages 3 and 4 are named *keratocone clissique*.

According to Amsler (1946) keratoconus develops through the four stages with the possibility of arrest anywhere on the way. The refractive properties are determined by radius of corneal curvature, which is a function of the corneal shape and apex location.

Edmund (1987) has demonstrated that the changes in the keratoconic refractive and refractive properties are more likely caused by changes in the corneal shape rather than by alteration in the location of the corneal apex. Thus the keratoconic pathogenesis may be expressed as a progressive alteration of the corneal shape. The basic mechanism for the maintenance of the normal corneal contour is not known. A hypothesis is that the final corneal shape is a passive consequence of distension of the corneal tissue by the IOP and by intense spikes of distension by eye rubbing. The distensibility of a membrane is determined by the membrane mass, the elastic properties of the membrane, the membrane's material, and the mechanical forces acting on the membrane. In a given point the membrane stress depends on the proportion between radius of curvature and corneal thickness. For a given IOP the central-peripheral stress distribution depends on the radius and thickness variation. An apex displacement introduces an alteration in the reflective properties of a reflective surface that is a function of the induced change in the radius of curvature. Consequently, if the reflecting surface is nearly spherical, a given apex displacement will introduce only a little change in the radius of the curvature and thus only a small alteration in the reflective properties. On the other hand, if the reflecting surface is very aspherical, a given apex displacement involves a large change in the radius of curvature and, consequently, a large alteration in the reflective properties. The bend in the horizontal line may be interpreted as either an increased apex displacement or a change in the corneal shape in an aspheric direction, or a combination of the two possibilities.

10.5   CLINICAL STUDIES OF KERATOCONUS

Keratoconus is a progressive disorder characterized by thinning and alteration of the corneal shape at least in the central area (Edmund, 1987). Presently, neither the etiology nor the pathogenesis of keratoconus is known in detail, but there is evidence that they may be associated with a variety of factors, including contact lens wear, eye rubbing, atopic disease, connective tissue disease, Down's syndrome, tapetoretinal degeneration, and inheritance (Edmund, 1987b). Depending on the stage of the disease, every layer and tissue of the cornea may become involved in the pathological process. According to Krachmer (Krachmer et al., 1984), many theories have been proposed regarding the pathogenesis of keratoconus. Among these are theories that implicate either alteration in the basal Bowman's layer and the anterior stroma as the site of the first change or the possible existence of primary pathology of keratocytes. However, the primary lesion seems to be in the anterior part of the cornea with secondary destruction toward a posterior direction (Teng, 1963). In this connection it is interesting to notice that the synthesis of the corneal glycossminoglycans (a matrix component) appears to be dependent on the corneal endothelium and/or epithelium (Klintworth, 1977).

The mechanism underlying this epithelial mesenchymal intersection is not fully understood. Further corneal collagen is arranged in regular lamella. This is most evident in the posterior corneal stroma, while the anteriorly situated collagen is less compactly interwoven into bundles. The collagen fibrils and adjacent lamella are interweaving and branching in the anterior third of the stroma. Some collagen lamella in the anterior stroma crisscross and terminate in Bowman's layer (Klintworth, 1977).

Considering the above, a possible hypothesis for the pathogenesis of keratoconus is that keratoconus may involve a primary lesion in the anterior part of the central cornea which affects Bowman's layer and the basal epithelial cells. This may result in reduced attachment of the anterior collagen lamella to Bowman's layer and increased sliding of the collagen bundles that form the lamella due to altered synthesis of matrix substance. The reduced attachment and the increased sliding of the collagen structures correspond to increased distensibility of the corneal tissue. The attachment and sliding of the corneal collagen structures may be influenced by constitutional genetics as well as external factors. Therefore, the reduced ocular rigidity and the association between keratoconus and connective tissue diseases such as Osteogenesis imperfecta, Marfan's syndrome, and Ehlers-Danlos syndrome may reflect a common constitution for decreased attachment and increase sliding of collagen structure. The frequency of the first-degree familial occurrence seems to be 7% to 20% and the mode of transmission may be autosomal dominant with incomplete penetrance, sex-linked recessive, or multifactorial (Krachmer et al., 1984; Ihalainen, 1986). The corneal structure and its metabolism are certainly under genetic control, but the details of such control are unknown. Perhaps the genetic influence is more subtle requiring also environmental stimuli to produce the phenotypic picture characteristic of keratoconus (Krachmer et al., 1984). The association of keratoconus to atopy and such external factors as contact lens wear and eye rubbing may be due to a damage of the basal corneal epithelium cells and perhaps Bowman's membrane, thus initiating the development of keratoconus.

10.6 MECHANICAL PROPERTIES OF KERATOCONIC AND NORMAL CORNEAS

Some previous Finite Elements (FE) models of the cornea assumed homogeneity and isotropy of the tissue, the latter stemming from the observation that, although the fiber bundles in the individual lamella are oriented (Fatt, 1978; Maurice, 1969), there is no overall fiber bundle orientation in the stroma, the major load-bearing layer of the cornea, at least in the central cornea. However, there is evidence that this apparent randomness gives way to a preferential circumferential orientation as one moves from the central cornea toward the limbus (Sayers et al., 1982). Fibers in the limbus have long been known to be circumferentially oriented (Fatt, 1978; Maurice, 1969). Also, fibers in the central cornea may be preferentially aligned in the medial-lateral and inferior-superior directions (Meek et al., 1987). Observations of preferential fiber orientation are inconsistent with the usual assumption of an isotropic constitutive law for the cornea. Moreover, the determination of the appropriate constitutive assumptions is critical to mechanical models.

10.7 EXPERIMENTAL STUDIES

Early experimental efforts were undertaken by Woo (Woo et al., 1972). In their experiments, whole corneas were pressure tested and the results showed a nonlinear material behavior with significant stiffening at higher pressure levels. However, the methods they used to monitor the displacement under pressure, which involved covering the corneas in ink, were thought to have affected their response to pressure. Similar tests were undertaken by Bryant and McDonnell (1996) and they gave further evidence of the nonlinear nature of the corneal material. The material was observed to behave linearly to a range of IOPs between 2 and 4 KPa. Beyond this pressure, the modulus of elasticity grew suddenly. Bryant and McDonnell (1996) used a fiber optic probe and a small dot of paint (1–2 mm) on the cornea's center to measure displacement—a method that was reported to have produced some inaccuracies in the results. The nonlinear behavior of the cornea was also confirmed by Nyquist as early as 1968 when he investigated the biomechanical behavior of porcine corneas using strip testing (Nyquist, 1968). In their research, twenty porcine corneal specimens were subjected to internal pressure increases while their performance was monitored. The specimens (also called buttons or trephinates) included the cornea and narrow ring of surrounding scleral tissue and they were no more than four hours post mortem when tested. They were mechanically separated from the rest of the eye globe using a sharp trephine cutting tool and then mounted onto a specially designed test rig that could provide watertight edge fixity for the specimens along their ring of scleral tissue. The specimens were subjected to gradually increasing posterior pressure caused by a column of saline water to simulate the effect of elevated IOP. In the meantime, a laser (Keyence, CCD laser displacement sensor, LK series) was used to continually monitor the displacement of the apex of the cornea. All corneas were subjected to a gradually increasing posterior pressure up to a maximum pressure of 14 kPa. This pressure was well above the level at which the corneas entered a stage of stable behavior that was expected to continue until bursting.

The results show a short initial inflating stage preceding a long phase of linear behavior, followed by sudden stiffening at about 4 kPa. Based on the results of earlier studies (Woo et al., 1972; Hjortdal, 1993, 1998) on the corneal microstructure and what has been found in the former testing, it is suggested that the stress-strain relationship is divided into two distinctive phases: a matrix regulated phase with low stiffness followed by a collagen regulated phase with much higher stiffness; in the first phase, the behavior is dominated by the corneal matrix, particularly within the stroma layer. As a result, the apical rise of the cornea increases almost linearly with pressure at a low stiffness. The collagen fibril layers in this phase remain loose and unable to contribute notably to the overall performance. Then, with the start of the second phase, it is expected that the fibril layers become taut and due to their much higher stiffness, they start to control the overall behavior and lead quickly to a much increased corneal stiffness.

To measure more directly the physical properties of the corneoscleral shell in keratoconus, mechanical stress-strain tests were performed by Nash (Nash et al., 1982) on strips of human cornea. Rectangular human corneal samples were glued to the arms of an extensometer, a technique that avoids the problem of slippage and compression found with conventional clamps. Strain was measured by using an electromagnetic displacement probe. The entire apparatus was immersed in a thermoregulated mineral oil bath to maintain constant corneal hydration. The resultant data obey the relation $\sigma = A[e^{\alpha x} - 1]$. The corneal stiffening constant α ranged from 34 to 82. It was found that there are significant differences in the parameters for the normal and keratoconic groups, with keratoconus corneas yielding lower α and higher A values than normal controls.

Edmund (1988) determined in a normal ($n = 29$) and a keratoconic group ($n = 27$) the ocular rigidity (E) based on measurements of IOP, corneal diameter, corneal shape and thickness profile. Data was gathered for the comparison between the normal and keratoconic group with respect to Y_s, the steady state corneal elasticity coefficient (10^6 N/mm^2); E, the ocular rigidity (10^{-2} mm^{-3}); and P_0 (mmHg). It appears that compared with the normal eye the keratoconic eye demonstrates a significant decrease in both Y_s and E. Thus, the tissue of the keratoconic eye seems to be more distensible than the tissue of the normal eye. Furthermore, no significant difference was found in the intraocular pressures between normal and keratoconic eyes. No significant correlation was observed between Y_s and E, neither for normal nor for keratoconic eyes. This means that the corneal steady state elastic response seems to be independent of the immediate elastic response of the ocular tunics.

Shin (Shin et al., 1997) assumed in their model that non-uniform fiber orientation within the cornea results in in-plane orthotropic moduli which vary as function of the radial distance from the cornea as shown in Figure 10.2.

In the past decade, ultrasound-based elastography became a major research topic in the medical ultrasound community. Most recently Tanter (Tanter et al., 2009) introduced a high-resolution quantitative imaging of cornea's elasticity using the supersonic shear imaging (SSI) technique. Based on the use of ultrafast echographic scanners that are able to reach very high frame rates (higher than a thousand images per second), the assessment of the local and quantitative value of the tissue's Young's modulus is enabled. Using this technique quantitative elasticity maps were acquired *ex vivo* on porcine cornea.

Quantitative maps of corneal elasticity were obtained in all fresh porcine eyes. A 190 kPa ± 32 kPa mean elasticity was obtained for four different specimens. Elasticity maps were also acquired after collagen induced cross-linking. A significant Young's modulus increase was obtained with a mean 890 kPa ± 250 kPa (460% increase). This 460% increase ratio, as quoted by the author, is in agreement with recent values provided in literature. In this study the corneal tissues were assumed to be isotropic. Therefore further work will concentrate on the influence of cornea elastic anisotropy on the shear wave propagation.

To this end, there is a need to better define the anisotropic characteristics of the cornea through the treatment of structure-function relations. As introduced earlier in this chapter, many studies have been undertaken to determine the orientation of collagen fibrils within the human cornea. These studies indicate that, in the human cornea, there is a preferred fibril orientation in the inferior-superior and nasal-temporal directions. This preferred orientation occurs at the center of the cornea and is maintained to within 2 mm of the limbus, where a gradual change to a tangential disposition occurs. However, the collagen fibril orientation and distribution at different depths within the

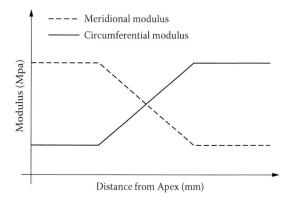

FIGURE 10.2   The assumed variation of orthotropic moduli for simulating the changing fiber orientation in the cornea. (Adapted from Shin, T.J., Vito, R.P., Johnson, L.W., McCarey, B.E. 1997. The distribution of strain in the human cornea. *Biomechanics* 30 (5): 497–503.)

human cornea has yet to be investigated. Abahussin (Abahussin et al., 2009) used femtosecond laser technology and wide-angle x-ray diffraction to study the distribution and predominant orientations of fibrillar collagen at different depths throughout the entire thickness of the human cornea. The results presented in this article indicate that the collagen fibrils are proportionally more aligned in the posterior two-thirds of the cornea whereas in the anterior third, the orientation of collagen is more isotropic. The quantitative information presented in this study may be helpful for improving understanding of the biomechanical properties of the cornea and may add further details about collagen fibril organization to computational finite element models.

10.8   INTRAOCULAR PRESSURE IN THE CORNEA

Emara (Emara et al., 1988) determined the relationship of intraocular pressure (IOP) and central corneal thickness (CCT) in normal myopic eyes. The IOP is measured by Goldmann applanation tonometry in which the cornea is subjected to both applanating and intraocular pressures. In clinical practice, the applanating pressure measured using an applanation tonometer is considered to be equal to the IOP (Orssengo and Pye, 1999). CCT is measured by ultrasonic pachymetry in which ultrasound energy is emitted from the probe tip acting as both the transmitter and the receiver. Some of the energy is reflected back toward the probe in the form of an echo. CCT was determined in a group of untreated corneas of 120 patients (203 eyes). Statistical analyses were performed with the Pearson correlation coefficient and paired Student t-test. In the untreated group of 288 eyes, mean CCT was 544.0 microns ± 37.3 (SD) (range 461 to 664 microns) and mean IOP was 15.6 ± 2.7 mmHg (range 10 to 24 mmHg). The correlation between IOP and CCT in this group was highly significant ($r = 0.44$; $P < 0.0001$). The slope was 0.032 mmHg/micron of CCT, or an approximate decrease of 1 mmHg, for a reduction in CCT of 31.3 microns.

10.9   SURFACE ELEVATION MAPS

Since surface shape is the primary determinant of corneal optics (Applegate, 1994; Applegate et al., 2000), a logical way to map the cornea is to show the surface elevation of each point, relative to a reference surface. With topographic land maps, elevations are measured from a reference "plane" at sea level. However, for the cornea, elevations measured from a plane are nearly useless because even minute changes in elevation (on the order of micrometers) can be optically significant, but these are lost in the larger total height of the cornea (Klyce and Wilson, 1989; van Saarloos and Constable, 1991; Leibowitz and Waring, 1998). A better method for presenting the true topography (surface elevation) is to measure from a reference sphere, ellipsoid, or other surface that approximates the general corneal shape (Salmon and Horner, 1995).

10.10   DIOPTRIC CURVATURE MAPS

Most corneal topography systems do not plot surface elevations but describe the surface in terms of dioptric values. These dioptric maps are popular because they use the terminology of keratometry, with which clinicians are familiar (Roberts, 1994a).

Just as different elevation maps of the same cornea can be drawn, dioptric data for the same surface can also be expressed in different ways (Klein, 1992; Mandell, 1992). In optometry, diopters are sometimes used to quantify surface curvature; in other cases diopters express surface refractive power. Near the corneal apex, surface curvature and power are so closely related that they are sometimes treated synonymously. When the data are appropriately scaled, this works for keratometry, since measurements are limited to the paraxial region. However, outside the paraxial zone, it is important to make a distinction between dioptric curvature and dioptric power. The axial and instantaneous maps are available on most commercial instruments used today.

10.11   COMPUTATIONAL SIMULATIONS

Orssengo and Pye (1999) and Emara (Emara et al., 2005) used a mathematical model to determine the true IOP and modulus of elasticity of the human cornea *in vivo* based on measurements obtained by applanation tonometry. Moreover the relationship between corneal mechanical properties and IOP was researched.

10.11.1   Dependence of IOP Readings on Thickness

According to the Emara (Emara et al., 1988) model, the IOP readings from applanation tonometry are dependent not only on the true IOP but also on the thickness, curvature, and elasticity of the cornea. Three simulations, which are the results of varying one parameter at a time while holding the other two constant, were done. In the simulation, Young's modulus, the curvature of the cornea, and the true IOP were kept at the following values: $E = 0.19$ MPa, $R = 7.8$ mm, and IOP = 10, 15, or 20 mmHg. The magnitude of Young's modulus that was taken was within the predicted range of normal elasticity. Corneal thickness was varied from 0.3 to 0.9 mm to demonstrate the overall trend of influence. The difference in the predicted IOP readings between the lower end $(0.536 - 3 \times 0.031$ mm$)$ and the upper end $(0.536 + 3 \times 0.031$ mm$)$ of corneal thickness in the normal population was 2.87 mmHg.

10.11.2   Dependence of IOP Readings on Radius of Curvature

The radius of curvature was varied from 3.0 mm to 11.0 mm to simulate the influence of curvature, while thickness was fixed at 0.536 mm and Young's modulus at 0.19 MPa. The difference in the predicted IOP readings between the lower end $(7.8 - 3 \times 0.27$ mm$)$ and the upper end $(7.8 + 3 \times 0.27$ mm$)$ of the corneal radius of curvature in the normal population was 1.76 mmHg (Liu and Roberts, 2005).

10.11.3   Dependence of IOP Readings on Young's Modulus

Keeping thickness, curvature, and IOP at normal values ($t = 0.536$ mm, $R = 7.8$ mm, IOP = 10, 15, or 20 mmHg), Young's modulus was varied from 0.1 to 0.9 MPa. Experimental data in the literature show that Young's modulus of human corneas can vary from 0.01 to 10 MPa; therefore, the normal human cornea may take any value in the simulation range. If this is true (i.e., the range for Young's modulus in the normal population is 0.1 to 0.9 MPa), the difference in the predicted IOP reading between the two ends is 17.26 mmHg (Liu and Roberts, 2005).

10.11.4 DEPENDENCE OF IOP ON CORNEAL THICKNESS AND ON MAGNITUDE OF YOUNG'S MODULUS

The corneal thickness was varied from 0.3 to 0.9 mm. Young's modulus was chosen to be 0.19 MPa or 0.58 MPa. The corneal radius of curvature was fixed at 7.8 mm. Different biomechanical properties resulted in different gradients of predicted IOP readings that were induced by variations in corneal thickness. A higher Young's modulus corresponded to a larger slope, while a lower Young's modulus resulted in a smaller slope. For example, with a Young's modulus of 0.19 MPa, the normal variation in corneal thickness (0.443 to 0.629 mm) would cause a 2.84 mmHg difference in predicted IOP readings; with a Young's modulus of 0.58 MPa, the difference would be 8.68 mmHg (Liu and Roberts, 2005).

Simulation with the Orssengo and Pye model (Orssengo and Pye, 1999) predicted IOP readings for a range of corneal thickness (0.3 to 0.9 mm) with a fixed corneal radius of curvature of 7.8 mm and corneal Young's modulus of 0.3 MPa. Three true IOP levels were theoretically studied: 10 mmHg, 15 mmHg, and 20 mmHg. The three predicted IOP readings corresponding to the three true IOPs for a corneal thickness of 0.536 mm were 12.5 mmHg, 15 mmHg, and 17.5 mmHg, respectively. It appears that the predicted IOP coincides with the true IOP only when the true IOP is 15 mmHg.

In a biomechanical analysis of the keratoconic cornea (Gefen et al., 2008) three-dimensional FE simulations were conducted to analyze the biomechanical factors contributing to the distorted shape of a keratoconic cornea. By employing a more realistic representation of the corneal geometry and anisotropic mechanical properties, Gefen et al. developed more accurate biomechanical models of normal and keratoconic corneas.

Cases of keratoconous were simulated by global or localized tissue weakening, as well as localized asymmetric thinning distortions of the cornea, considered separately or together in the models, to determine their relative individual or combined influences on the shape of the cornea. In addition, the relationship between corneal topography due to mechanical deformations and the dioptric power maps, which are the relevant clinical imaging method for diagnosis and severity assessment, was also explored (Gefen et al., 2008).

The parameters that were used to classify the keratoconus cases according to their severity are displacement and the dioptric power. The corneal displacements are given from the FE model, but another computational method was developed to calculate the dioptric power. A MATLAB® code using the FE results as input calculated the dioptric power for each particular node on the cornea anterior surface and plotted a dioptric power map. The FE model and the MATLAB program together made it possible to perform a full simulation of the corneal model under various mechanical and pathological conditions and in this way to better understand the factors that are involved in the pathogenesis of keratoconus (Gefen et al., 2008).

The complexity of the structure and the form of the cornea at both the micro and macro levels presented a particular challenge during the development of the models. On one hand, there was a desire to simulate the real structure and form of the cornea to improve accuracy, and on the other, there was a practical requirement to simplify the models and keep them at a reasonable level of complexity. Several parameters were considered, including the density of the finite elements mesh, the composite structure of the cornea and the significance of the out-of-plane flexural and torsional resistance of the cornea. Parameters that were found to have smaller or negligible effect (with an effect on accuracy below 2%) were not considered in the final construction of the model (Gefen et al., 2008).

The material properties and corneal topography were taken from the literature based on experimental testing that was carried out on corneal specimens. The normal cornea without any load was treated as a symmetric sphere and the corneal tissue was considered an elastic linear material with 3D orthotropic mechanical properties. The out-plane Young's modulus (E_{rr}) was assumed to be a constant 5.0 MPa and the meridional modulus of elasticity was assumed to be a constant 2.0 MPa. Poisson's ratio was assumed to be 0.46 (Gefen et al., 2008). Poisson's ratio is a material property that characterizes the deformation perpendicular to the direction of the load. The range of Poisson's ratio is 0.0 to 0.5 for most engineering materials. For a perfectly incompressible material, Poisson's ratio is 0.5. Most soft biological tissues are nearly incompressible (because they contain water as their dominant substance), so it is common practice to use a Poisson's ratio close to 0.5 for modeling soft tissue (Liu and Roberts, 2005). Battaglioli and Kamm (1984) found that the Poisson's ratio of the sclera varies between the relatively narrow range of 0.46 to 0.5.

Also this value (0.46) provides numerical stability in all simulation cases. The simulations that were carried out in this study (Gefen et al., 2008) are divided into four major groups:

1. Normal cornea model (Case 1)
2. Models with degraded mechanical properties (Cases 2–5)
3. Models with thinning tissue geometry (Cases 6–8)
4. Models with a combination of both degraded mechanical properties and thinning tissue (Cases 9–10)

Most of the analysis cases were simulated for two IOPs: 15 mmHg, which is considered a normal value, and 25 mmHg, which is considered a high value. Case 1 (normal cornea model) and Case 9 (represents an advanced condition of keratoconus) were simulated for two additional IOP levels—10 and 20 mmHg—to examine the influence of the IOP change on both normal and keratoconic corneas.

The meridional modulus of elasticity $E_{\varphi\varphi}$ and shear modulus perpendicular to the corneal surface $G_{r\varphi}$ (analysis Cases 2–3) were found to have an influence on the conical shape of a keratoconic cornea. Degradation of modulus of elasticity has a higher influence on the cornea's conical shape than shear modulus degradation, but there is no doubt that thinning tissue has the highest influence on the cornea's conical shape as an individual factor (Gefen et al., 2008).

To demonstrate the influence of the thinning tissue factor, three different FE models were developed: one with thinnest point of 0.35 (Case 6), the second with thinnest point of 0.2 mm (Cases 9–10), and the third with two thinning regions (Case 8). Their results were compared with those that were obtained from the normal cornea analysis (Case 1). It was obvious that the change of maximal displacement and dioptric power as a function of the corneal minimum thickness is not linear. This demonstrates the significant contribution of tissue thinning on pathogenesis of keratoconus. It means that in advanced condition of keratoconus even minimal change within the tissue thickness bears an additional significant alteration in the corneal shape. Examining Case 7, in which minimum cornea thickness of 0.2 mm was assumed demonstrating an advanced condition of keratoconus, maximal displacement and dioptric power of 103 μm and 48.0 D, respectively were achieved. Even though the maximal displacement is very close to the mean elevation value that was reported in the literature (mean value of 0.117 ± 0.076 mm), the dioptric power is relatively low (according to the literature the mean value of keratoconic corneas is 56.2 ± 8.5 D) (Gefen et al., 2008).

In addition, it has been shown that in most of the keratoconus cases, the cone center is obtained in the inferior temporal quadrant, just where the thinnest point is located. It may be concluded that the keratoconus asymmetry is derived from the thinning tissue location. Indeed, in all analysis cases in which the thinnest point was located in a different region than the corneal apex, the maximal displacement and dioptric power were not obtained near the corneal apex, but near the thinnest point (Gefen et al., 2008).

The obtained dioptric power and maximal displacements, for analysis cases in which tissue thinning only was assumed as an individual factor with no degradation of mechanical properties, do not match the values that were observed in the literature. Actually, both tissue thinning and degraded mechanical properties alone did not yield a topography of keratoconus when they were applied as an individual factor in the FE model (Figure 10.3). However, integrating them in the FE model, as demonstrated in Case 9, yielded maximal displacement of 230 μm and dioptric power of 54.3 D under a normal IOP of 15 mmHg. Those are certainly corresponding to the mean values that were observed in the literature (56.2 ± 8.5 diopters). If we assume that the condition to pathogenesis of keratoconus is a presence of those two factors, it is reasonable also to assume that it is not coincidence. It certainly is possible that a decrease in one of them may cause a decrease in the second. Still, the questions of which of them starts the whole process and what is the relationship between them remain open (Gefen et al., 2008).

The intraocular pressure (IOP) has an important role in the mechanical behavior of the normal and keratoconic corneas. In the normal cornea model, a change of 5.0 μm in the radius of curvature was achieved for 1.0 mmHg IOP increase, whereas in the keratoconic cornea, a change of 39.0 μm in the radius of curvature was achieved for 1.0 mmHg increase. This fact is very reasonable considering that the keratoconic cornea has more elastic mechanical properties due to the thinning and degradation. Generally, the increase of IOP in all analysis cases yielded an increase in the maximal dioptric power. The more elastic the cornea tissue is, the higher the change in the maximal displacement and dioptric power per IOP is achieved (Gefen et al., 2008).

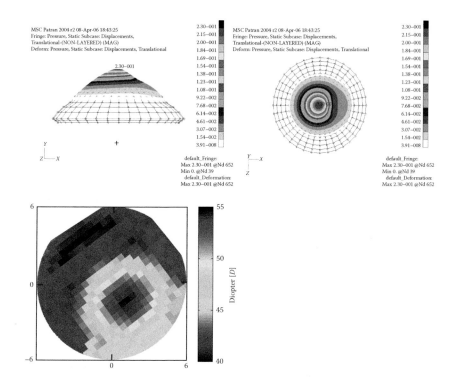

FIGURE 10.3 Analysis results corresponding to Case 9 with IOP = 15 mmHg. Maximum displacement of 230 μm, with Maximum Diopter of 54.3 D. (Adapted from Gefen et al., 2008.) (Please see color insert.)

The stress distribution has an importance in the research of the pathology of keratoconus. Thus, the stress distribution through the corneal center was calculated for all corneal conditions in which an average IOP of 15 mmHg was assumed. Special attention should be paid to the location of the maximal stress point. In all cases it was obtained at the tissue's thinnest point. In the normal cornea model (Case 1) the thinnest point and the maximal stress region are located at the corneal apex, but in Cases 6–10 the thinnest point was located at a small distance from the corneal apex. The maximal stress region like the cone center was obtained at the cornea's thinnest point.

The minimum thickness of the cornea tissue has a significant influence on the stress level. The maximal stress value changes exponentially to the tissue thickness. It means that in an advanced condition of keratoconus as demonstrated in Case 9, every small IOP increase bears a significant increase in the stress level. Based on this, an optional explanation as to how the IOP value may have a major role in the pathogenesis of keratoconus was offered. The hypothetic mechanism in the genesis of keratoconus may include the following scenario: IOP increase bears a high stress level at the thinnest point of the cornea tissue. Some of the tissue fibers cannot withstand this stress level and start to fail. As a result, tissue degradation and a decrease in mechanical properties occur and then a high stress level is obtained even under lower IOPs and so on and so forth. Other scenarios may support the possibility that the whole process begins with tissue degradation and the IOP actually remains stable. While this may provide some basis for further examination, the factor that is responsible for the keratoconus initiation is yet unknown (Gefen et al., 2008).

The analyses revealed that three factors affect the shape distortion of keratoconic corneas:

1. Localized tissue thinning
2. Reduction in the tissue's meridian elastic modulus E''
3. Reduction in the shear modulus perpendicular to the corneal surface Gr'

Tissue thinning was found to be the most influential factor contributing to the bulged shape of the keratoconic cornea, and the center of the bulge closely followed the thinnest tissue region. Maximal stress levels also occurred at the center of the bulged region, where the tissue is thinnest, and this may be the mechanism responsible for the progressive nature of the disease. Finally, the IOP levels had little influence on dioptric power in the healthy cornea, but a substantial influence in keratoconic conditions, particularly the more severe ones, and so regulation of IOP levels in keratoconus may be an important aspect in managing this disease.

Grytz (Grytz et al., 2010) introduced a computational remodeling approach to predict the physiological architecture of the collagen fibril network in corneoscleral shells.

The strong relation between structure and function was discussed earlier in this chapter; organized collagen fibrils form complex networks that introduce strong anisotropic and highly nonlinear attributes into the constitutive response of human eye tissues. When trying to construct a more accurate model of the cornea to better understand the influence of mechanical properties on corneal diseases one may want to take into consideration that the living tissue is ever subjected to remodeling processes that are affected by numerous factors including the mechanical properties themselves. Physiological adaptation of the collagen network and the mechanical condition within biological tissues are complex and mutually dependent phenomena. The biomechanical properties of eye tissues are derived from the single crimped fibril at the microscale via the collagen network of distributed fibrils at the mesoscale to the incompressible and anisotropic soft tissue at the macroscale.

The computational model that was presented in this study was used for investigating the interaction between the collagen fibril architecture and mechanical loading conditions in the corneoscleral shell. It was based on an algorithm that is based on the hypothesis that collagen fibrils adapt their orientation with respect to the local stress environment of the tissue. It has already been shown lately in an investigation of the different approaches for the stimulus (stress or strain) that the Cauchy stress seems to be a reasonable candidate to drive the remodeling process in tissues such as cardiovascular tissues.

The numerical findings agreed qualitatively well with experimental observations. The concentration of the collagen fibril orientations toward the circumferential direction at the limbus predicted by the remodeling algorithm can be interpreted as the development of a fibrillar annulus. From synchrotron x-ray diffraction data, the existence of a circumcorneal annulus of collagen fibrils at the limbus is well known (Newton and Meek, 1998).

In a recent study, Pandolfi et al. (2008) proposed 3D modeling and computational analysis of the human cornea considering distributed collagen fibril orientations. Their model was able to provide the refractive power by analyzing the structural mechanical response with the nonlinear regime and the effect the intraocular pressure has. It was concluded that a model for the human cornea must not disregard the peculiar collagen fibrillar structure, which equips the cornea with the unique biophysical, mechanical, and optical properties.

Most recently, a patient-specific modeling of corneal refractive surgery outcomes was done by Roy et al. (2011). The purpose of this study was to develop a 3D patient-specific finite element (FE) model of the cornea and sclera to compare predicted and *in vivo* refractive outcomes and to estimate the corneal elastic property changes associated with each procedure. The model allowed an analysis of the biomechanical changes associated with a specific laser-assisted *in situ* keratomileusis (LASIK) treatment plan and their impact on the accuracy of the postoperative optical result. In addition, the model was used to estimate the magnitude of corneal elastic property reductions based on clinical topographic changes between the preoperative and one-week postoperative examinations. Preoperative and postoperative clinical characteristics of a 35-year-old female were recorded and used with the FE model. In both eyes, a reduction in corneal elastic properties or weakening of the cornea from the preoperative state resulted in more accurate axial power estimates by the FE model compared with *in vivo*. These results suggested that the anterior corneal flattening associated with a myopic correction is overestimated if elastic properties are assumed to be as high after surgery as before surgery; conversely, weakening of the cornea, which favors less biomechanical flattening by allowing more forward-directed central corneal displacement after LASIK, is required to produce the best match to the clinical response.

In the future, the equivalency of the FE model results to the *in vivo* measurements may allow the use of a more accurate patient-specific 3D computational modeling of the cornea to better understand the surgical impact on corneal elastic properties and thus refine surgical results in any corneal surgery.

10.12 CONCLUDING REMARKS

The geometry, mechanical properties that are derived from the tissue structure, the IOP, and histological evaluation of the cornea are fundamental to our understanding of corneal behavior in the normal condition and in keratoconus pathogenesis. The literature, taken together, assumes the cornea geometry to be spherical, and thickness variations from 0.52 mm at the center to 0.65 mm near the limbus.

It was shown that fibers in the central cornea are preferentially aligned in the medial-lateral and inferior-superior directions. There is also a preferential circumferential orientation as one moves from the central cornea toward the limbus. According to these findings the cornea tissue may not have isotropic homogeneous mechanical properties. This non-uniformity has been previously observed in Shin, Vito, Johnson and McCarey's (1997) work and may explain the cornea flattening in the limbal region when the cornea is subjected to IOP.

It has been shown that keratoconus is characterized by deterioration of the structure of the cornea mainly in the form of localized loss of up to 75% of the corneal tissue. As a result, the cornea changes shape under IOP, with serious implications on its refractive power. To research the involved factors in the pathogenesis of keratoconus, computational models should take them into account and enable us to perform a sensitivity analysis, while only one factor is modified and the rest remain constant. There is evidence of a decrease in tissue mass and mechanical properties in the keratoconic cornea which are reflected in the cornea's change in shape compared with a normal cornea.

It has been observed that keratoconus severity is determined by measuring the corneal power and maximum elevation which occurs, in most of the keratoconic cases, in the cone center, and not in the corneal optic axis. Accordingly the output from a computational model should be cornea elevation and power maps.

Measurements of the elastic modulus of the cornea show that radially, the cornea is stiffer at the center, whereas moving further from the center involves some mechanical weakening. Circumferentially, the cornea is strongest at the limbus and the mechanical properties degrade when moving toward the center. Yet most of the models developed for the cornea in the literature assume homogeneity and isotropy of the tissue. On the other hand, several studies such as the one done by Shin et al. (1997) assumed in their model that a non-uniform fiber orientation within the cornea results in in-plane orthotropic moduli which vary as a function of the radial distance from the corneal apex. Nevertheless, orthotropic mechanical properties should be assumed in computational models as shown in recent studies (Gefen et al., 2008; Anna Pandolfi et al., 2008).

The mean modulus of elasticity of a normal cornea was found to be 2.5 MPa with SD of 0.55, while in keratoconic cornea it is 1.35 MPa with SD of 0.91. No experimental information was found about the shear modulus of the cornea, but the computational simulations show that like other elastic material it is one size lower than the modulus of elasticity. The mean ocular pressure observed in the human cornea is 15.6 ± 2.7 mmHg. The cornea tissue was observed to behave linearly to a range of IOPs between 2 and 4 KPa. Beyond this pressure, the modulus of elasticity grew suddenly. No significant difference was found in the IOPs between normal and keratoconic eyes. There is a decrease in the corneal radius of curvature as a result of IOP increase. The relationship between IOP and apex elevation, dioptric power, and maximal stress should be further examined.

REFERENCES

Abahussin, M., Hayes, S., Knox Cartwright, N. E. 2009. 3D collagen orientation study of the human cornea using x-ray diffraction and femtosecond laser technology. *Invest. Ophthal. Vis. Sci.*, 50: 11.

Aghamohammadzadeh, H., Newton, R. H., Meek, K. M. 2004. X-ray scattering used to map the preferred collagen orientation in the human cornea and limbus. *Structure*. Feb; 12(2): 249–256.

Amsler, M. 1937. Le keratocone frusta. *Bull. Soc. Fr. Ophthalmology* 50: 100–114.

Amsler, M. 1938. Le keratocone frusta au Javel. *Ophthalmologica* 96: 77–83.

Amsler, M. 1946. Keratocone classique et keratocone frusta; arguments unitaires. *Ophthalmologica* 111: 96–101.

Anderson, K., El-Sheikh, A., Newson, T. 2004. Application of structural analysis to the mechanical behavior of the cornea. *The Royal Society* 1: 1–13.

Andreassen, T. T., Simonsen, A. H., Oxlund, H. 1980. Biomechanical properties of keratoconus and normal corneas. *Exp. Eye Res.* Oct; 31(4): 435–441.

Auffarth, G. U., Wang, L., Völcker, H. E. 2000. Keratoconus evaluation using the Orbscan Topography System. *J Cataract Refract. Surg.* Feb; 26(2): 222–228.

Battaglioli, J. L., Kamm, R. D. 1984. Measurements of the compressive properties of scleral tissue. *Invest. Ophthalmol. Vis. Sci.* 25: 59–65.

Bron, A. J. 1988. Keratoconus. *Cornea* 7(3): 163–169.

Bryant, M. R., McDonnell, P. J. 1996. Constitutive laws for biomechanical modeling of refractive surgery. *Mech. Eng.* 118: 473–481.

Daxer, A., Fratzl, P. 1997. *Invest. Ophthalmol. Vis. Sci.* 38: 121–129.

Edmund, C. 1987a. Corneal apex in keratoconic patients. *Optom. Physiol. Opt.* 64 (12): 905–908.

Edmund, C. 1987b. The corneal apex in keratoconic patients. *Am. J. Optom. Physiol. Opt.* In press.

Edmund, C. 1988. Corneal tissue mass in normal and keratoconic eyes in vivo estimation based on area of horizontal optical sections. *Acta Ophthalmol.* 66: 305–308.

Edmund, C. 1989. Corneal topography and elasticity in normal and keratoconic eyes. *Acta Ophthalmol.* 67(193).

Emara, B., Probst, L. E., Tingey, D. P., Kennedy, D. W., Willms, L. J., Machat, J. 1998. Correlation of intraocular pressure and central corneal thickness in normal myopic eyes and after laser in situ keratomileusis. *J. Cataract Refract. Surg.* 10: 1320–1325.

Emara, B., Probst, L. E., Tingey, D. P., Kennedy, D. W., Willms, L. J., Machat, J. 2005. Relationship between central corneal thickness and retinal fiber layer thickness in ocular hypertensive patients. *Ophthalmology* 112: 251–256.

Fatt, I. 1978. Measurement of oxygen flux into the cornea by pressing a sensor onto a soft contact lens on the eye. *Am. J. Optom. Physiol. Opth.* May; 55(5): 294–301.

Foster, C. S., Yamamoto, G. K. 1978. Ocular rigidity in keratoconus. *Am. J. Ophthalmol.* 86: 802–806.

Gallagher, B., Maurice, D. M. 1977. Striations of light scattering in the corneal stroma. *J. Ultrastruct. Res.* 61: 100–114.

Gefen, A., Shalom, R., Elad, D., Mandel, Y. 2009. Biomechanical analysis of the keratoconic cornea. *J. Mech. Behav. Biomed. Mater.* Jul; 2(3): 224–236.

Grytz, R., Meschke, G. 2010. A computational remodeling approach to predict the physiological architecture of the collagen fibril network in corneo-scleral shells. *Biomech. Model Mechanobiol.* 9: 225–235.

Hjortdal, J. O. 1996. Regional elastic performance of the human cornea. *J. Biomechanics* 29: 931–942.

Hjortdal, J. O. 1998. On the biomechanical properties of the cornea with particular reference to refractive surgery. *Ophthalmol. J. Nordic Countries* 76(225): 1–23.

Hjortdal, J. O. 1993. Regional elastic performance of the human cornea. *J. Biomechanics* 29(7): 931–942.

Ihalainen, A. 1986. Clinical and epidemiological features of keratoconus. Genetic and external factors in the pathogenesis of the disease. *Acta Opthalmol. (Copenh).* Suppl 178.

Klintworth, G. K. 1977. The cornea structure and macromolecules and health and disease. *Am. J. Pathol.* 89: 717–808.

Klyce, S. D., Wilson, S. E. 1989. Methods of analysis of corneal topography. *Refract. Corneal Surg.* Nov-Dec; 5(6): 368–371.

Krachmer, J. H., Feder, R. S., Belin, M. W. 1984. Keratoconus and related noninflammatory corneal thinning disorders. *Surv. Opthalmol.* 82: 182–188.

Leibowitz, H. M., Waring, G. O. 1998. *Corneal disorders: Clinical diagnosis and management*, 2nd ed. Saunders; pp. 1–1172.

Liu, J., Roberts, C. J. 2005. Influence of corneal biomechanical properties on intraocular pressure measurement. *J. Cataract Refract. Surg.* 31: 146–155.

Mandell, R. B., Polse, K. A. 1969. Keratoconus. Spatial variation of corneal thickness as diagnostic test. *Arch. Ophtalmol.* 82: 182–188.

Maurice, D. M. 1969. The cornea and sclera, in *The Eye*, Davson, H. (ed.). Academic Press: New York and London, pp. 489–600.

Maurice, D. M. 1988. *Mechanics of the cornea*. Trans, World Congr. Cornea III, Washington D.C. Raven Press, NY.

Meek, K. M., Blamires, T., Elliott, G.F., Gyi, T. J., Nave, C. 1987. The organisation of collagen fibrils in the human corneal stroma: a synchrotron x-ray diffraction study, *Curr. Eye Res.*, 841–846.

Nash, I. S., Greene, P. R., Foster, C. S. 1982. Comparison of mechanical properties of keratoconus and normal corneas. *Exp. Eye Res.* 35: 413–423.

Newton, R. H., Meek, K. M. 1998. *Biophys. J.* 75: 2508–2512.

Nyquist, G. W. 1968. Rheology of the cornea: experimental techniques and results. *Exp. Eye Res.* 7. 183–188.

Orssengo, G. J., Pye, D. C. 1999. Determination of the true intraocular pressure and modulus of elasticity of the human cornea in vivo. *Bull. Math. Biol.* 61: 551–572.

Pandolfi, A., Holzapfel, G. A. 2008. Three-dimensional modeling and computational analysis of the human cornea considering distributed collagen fibril orientations. *J. Biomech. Eng.* 130.

Pinsky, P. M., Dayte, D.V. 1991. A microstructurally based finite elements model of the incised human cornea. *Biomechanics* 24: 907–922.

Pouliquen, Y. B., Graf, Y., Kozak, J., Bisson, J., Faure, F., 1970. Bourles, Frouin. Etude morphologique et biochimique de kératocone. I. Etude morphologique, *Arch. Ophtalmol.* 30: 497–532.

Rabinowitz, Y. S. 1998. Keratoconus. *Surv. Opthalmol.* 42: 297–319.

Roy, A. S., Dupps, W. J., Jr. 2011. Patient-specific modeling of corneal refractive surgery outcomes and inverse estimation of elastic property changes. *J. Biomech. Eng.* 133.

Sayers, Z., Koch, M. H. J., Whitburn, S. B., Meek, K. M. 1982. Synchrotron x-ray diffraction study of corneal stroma. *J. Molec. Biol.*, 593–607.

Shin, T. J., Vito, R. P., Johnson, L. W., McCarey, B. E. 1997. The distribution of strain in the human cornea. *Biomechanics* 30 (5): 497–503.

Smolek, M. K. 1993. Interlamellar cohesive strength in the vertical meridian of human eye bank corneas. *Invest. Ophthalmol. Vis. Sci.* 34: 2962–2969.

Tanter, M., Touboul, D., Gennisson, J.-L. 2009. High-resolution quantitative imaging of cornea elasticity using supersonic shear imaging. *IEEE Transactions on Medical Imaging*, Vol. 28, No. 12.

Teng, C. C. 1963. Electron microscope study of the pathology of keratoconus. Part 1. *Am. J. Opthalmol.* 55: 18–47.

van Saarloos, P. P. Constable, I. J. 1991. Improved method for calculation of corneal topography for any photokeratoscope geometry. *Optom. Vis. Sci.* Dec; 68(12): 960–965.

Woo, S. L. Y., Kobayashi, A. S., Schlegel, W. A., Lawrence, C. 1972. Non-linear properties of intact cornea and sclera. *Exp. Eye Res.* 14: 29–39.

Yaylali, V., Kaufman, S. C, Thompson, H. W. 1977. Corneal thickness measurements with the Orbscan Topography System and ultrasonic pachymetry. *J. Cataract Refract. Surg.* 23: 1345–1350.

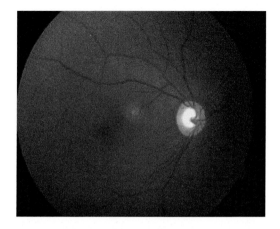

FIGURE 1.2 Location of macula, fovea, and optic disc.

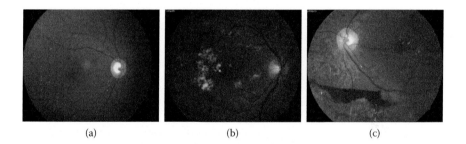

(a)   (b)   (c)

FIGURE 1.3 Typical images of (a) normal, (b) NPDR, and (c) PDR.

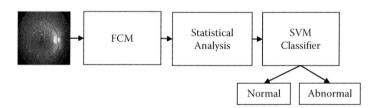

FIGURE 1.4 Block diagram of automated DR detection system.

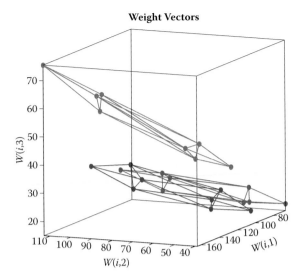

FIGURE 1.6 Weight vectors of SOM: Green indicates normal; red and blue indicate NPDR and PDR classes, respectively.

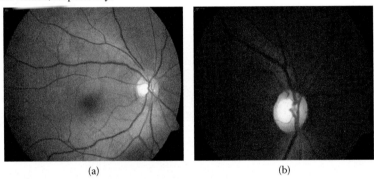

(a)   (b)

FIGURE 3.3 (a) Normal retina; (b) glaucoma retina.

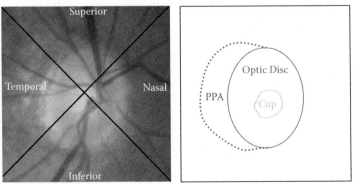

FIGURE 4.1 A retinal fundus image of a right eye shown on the left-hand side. Annotations describe the four different zones of a retina. The temporal and nasal zones are flipped for a left eye. A sketch map, shown on the right-hand side, illustrates the position of optic nerve areas, such as the optic disk (OD), optic cup (Cup), and parapapillary atrophy (PPA).

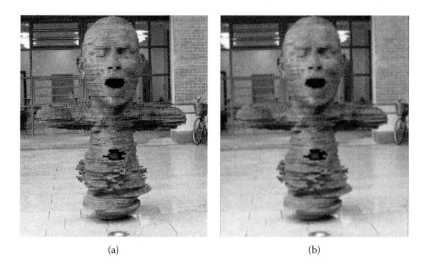

(a)   (b)

FIGURE 4.5   (a) Original image. (b) Image after convolution filtering.

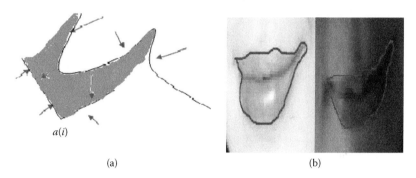

a(i)

(a)   (b)

FIGURE 4.6   (a) The sketch map of the motion of segmenting anchor by snakes. (b) The lips segmentation by the snake.

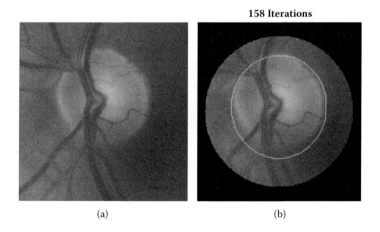

(a)   (b)

FIGURE 4.11   (a) Original fundus image. (b) A segmentation result of the optic disk using Tang's model.

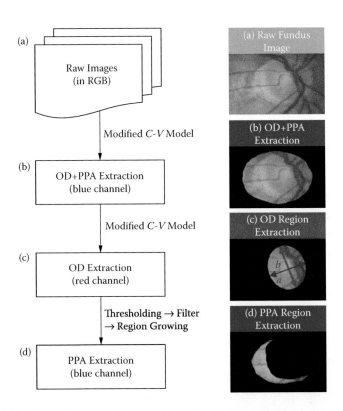

FIGURE 4.12 Flow chart shows the extraction of the PPA and the OD region.

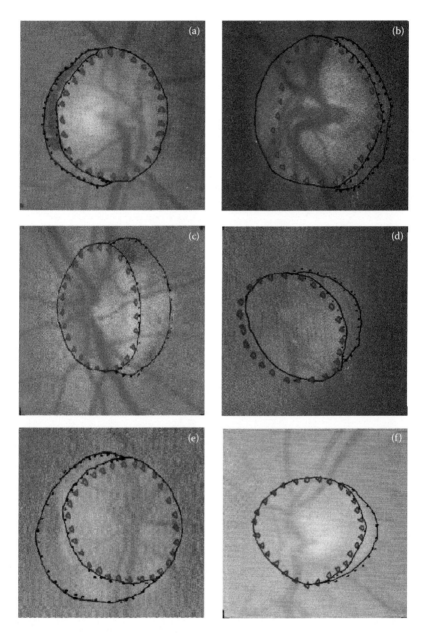

FIGURE 4.13 Segmentation results from the proposed algorithm. First column (a), (c), (e): Results from good-quality images. Second column (b), (d), (f): Results from poor-quality images. The ground estimate is drawn on the black solid line while the estimated PPA and OD regions are enclosed by the spots and the triangles, respectively.

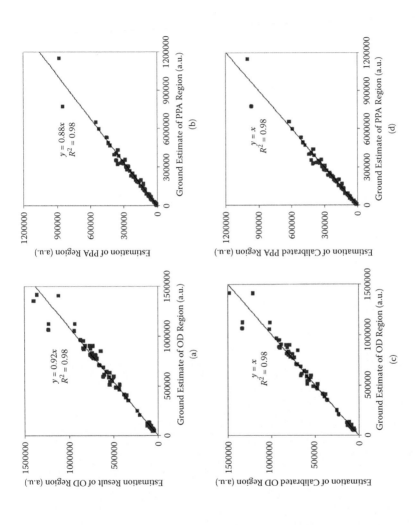

FIGURE 4.14 The correlation between the ground estimate (*x*-axis) and the results obtained by the proposed tool (*y*-axis) in quantifying the size of each region, in arbitrary pixel unit. First column (a), (b): direct estimation results from the tool; second column (c), (d): estimation results of the OD and PPA regions after calibration such that $y = x$. The correlation coefficient was found to be 0.98 in all cases.

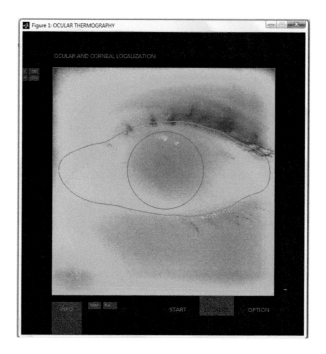

FIGURE 7.1 Ocular and corneal localization by snake algorithm.

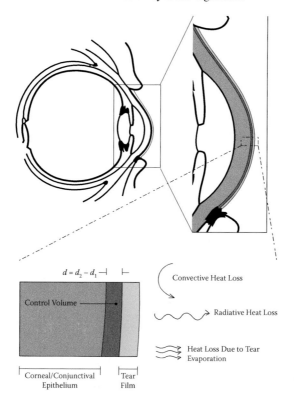

FIGURE 8.1 Tear film layer, the control volume of interest and the heat loss.

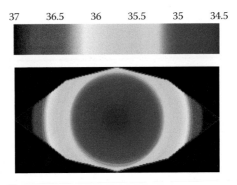

FIGURE 8.2 OST stimulated according to a 3D ocular model.

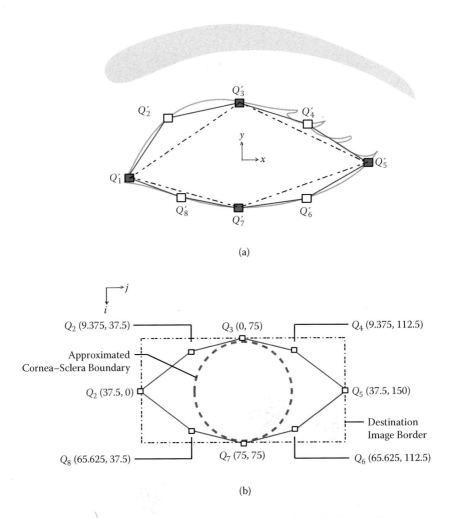

FIGURE 8.5 Points and lines defined in the source and the destination images in the warping of ocular thermal images.

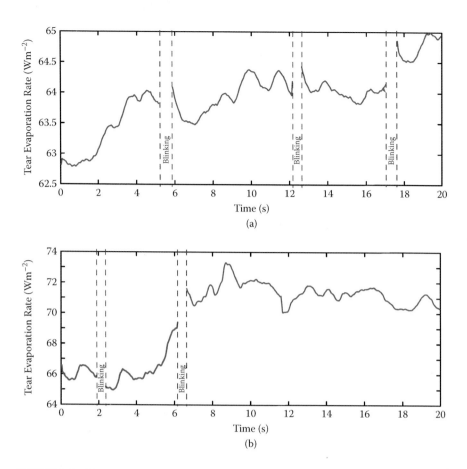

FIGURE 8.6 Tear evaporation rate of a normal subject: (a) left eye; (b) right eye.

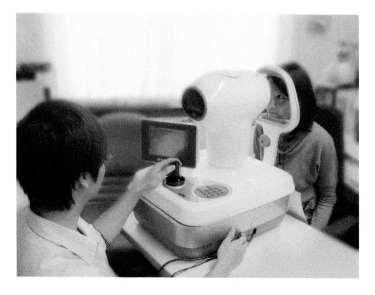

FIGURE 9.3 The tear film thermal image measurement system.

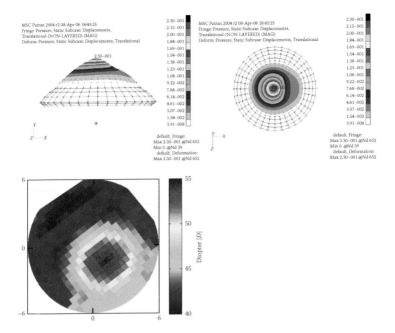

FIGURE 10.3 Analysis results corresponding to Case 9 with IOP = 15 mmHg. Maximum displacement of 230 µm, with Maximum Diopter of 54.3 D. (Adapted from Gefen et al., 2008.)

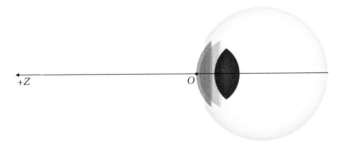

FIGURE 12.1 Position of the Virtual Eye in the Cartesian coordinate system. The x-axis is going out from the paper and the origin is the apex of the anterior cornea.

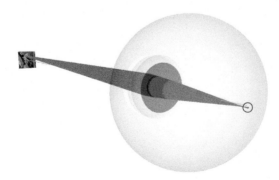

FIGURE 12.7 Projection of cones and set of points Ω on the retina.

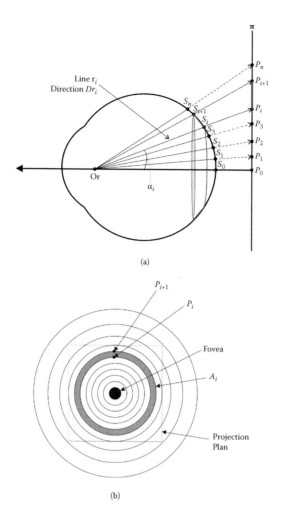

(a)

(b)

FIGURE 12.13 (a) Concentric rings on the surface of the retina. (b) Concentric rings in the projection plane image PGM image (mxn).

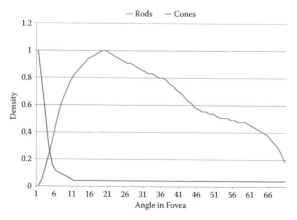

FIGURE 12.14 Discrete values for density of receptor cells in the retinal eccentricity.

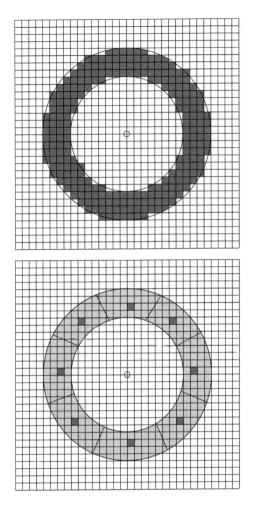

FIGURE 12.15 (a) Ring with maximum density; all the incident light will be detected in this ring. (b) Ring with lower density; much of the incident light in this ring is lost, because there is no receptor to detect it.

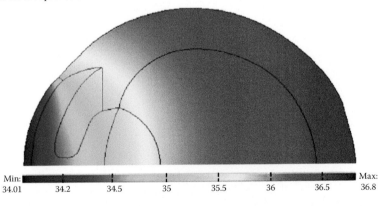

Min: 34.01   34.2   34.5   35   35.5   36   36.5   Max: 36.8

FIGURE 13.7 Thermal pattern of the 2D model without exposure to radiation.

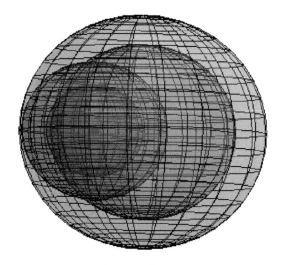

FIGURE 13.9   The 3D human eye model.

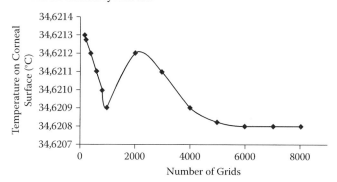

FIGURE 13.10   Grid convergence for the 3D web-spline model.

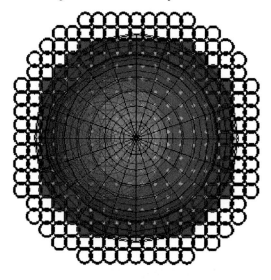

FIGURE 13.11   Grid representation for the 3D human eye model.

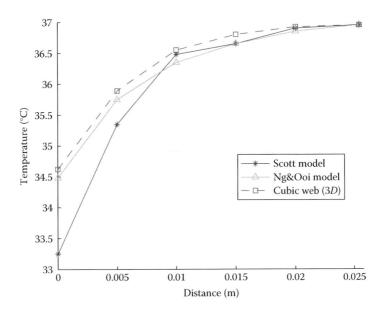

FIGURE 13.12 Comparison of the results for the 3D model using the methods in [35], [38] and the cubic web-spline method.

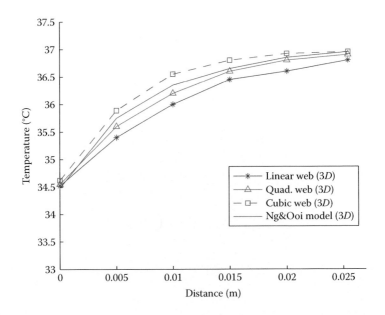

FIGURE 13.13 Comparison of the results for the 3D model using the method in [38] and the linear, quadratic, and cubic web-spline method.

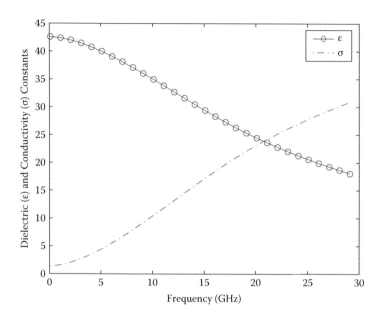

FIGURE 13.14 Dielectric and conductivity variations of cornea tissue.

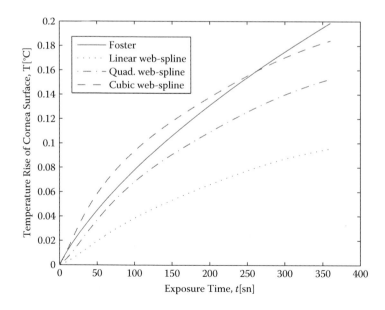

FIGURE 13.17 Temperature rise on the cornea surface at 6 min. duration at 10 mW/cm².

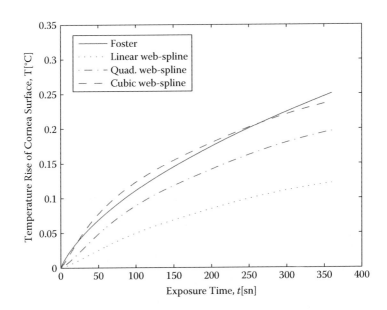

FIGURE 13.18 Temperature rise of cornea surface at 6 min. duration at 6 GHz.

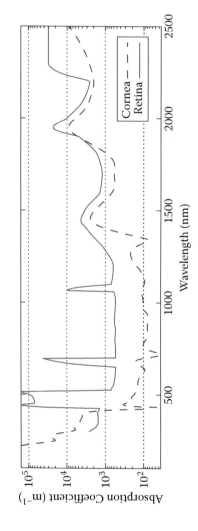

FIGURE 14.4 Wavelength dependence of the absorption coefficient of retina and cornea.

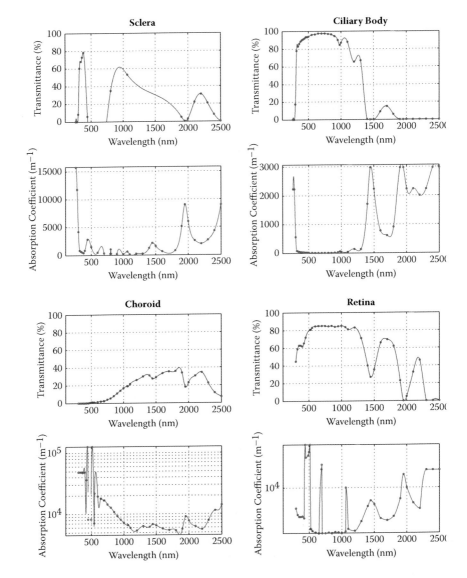

FIGURE 14.5 Transmittances and absorption coefficients of sclera, ciliary body, choroid, and retina.

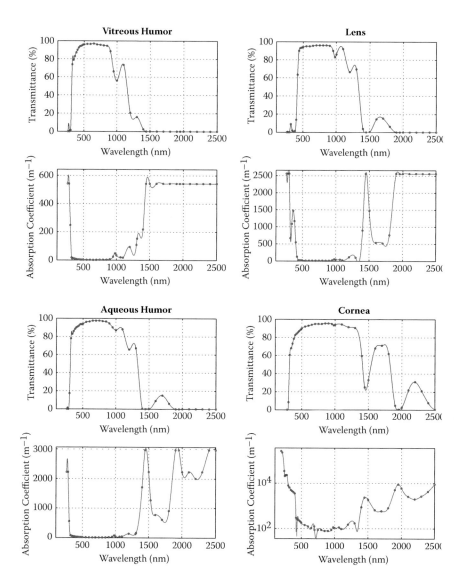

FIGURE 14.6 Transmittances and absorption coefficients of vitreous humor, lens, aqueous humor, and cornea.

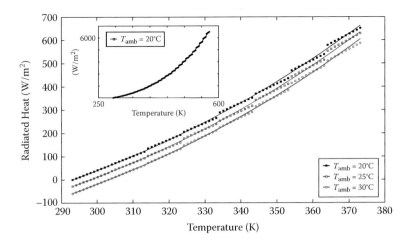

FIGURE 14.7 Approximation of radiation term by segments of 10 K.

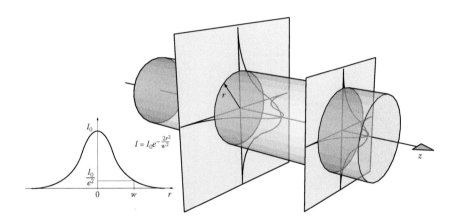

FIGURE 14.8 Gaussian beam propagation along z-axis.

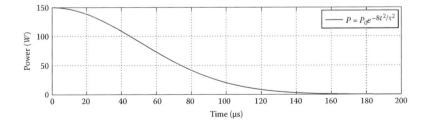

FIGURE 14.9 Laser pulse temporal profile.

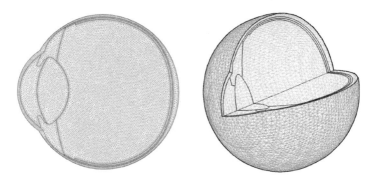

FIGURE 14.10 Finite element mesh: (a) 2D model, (b) 3D model.

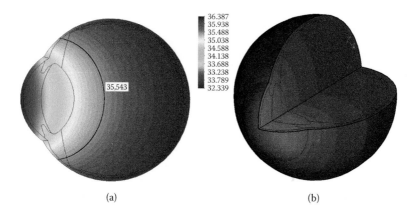

(a)   (b)

FIGURE 14.11 Steady state temperature distribution in the human eye: (a) 2D model, (b) 3D model.

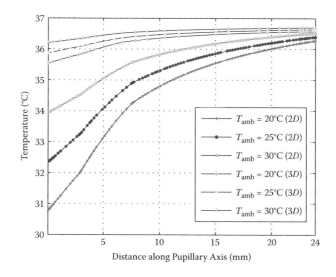

FIGURE 14.12 Steady state temperature along the pupillary axis. Dependence on ambient temperature.

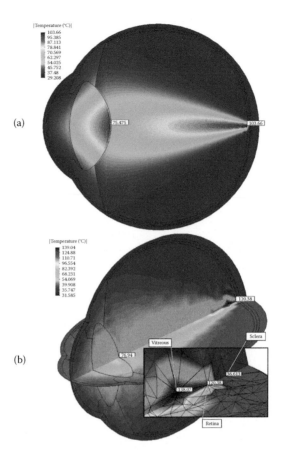

FIGURE 14.13 Comparison between temperature field distribution in the eye: (a) 2D model, (b) 3D model (horizontal and vertical slice). Nd:YAG laser parameters: pulse duration 1 ms, laser power 0.16 W, beam diameter on the cornea 2 mm, and pupil diameter 7.3 mm.

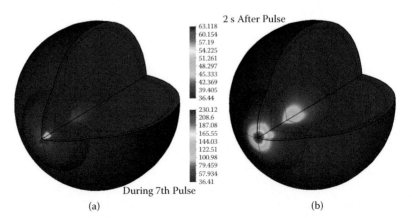

FIGURE 14.14 The temperature field distribution in the human eye; including horizontal and vertical half-slices: (a) at the end of the last pulse, (b) 2 seconds after the last pulse. Ho:YAG laser parameters: 7 pulses of 200 μs duration, laser off time 2 sec, laser power 150 W, beam diameter on the cornea 0.6 mm, and pupil diameter 1.5 mm.

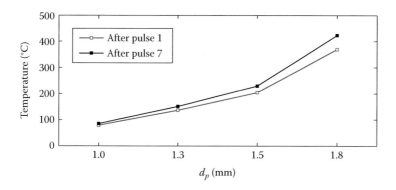

FIGURE 14.17   Ho:YAG laser: The effect of the pupillary opening on the temperature.

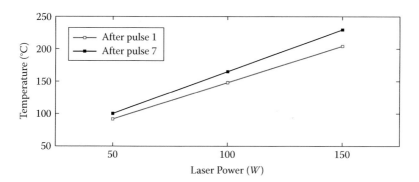

FIGURE 14.18   Ho:YAG laser: The effect of the applied laser power on the temperature.

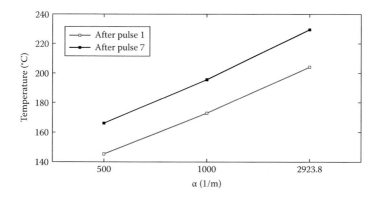

FIGURE 14.19   Ho:YAG laser: The effect of the absorption coefficient of cornea on the temperature.

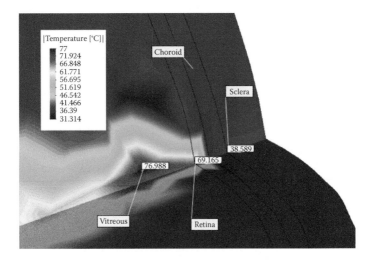

FIGURE 14.20 The temperature field around posterior part of the eye and temperature values for the selected nodes. Ruby laser parameters: pulse duration 10 ms, laser power 0.15 W, beam diameter on the cornea 8 mm, and pupil diameter 7.3 mm.

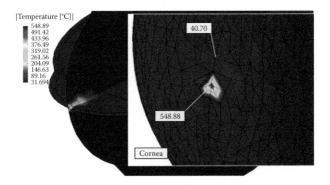

FIGURE 14.21 The temperature around anterior of the eye and detail of the corneal surface. ArF laser parameters: pulse duration 15 ns, laser energy 450 µJ, beam diameter on the cornea 0.2 mm, and pupil diameter 1 mm.

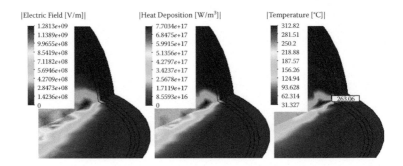

FIGURE 14.22 Distribution of the electric field, deposited laser energy and the temperature. Nd:YLF laser parameters: pulse duration 30 ps, pulse energy 100 µJ, beam diameter on the cornea 1 mm, and pupil diameter 7.3 mm.

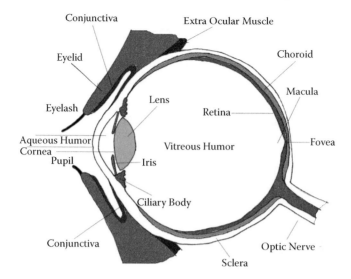

FIGURE 15.1 Schematic diagram of the physiology of the human eye. (From http://www.
lookupinfo.org/eye_care/eye_conditions.aspx)

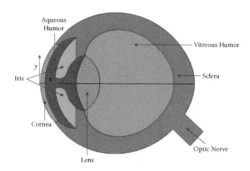

FIGURE 16.1 Anatomy of 2D model of eye [2]. (a) Edge-based smoothing domains in 2D
problem for gradient smoothing and integration are created by sequentially connecting the
centroids of the adjacent triangles with the end-points of the edge. (b) For 3D problems, the
smoothing domain is created using the neighbor tetrahedral elements by connecting vertexes
of the triangle (face k) to the centroids of two adjacent elements.

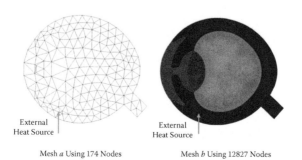

Mesh *a* Using 174 Nodes   Mesh *b* Using 12827 Nodes

FIGURE 16.3 Four sets of different mesh with heat source distributed in a small circle.
Center of heat source: x = 8.5 mm, y = −9.2 mm.

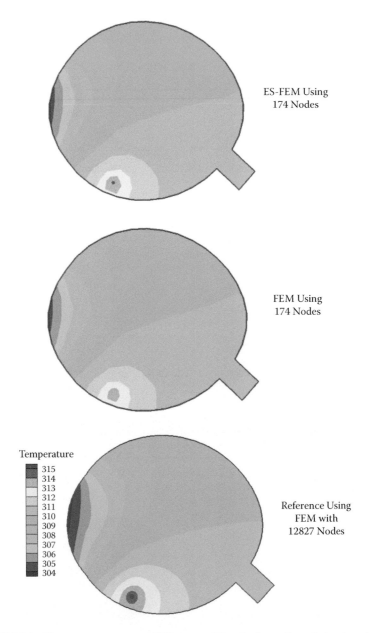

FIGURE 16.4 Temperature contour of 2D eye model under hyperthermia treatment.

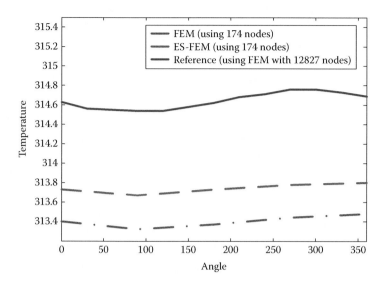

FIGURE 16.5 Temperature distribution at the heating source.

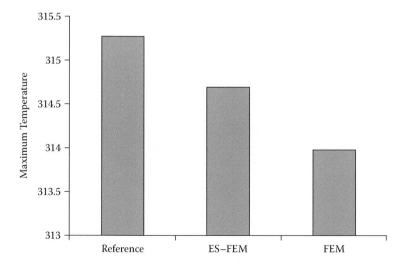

FIGURE 16.6 Comparison for maximum temperature at the heating source.

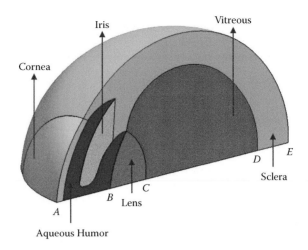

FIGURE 16.7 3D quarter model of human eye.

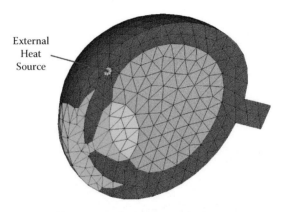

(a) Coarse mesh with 1292 nodes for section *Y-Y*

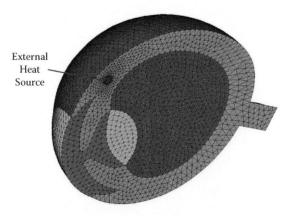

(b) Very fine mesh with 17867 nodes for section *Y-Y*

FIGURE 16.8 Two sets of different mesh with heat source distributed in a small sphere.

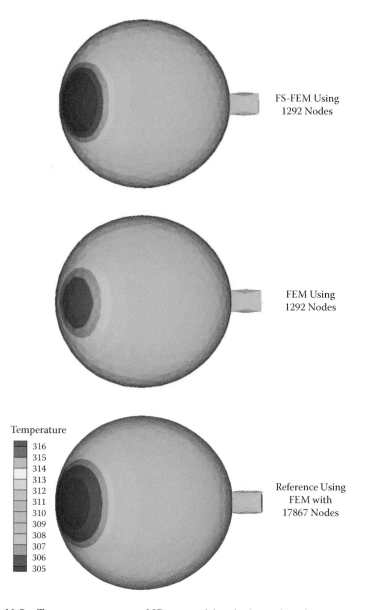

FIGURE 16.9 Temperature contour of 3D eye model under hyperthermia treatment.

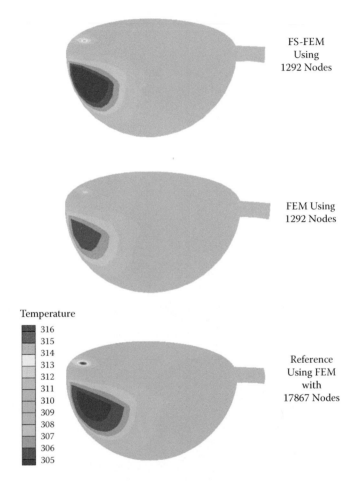

FIGURE 16.10 Temperature contour of 3D eye model for section Y-Y.

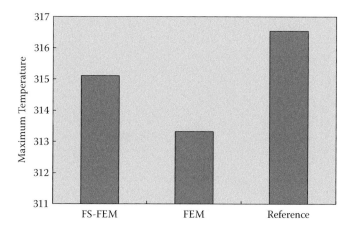

FIGURE 16.11 Comparison for maximum temperature at the heating source.

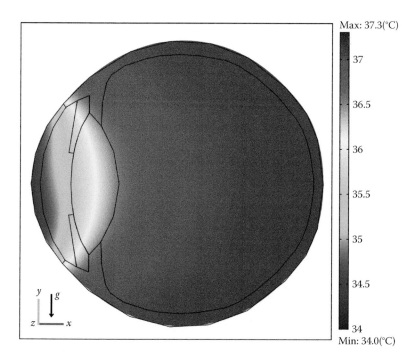

FIGURE 17.2 Temperature distribution on the $z = 0$ plane, including the AH flow, for the standing position.

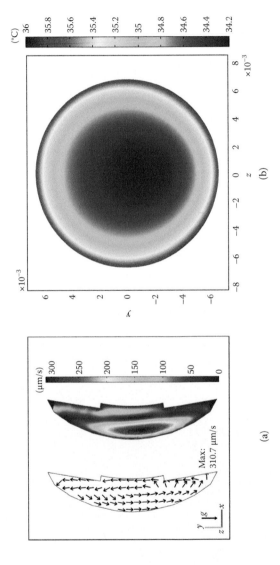

FIGURE 17.3 (a) Direction and magnitude of the velocity field inside the anterior chamber at standing position. (b) Temperature distribution on the corneal surface with consideration of the AH flow.

11 Modeling Retinal Laser Surgery in Human Eye

Arunn Narasimhan and Lingam Gopal

CONTENTS

11.1 INTRODUCTION

11.1.1 LASER IN OPHTHALMOLOGY

Ophthalmology has used laser extensively for diagnosis and treatment of many maladies of the eye since the 1960s [1,2]. The first significant biomedical study dates back to 1961, with experiments on ruby laser-induced photocoagulation in the eyes of rabbits [3]. Laser is now used in the treatment of a range of eye diseases including nearsightedness, farsightedness and astigmatism, and complex conditions such as age-related macular degeneration, diabetic maculopathy, retinopathy, choroidal neovascularization, and glaucoma. Laser eye therapies range from continuous wave (cw) photocoagulation to more recent techniques such as selective retinal pigment epithelium (RPE) treatment (SRT) [4], photodynamic therapy (PDT) [5], and trans-pupillary thermotherapy (TTT) [6]. Argon, krypton, argon pumped dye, Nd:YAG, and most recently, near-IR diode lasers are commonly used for ophthalmic laser treatments.

The interaction between laser and the biological tissue depends on the conditions of irradiation. The wavelength of laser radiation, the absorption coefficient of the tissue, the power (or energy) density, and the duration of laser radiation determine the type of effect laser has on ocular tissue. Understanding the type of interaction of laser with biological tissues is of fundamental importance in developing therapies for eye diseases and establishing safety standards. The principles of laser–tissue interaction are now fairly understood. It is known that an intense and collimated beam of laser, when focused on a particular spot on the retina or any other absorbing eye tissue, causes heating effects. Not all parts of the eye absorb the laser radiation equally. Only parts such as the retina and iris that contain chromophores like melanin, hemoglobin, and xanthophylls absorb laser radiation in the visible and IR wavelengths. The biophysical/biochemical effect of laser on these tissues depends on the magnitude and rate of laser-induced heating. The effects can be photo-ablative, photo-thermal or photo-acoustic, depending on the conditions of irradiation.

11.1.2 Laser–Tissue Interaction

Less than 10°C rise in temperature of the laser-absorbing tissue over a period of a few seconds to minutes causes heat-induced cell damage or death without causing structural alterations to the tissue. The time scale for large-scale protein molecular rearrangement, such as folding or unfolding, is on the order of milliseconds to seconds and laser-induced heating to such time scales can cause photothermal denaturation [7,8]. The damaged molecules may be biochemically active and react with other chemicals in the cell to produce secondary damage [9]. A 20–30°C rise of temperature over time periods ~ 1 s causes photocoagulation (denaturation of tissue proteins) [10] through a cascade of chemical changes initiated by interaction of laser with specific biomolecules in the cells. Receptor photopigments, retinal pigment epithelial (RPE) melanin granules, and RPE lipofuscin granules can undergo photochemical reactions on laser exposure, these reactions involving free radicals and active oxygen species. It has been experimentally proven that melanin from RPE cells formed free radicals during illumination as identified by their rapid oxidation of ascorbic acid added as a marker [11,12]. Free radicals and secondary active oxygen species can damage intracellular components in the absence of radical scavengers. Free radicals are also known to promote inflammation in tissues. The inflammation triggers neovascular events by stimulating cell proliferation in fibroblasts and RPE cells, two cell types implicated in the recurrence of neovascularization in the eye [13,14,15].

From microsecond to nanosecond exposure times, RPE damage is induced by intracellular microbubble formation around the melanosomes inside the RPE cell as discussed in [16] and [17]. These bubbles expand and collapse rapidly and generate plasma that can disintegrate the RPE cell structure or disrupt the cell membrane. At subnanosecond exposures, other nonlinear damage mechanisms appear, such as shock waves and laser-induced breakdown. Very rapid temperature rise can cause nonlinear effects such as photovaporization, that is, explosive vaporization of tissue. Rapid pulsing of laser at rates of picoseconds or nanoseconds can cause mechanical damage due to rapid heating with no interval for heat dissipation. Such nonlinear processes that occur above a certain ("optical breakdown") threshold of irradiance are difficult to predict [18] and can cause severe damage including retinal perforation, disruption of choroidal blood vessels with subretinal hemorrhage, and in severe cases, vitreous hemorrhage.

The photo-thermal effect of laser on tissue is used in ophthalmology to treat retinopathy and macular degeneration maladies of the eye [19–21]. Pan Retinal Photocoagulation (PRP), for example, relies on the photothermal effects of laser [20–27]. During PRP, the laser beam is focused on one or more spots on the retina to cause a controlled burn or photocoagulation at that spot. Since at ~60°C, the retinal region must physiologically cope with temperatures almost twice that of the core body temperature of 37°C [28] during such laser treatment. The risk of laser PRP treatment is that visible and near-IR radiations can damage the retina in doses at or above a certain threshold value [29]. When an intense and collimated laser beam is focused on a particular spot on the retina, the irradiated spot can be heated to temperatures higher than that required to coagulate the diseased tissue. This is true even with low-power lasers; a 1 mW (0.001 W) laser can result in a retinal irradiance (energy per time unit per unit area) higher than 300 W/cm^2 when incident on the retina as an intensely collimated beam. Overheating could disrupt cellular mechanism in regions adjoining the target retinal zone, resulting in damage to the retina [30]. Limited blood flow in the eye aggravates this situation [31]. Local transfer of heat to surrounding healthy tissues during retinal photocoagulation may cause rupture of Bruch's membrane with choroidal hemorrhage, or damage to the nerve fiber layer [32].

There have been many reports of damage to ocular components such as lens, cornea, and retina due to laser treatment. Whitachre and Mainster [33] reported three cases of laser injury to healthy retinal areas during photocoagulation in eyes containing gas, caused by reflection of the beam at the gas-fluid interface. Jampol et al. reported retinal detachment during Nd:YAG laser irradiation treatments applied 2 to 3 mm from the retina due to microperforation of a superficial retinal vein and a focal area of damage to the RPE [34].

11.1.3 COMPUTER MODELING AND SIMULATION OF LASER SURGERY

It is important to know the levels of laser irradiation that can produce the required photo-thermal effects without causing damage to healthy eye tissues. There have been a few experimental studies to establish laser threshold values (reference table). Most of these studies were made on animals, although there are one or two studies on live human eyes (e.g., [35]) where a thermopile was used to measure the temperature rise in the cone as it was irradiated with a ruby laser. Table 11.1 compiles the available data on the threshold levels for laser exposure for humans and animals.

The experimental studies on live human eye are more than half a century old, and further direct measurements in specific eye regions have subsequently become impossible due to clinical study regulations and ethical considerations. There are also practical difficulties involved in directly monitoring the temperature in the interior of a live human eye.

Computer modeling and simulation studies can help understand the temperature evolution during laser irradiation and set optimum parameters for safe and effective treatments. Indeed, much knowledge has been gained in the recent past from simulation and modeling studies of laser eye treatment.

TABLE 11.1
Threshold Levels for Laser Exposure

Species	Laser	Pulse Duration	Energy µJ	Effect	Reference
Rabbits	Ruby	500 µs	80	Threshold lesion	[65]
-do-	-do-	80 ns	2.2	Threshold lesion	[35]
Humans	Ruby	700 µs	1,110	Threshold lesion	[35]
Humans	Nd:YAG	150 µs	1,550	Threshold lesion	[66]
Rhesus monkeys	-do-	-do-	259	Threshold lesion	
Humans	Ruby	200 µs	950	Threshold lesion	[67]
Rhesus monkeys	Ruby	200 µs	80	Threshold lesion	[18]
Rhesus monkeys	Nd:YAG	30 ps	13×10^3	Threshold lesion	[18]
Rhesus monkeys	Dye	4 ns(532 nm)	0.9	Threshold lesion	[68]
Rhesus monkeys	Nd:YAG	30 ns	1,700	Subretinal hemorrhage	[69]
Rhesus monkeys	Frequency-doubled Nd:YAG	20 ns	156	Vitreous hemorrhage	[70]

Source: Adapted from Y. Barkana, M. Belkin, Laser Eye Injuries, *Survey of Ophthalmology* 44 (6) (2000) 459–478.

11.2 MATHEMATICAL FORMULATION

11.2.1 GEOMETRY AND PROPERTIES

Numerical modeling of the eye involves solving discretized governing equations over control volumes that pave and fill the chosen computational domain. The computational domain can be local—pertaining to a single component of the eye like the retina—or the entire volume in three dimensions. Differences exist in the geometry and typical dimensions of components chosen by different researchers but can be considered minor. The diameter of the eye along the pupillary axis is about 24 mm, while the vertical diameter is about 23 mm (from [36]). The posterior half of the human eyeball is almost spherical [37]. In most of the modeling studies in literature, each eye region is assumed to be homogeneous and the eye is assumed to be symmetrical about the pupillary axis, shown in Figure 11.1.

The thickness of sclera varies from 0.6 mm at the limbus to 0.5 mm at the equator and 1 mm at the exit of optic nerve. The retina varies in thickness from 0.5 mm to 0.1 mm, being thick around the optical disk and thinning at the equator. The retina has ten layers; the inner nine layers are considered neural retina and the outermost layer comprises pigmented epithelium also known as RPE.

RPE cells have multiple essential functions and serve as "nurse cells" for the retina. RPE absorbs and delivers nutrients to the neurosensory retina and transports the metabolic end products and waste to the choroid. The RPE cells have the pigment, melanin, that protects the photoreceptors from short-wavelength light damage and shields scattered light from the sclera. The thickness of the RPE layer varies from 6 µm to 15 µm as reported in [30].

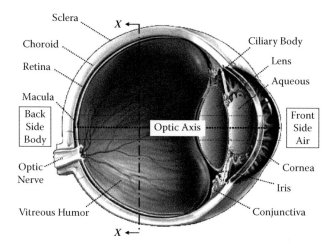

Sclera

Choroid

Retina

Macula

Back Side Body

Optic Nerve

Vitreous Humor

X

Optic Axis

Ciliary Body

Lens

Aqueous

Front Side Air

Cornea

Iris

Conjunctiva

X

FIGURE 11.1   Three-dimensional schematic of the physiology of the human eye.

The eye's cooling mechanisms involving convection, radiation, and evaporation mode of heat transfer are located at the corneal surface of the eyeball. The characteristic cooling mechanism of bio-tissues is convection and perfusion of blood flow. The choroid, present between the sclera and retina, facilitates blood flow at the back of the eye and cools the rest of the eye. It is assumed that RPE absorbs all the energy at the wavelength of argon laser.

The values for the required thermo-physical material properties for all ocular regions mentioned in Figure 11.1 are available from literature. Some primary sources published between 1962 and 2006 are provided in the references [29,38–43].

Usually an argon laser with power $Q = 0.2$ W irradiating a spot size of 500 μm is used in retinal surgery and has been used in numerical simulations. But the power range and spot size are variables that are patient (disease) specific. Also, the percentage heat generation due to the irradiation in different regions of the laser path are also different. Different laser irradiation spot sizes have been used in the actual surgery, leading to difference in the laser power input. These values are available in several recent studies (spot size [42,44,45]; heat generation percentage [44,46]; laser power [42,43,45]).

11.2.2   HEAT AND BIOHEAT EQUATIONS

Thermal damage to the eye during laser surgery depends on the rate of heat generation and transfer. The nature of heat transfer inside the human eye tissue has to be understood clearly to predict temperature distribution during laser surgery. In all the discussed numerical modeling studies, to obtain temperature distribution resulting from laser irradiation, a suitable energy equation in the eye domain is solved with its boundary conditions. Since most regions of the eye can be treated as solid or stagnant fluid, the conventional Fourier heat equation is sufficient as the governing energy equation. However, when blood flow is involved, it results in blood perfusion in the tissues, the effect of which cannot be properly captured in the conventional heat equation as shown by Pennes [47] in 1948. Such a blood perfusion situation exists in the choroidal regions of the eye. To model this in numerical simulations, the authors have adopted the Pennes bioheat transfer equation, which can be written as

$$\rho c_t \frac{\partial T_t}{\partial t} = \lambda \left(\frac{\partial^2 T_t}{\partial x^2} + \frac{\partial^2 T_t}{\partial y^2} + \frac{\partial^2 T_t}{\partial z^2} \right) + Q''' + \dot{m}_b c_b (T_b - T_t) \tag{11.1}$$

Here λ is the thermal conductivity of the region where heat transfer is taking place, while c and ρ are corresponding regional material specific heat capacity and density.

The last term of the equation models blood perfusion in tissues, where $\dot{m}_b$ is the local blood flow rate in kg/s, T_b is the blood temperature and T_t is the tissue temperature. The second-to-last term, Q''', identified as the source term, is used to account for the metabolic heat generation and also the laser irradiation, when the incident radiation in an eye region (like retina) is accounted as volumetric heat generation (in W/m³).

When compared with the cross sections of the eye (24 mm), the retinal and scleral regions are very small (around or less than 1 mm). In this, the RPE thickness is about 10 µm. Since this is where most of the laser irradiation is absorbed, a reasoning followed in [48] and [49] is to treat this RPE region as a lumped system. Such a treatment does not affect overall temperature distribution in the other section of the eye during simulations for interpreting the results. The RPE region properties, radiation absorption coefficients in particular, are available primarily from [29] and [42]. Using the thermo-physical properties and laser irradiation absorption coefficients, the total incident energy can be converted as a volumetric heat generation rate (Q''', in the above equation) for each region of the eye, including the retina.

An observation to highlight here is that the metabolic heat generation rate in eye tissue is on the order of 10^3 Wm⁻³, whereas the resulting volumetric heat generation rate in the RPE resulting from a typically applied laser power of 200 mW is on the order of 10^{10} Wm⁻³. Thus error incurred in the numerical modeling even by neglecting metabolic heat generation rate is observed to be negligible. Since the blood perfusion term represents choroidal blood flow that cools the eye from the rear, the choroidal blood mass flow rate needs to be measured. It is usually calculated from

$$\dot{m}_b = \omega \times V_c \tag{11.2}$$

where ω is the blood perfusion rate and V_c is the volume of the choroid in the interior of the eyeball. Based on available measurements of volumetric blood flow rate in the human body, suitable values for ω are available in literature, for instance in [43].

Even when choroidal blood flow is present, the rear of the interior layer of sclera toward the body is assumed in general in literature [43,48–51] to be at 37°C, the core body temperature. Depending on the extent of the eye domain that is used in the computational domain, different boundary conditions are used in the corneal (front) side. When the cross section of the entire eye is used, a modified convection-radiation boundary condition that also accounts for corneal evaporation has been used. In a recent truncated three-dimensional model, since the computational domain ends well within the vitreous, an adiabatic boundary condition of the form

$$\lambda \frac{\partial T_t}{\partial \eta} = 0 \tag{11.3}$$

has been applied at the truncated viterous plane.

The alternative of modeling the blood perfusion through the choroid has also been invoked in the literature, for instance in [43]. For enabling this, a convection-type boundary condition is imposed at the sclera (see Figure 11.2), written as

$$\lambda \frac{\partial T_t}{\partial \eta} = h_s (T_t - T_{body}) \tag{11.4}$$

Here h_s is the convection heat transfer coefficient at the sclera, which accounts for the convective cooling of the choroidal blood flow. Typical values of h_s range in literature between 26 and 300 W/m^{2}K, the low value corresponding to no blood flow and the high value corresponding to the maximum possible choroidal blood flow.

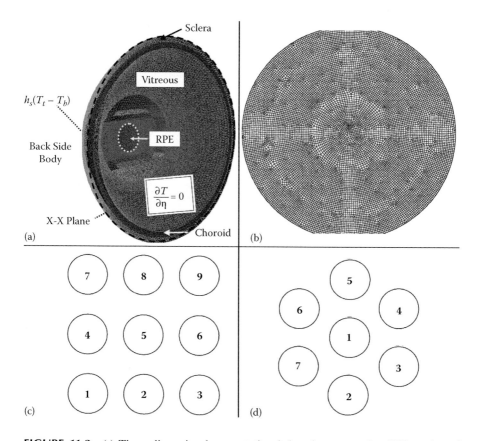

FIGURE 11.2 (a) Three-dimensional computational domain truncated at X-X section of Figure 11.1; (b) grid structure at RPE plane; (c) square array of 3 × 3 spots marked with sequence of heating; (d) circular array with seven sequential heating spots.

When blood perfusion effect is simplified this way, using the Pennes bioheat equation in numerical modeling is superfluous. The conventional Fourier heat equation (the above Pennes heat equation minus the last term) is sufficient to predict the temperature distribution and evolution in the eye domain.

11.2.3 EARLY (BEFORE 2000) NUMERICAL MODELING OF LASER SURGERY

Heat transport in the human eye has been studied by analytical techniques and numerical simulations. These have been compared and complemented by experimental studies using animal eyes that closely match human eyes in thermophysical properties. An early model of heat transport in the human eye was presented by Cain and Welch [52] using the bioheat transfer equation and corroborated with experiments conducted on the rabbit eye. Emery et al. [38] presented a numerical heat transport model for the rabbit eye and used finite element analysis. Taflove and Brodwin [53] considered the eye as a homogeneous tissue with constant convection heat transfer coefficient over the entire surface of the eyeball and developed a model using a finite difference method of solution. In such a model, the frontal sections of the eye such as cornea (see Figure 11.1) are indistinguishable from the anterior sections such as sclera and the body core. The thermal barrier property of the lens is also lost in the homogeneity. Furthermore, the assumption of uniform initial ($t = 0$ seconds) temperature (37°C) of the entire eye is unrealistic since the transient solution depends on the initial temperature distribution between the sclera and cornea.

Al-Badwaihy and Youssef [54] used the Fourier heat equation in an analytical model with combined convection and radiation heat transfer coefficients of the rabbit eye to understand the thermal effects of microwave radiation. Lagendijk [40] used a computational grid that approximated the shape of the lens and other ocular structures to present models of human and rabbit eyes. Scott [41] used the bioheat transfer equation to develop a two-dimensional finite element model of heat transport in the human eye. In this study, the steady state temperature variation in the eye on exposure to IR radiation was considered. In another two-dimensional finite element model, Scott [55] calculated temperature change in the intraocular media of the human eye exposed to infrared radiation. This model considered both transient and steady state situations and showed that temperature variation can occur in the anterior segment of the eye if there is simultaneous increase in evaporation from the anterior corneal surface and rapid blinking. However, these models are not developed with region- or treatment-specific objectives.

Amara [56] studied laser-ocular media interaction through a numerical heat transport model. Thompson et al. [57] reported a numerical granule model of laser absorbance in RPE, assuming cone and receptors to be spherical, which deviates from the realistic conical shape. The model does not consider the bulk of the eye affected by laser.

11.2.4 RECENT NUMERICAL MODELS OF LASER SURGERY

A model similar to that studied by [56] was presented by Cvetkovic et al. [58]. Their models were aimed at compliance to laser safety regulations and do not pertain specifically to clinical applications such as laser eye surgery. Chua et al. [59] developed a numerical model to predict laser-induced temperature distribution in four ocular tissues along the central pupillary axis (see Figure 11.1). In this study, the initial temperature of the eye was assumed to be constant throughout the eye and the complete geometry of the eye was not considered. Kandula et al. [60] reported a study to monitor temperature of the eye during long-duration surgery, but the study was not extended to short-duration laser treatment such as retinopathy. Sandeau et al. [61] extended the study through numerical simulations of rabbit eye using bioheat transfer equations and subsequent experimental work.

Flyckt et al. [43] studied the effect of choroidal convection, the principal cooling technique of the eye, on heat transfer characteristics. Higher values of choroidal heat transfer coefficients were obtained during numerical simulation along a simple three-dimensional geometry of the eye than in earlier work by one of the authors [40]. Hirata [62] performed steady state simulation on the effect of microwave radiation on the human eye using an improved numerical model of the irradiated eye. Ng et al. [50,63] reported steady state simulation of a two-dimensional model of the eye, which was followed by a three-dimensional model by Ng and Ooi [51].

11.3   TRANSIENT SIMULATIONS OF RETINAL SURGERY

11.3.1   2D AND 3D FVM MODELS

A geometrically identical, full-scale two-dimensional finite volume method (FVM)-based numerical model of the human eye has been developed by the authors to understand transient temperature evolution and its effects inside the human eye subjected to laser irradiation [49]. The cooling effect of blood flow in the choroid was modeled using a perfusion source term in the energy equation and also by using a suitable convection boundary condition at the sclera. Under steady state the choroidal blood flow was found to reduce the retinal temperature. However, during transient evolution that resembles the actual laser surgical process, the retinal temperature was found to be unaffected by choroidal blood flow. This is attributed to the larger time scale required for the heat diffusion from retina to choroid compared to the time of laser surgical operation (100 ms).

Results from the two-dimensional model were used to develop a transient numerical simulation of multi-spot retinal laser irradiation in a three-dimensional model [48,64]. The retinal and adjacent regions were included for analysis in a truncated three-dimensional computational domain. Resembling an actual surgery, a 3 × 3 square array formed by nine laser spots, each heated sequentially with 0.2 W power, was considered and evolution of the temperature distribution for 100 ms studied for several spot distribution and laser power conditions. It was found that when the photocoagulation temperature was around 60°C, excessive heating of the RPE by laser irradiation causes long-term thermal damage. It is therefore essential the RPE temperature quickly reduce well below 60°C within the duration of irradiation of each spot (~ 200 ms). When the distance between two consecutive spots was small (i.e., $D \leq 0.375$ mm), unheated RPE regions are overheated to 60°C due to the ongoing irradiation of a neighboring spot. A gradual increase in peak temperature of consecutive spots in a row (up to 10°C within ~ 400 ms) was another observed disadvantage. It was also shown that for $D \geq 0.6$ mm, the transient heat diffusion from the RPE to the adjacent scleral, choroidal, and vitreous humor regions was sufficient to reduce RPE close to core body temperature of 37°C during the sequential irradiation process. Irrespective of the distance between two consecutive spots in an array, pulsating the laser power about an average of 0.2 W was found to reduce the excess heating of RPE. Pulsating the laser irradiation with a frequency determined to maintain the maximum temperature within ±5°C of 60°C has been proposed as a method to reduce long-term thermal damage of RPE due to excess heating.

The authors have also numerically simulated multi-spot retinal laser surgery using a truncated three-dimensional model of the human eye. Two different arrays are studied—a square array of nine spots and a circular array of seven spots. The spots are distributed uniformly within the array and irradiated sequentially. The computational domain involves only the posterior section of the eye comprising the vitreous humor, RPE, choroid, and sclera. An argon laser with power $Q = 0.2$ W irradiating a spot size of 500 μm is selected for the numerical simulation. Finite volume formulation of Pennes bioheat transfer is employed as the governing equation to simulate the transient temperature distribution. Transient simulations of pulsatile irradiation and reduced laser power are also performed for both arrays and shown to prevent thermal damage of the eye by overheating.

Figure 11.3 shows the isotherms for spots 2, 4, and 6 of square array (Figure 11.3a) and circular array (Figure 11.3b) at 300, 700, and 1100 ms heating, respectively for a value of $D = 0.625$ mm. The temperature profile of the heat-affected zone evolves with duration of irradiation. During the initial stages of laser heating, the isotherms of both arrays are similar. As heating progresses, distinct changes in the isotherms are seen, which can be attributed to two factors. (1) In the square array, heating commences at the outermost spot and proceeds along the rows, while in the circular array, heating starts at the central spot. (2) As mentioned earlier, the effective center-to-center distance between the corner spots (spots 1, 3, 7, and 9) and central spot is $\sqrt{2}\,D$ compared to the inter-spot distance of D between any other two adjacent spots in the array. In the circular array, on the other hand, all spots are placed equidistant (D) from the central spot and from neighboring spots.

In Figure 11.3, at the end of the 100 ms heating of spot 2, the peak temperature attained by the spot is almost the same in both arrays. But by the time the fourth spot is heated, the peak temperature of spot 4 is higher for the circular array than for the square. The situation is reversed at the end of heating cycle of spot 6. But the difference in peak temperatures is less than 1°C between corresponding spots of the two arrays.

To ascertain the effect of sequence of irradiation, the histories of peak temperature evolution of the central spot in both arrays are presented in Figure 11.4a and b, respectively for the values of D considered. By virtue of being surrounded on all sides by other spots, the central spot has the least diffusion space available in both cases. For the square array, as the value of D increases, peak temperature of the central spot of the square array decreases as seen in Figure 11.4a.

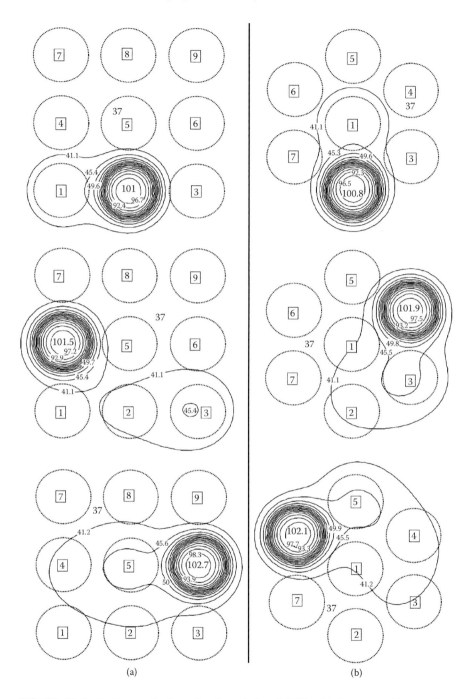

FIGURE 11.3 Isotherms for laser heating of $Q = 0.2$ W with inter-spot distance $D = 0.625$ mm for spot 2 (at 300 ms), spot 4 (at 700 ms), and spot 6 (at 1100 ms): (a) square array; (b) circular array. All the temperatures are in °C.

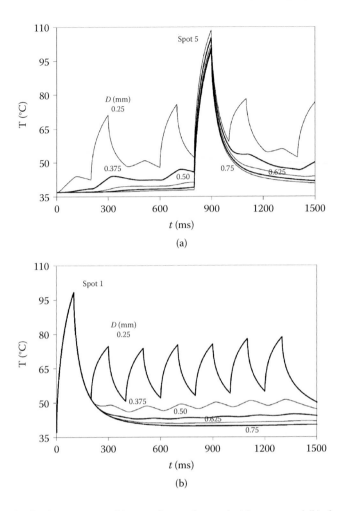

FIGURE 11.4 Peak temperature history of central spots in (a) square and (b) circular array.

After a certain value of D (say 0.625 mm), there is negligible change in peak temperature of the central spot. For a smaller value of D, the remnant heat from neighboring pre-irradiated spots (spots 1 to 4) diffuses to the central region and thus preheats the spot. The pre-irradiated neighboring spots pose an unfavorable temperature gradient and thus suppress diffusional cooling. In the circular array (Figure 11.4b), the central spot is irradiated first and therefore is not preheated by neighboring spots.

As irradiation of other spots proceeds, the central spot in the circular array is at a higher temperature than its counterpart in the square array since spots on all sides of the central spot in the former are heated sequentially and there is diffusion of heat from the peripheral spots to the central spot. It is surmised that the spots with least diffusion space should be irradiated in the initial part of the irradiation sequence. However, this keeps these spots at elevated temperatures longer.

11.3.2 METHODS TO MITIGATE THERMAL DAMAGE DUE TO EXCESS HEATING

In PRP treatment, a temperature of 60°C is sufficient to coagulate the diseased tissue. Temperatures beyond this level may damage the surrounding healthy tissue by diffusion of heat that can cause short- and long-term side effects. In practice, employing the present setting of power, pulse duration, and $D = 0.625$ mm, the peak temperature at RPE reaches 103°C (see Figures 11.3 and 11.4), a situation that has to be avoided to prevent irreversible damage to the eye.

One feasible solution is to pulsate the irradiation, as proposed in [49], an approach that reduces the peak temperature of the domain. An alternate approach to reduce the peak temperature to photocoagulation temperatures is to reduce the laser power. To maintain the temperature at around 60°C, accurate prediction of laser power is essential, as shown in [64].

The isotherms for the square and circular arrays, using reduced power setting of 0.072 W, are presented in Figure 11.5a and b. As with the pulsatile case, the isotherms of the reduced power irradiation are similar to full power (0.2 W) settings in both arrays, but peak temperatures of the spots are maintained around 60°C with minor deviations.

Peak temperature evolutions of spots 1 and 7 of the square and circular arrays for a value of $D = 0.625$ mm are presented in Figure 11.6a and b, respectively. These results are for simultaneous heating of all the spots and are obtained under different conditions, namely (1) heating with full laser power of 0.2 W, (2) pulsatile heating with a time period of 10 ms, (3) pulsatile heating with a time period of 5 ms, and (4) heating with reduced laser power of 0.072 W. During heating with full laser power of 0.2 W the peak temperatures attained by spots 1 and 7 of square array at 100 ms and 1300 ms are 100.3°C and 101.4°C, respectively. The peak temperatures of corresponding spots of the circular array attain 100.5°C and 102.8°C, respectively. When the laser is pulsated, the average peak temperature of spots of both arrays reduces to 70°C with minor deviations at the end of each heating cycle of 100 ms. When laser power is reduced to 0.072 W, the peak temperatures of spots are maintained around 60°C at the end of heating cycle.

Figure 11.7 shows the comparison between peak temperature attained by RPE during laser irradiation without (a) and with (b) pulsation, for an inter-spot distance $D = 0.625$ mm. These results are for sequential heating of the spots, however, with identical laser power as that of simultaneous irradiation.

Figure 11.7b shows the peak temperatures of spots 1, 2, and 3 for $D = 0.25$ mm when peak temperatures of spots are controlled within ± 10% of the photocoagulation temperature of 60°C through controlled pulsation. As $D = 0.25$ mm, this case refers to overlapping of spots in square array. The effect of diffusion and thus back heating is dominant compared to the case where $D \geq 0.50$ mm (non-overlapping cases). However, comparing with continuous mode of irradiation (Figure 11.7a), it is evident from Figure 11.7b that pulsating incident irradiation on a spot reduces the average temperature of the adjacent spots below 60°C. Controlled pulsation not only reduces the peak temperature of the RPE region (cells) but also reduces the back heating due to overlapping. This result is independent of the distance between two consecutive spots.

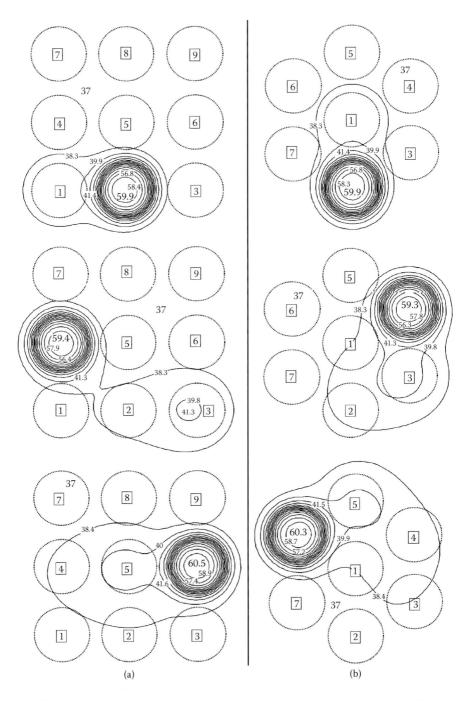

FIGURE 11.5 Comparison of isotherms evolution for three spots with $D = 0.625$ mm: (a) square array of 3×3 spots; (b) circular array with seven spots, with laser heating of reduced laser power of $Q = 0.072$ W.

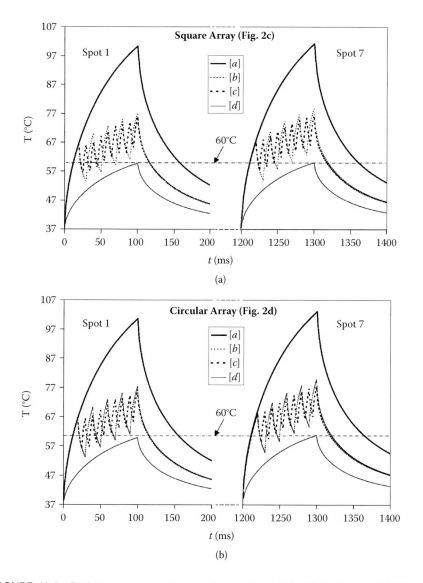

FIGURE 11.6 Peak temperature evolution of spots 1 and 7 for [a] heating with full laser power of 0.2 W, [b] pulsatile heating with a time period of 10 ms, [c] pulsatile heating with a time period of 5 ms, and [d] heating with reduced laser power of 0.072 W.

It is worth noting that in the continuous mode of heating, the time taken to reach a temperature of 66°C (+10% of photocoagulation temperature) also reduces gradually from spot 1 to spot 3. Spot 1 takes 19 ms, while spot 2 and spot 3 take 15.5 ms and 15 ms, respectively. Once pulsation starts, time for the heating cycle reduces from 6 ms to 4.5 ms gradually while time for the cooling cycle increases from 7 ms to 15 ms with a gradual increase of 2 ms for subsequent cycles.

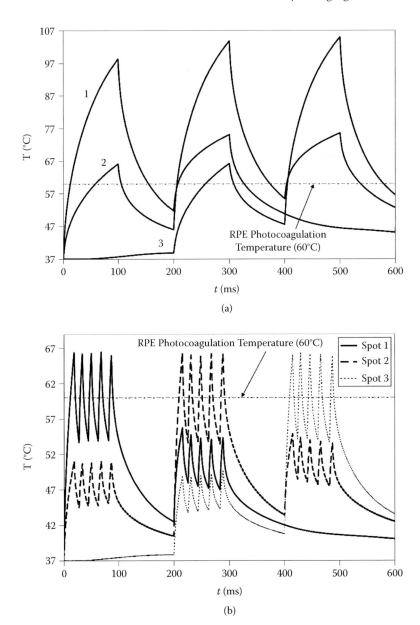

FIGURE 11.7 Peak temperature evolution of spots 1, 2, and 3 using square array during sequential heating for inter-spot distance of $D = 0.25$ mm with continuous heating (a) and pulsatile heating (b) at $Q = 0.072$ W.

11.4 CONCLUSIONS

The discussed literature available on numerical modeling of retinal laser surgery allows one to summarize certain aspects. The complexity of the geometry of the human eye at the continuum level has been captured with enough precision using the available computational tools. Both Finite Element (FEM) and Finite Volume Method (FVM)-based models invoke continuum physics. This is valid irrespective of whether the bioheat equation is invoked. To study the thermal aspects of laser surgery in local regions at a micro-scale resolution, further modeling involving molecular-level simulations, lattice Boltzmann method (LBM)-based approach, and so on, is required. Similarly, as the blood perfusion effect in the Pennes bioheat equation is macroscopic in nature, micro-scale detailing of local eye regions would also require more sophisticated bioheat transfer models to be adopted in the simulations.

Experimental measurements of temperature during laser surgery in a functioning human eye are also currently not available. Notwithstanding the obvious difficulties in performing such experiments, much of the numerical analysis performed and solution methods proposed to limit thermal damage during surgery requires corresponding experimental verification to make a direct impact in the medical practitioner's surgical process. Only interdisciplinary teams of practicing medical doctors, computational engineers, and experimental biologists can contribute in that direction.

REFERENCES

1. D. Ross, G. Zeidler, Pumping new life into ruby lasers, *Electronics* 39 (1966) 115–118.
2. K. P. Thompson, Q. S. Ren, H.-M. Parel, Therapeutic and diagnostic application of lasers in ophthalmology, *Proceedings of the IEEE* 80 (6) (1992) 838–860.
3. M. Zaret, G. Breinin, R. H. Schmidt, Ocular lesions produced by an optical maser (laser), *Science* 134 (1961) 1525–1526.
4. R. J. Brinkman, C. E. A. Wirebelauer, Photodynamic therapy of sub-foveal choroidal neovascularization in age-related macular degeneration with verteporfin: one-year results of 2 randomized clinical trials—TAP report, *Arch. Ophthalmol.* 117 (1999) 1329–1345.
5. TAP Study Group, Treatment of age-related mcular degeneration with photodynamic therapy (TAP) study group, subthreshold retinal pigment epithelium photocoagulation in macular diseases: a pilot study, *Br. J. Ophthalmol.* 84 (2000) 40–47.
6. R. Berrocal, M. E. A. Ip, Transpupillary thermotherapy of occult subfoveal choroidal neovascularization in patients with age-related macular degeneration, *Ophthalmology* 117 (1999) 1329–1345.
7. R. Birngruber, Choroidal circulation and heat convection at the fundus of the eye, chap. 5, *Laser Appl. Med. Biol.*, Plenum, New York, 277–361, 1991.
8. D. Sliney, J. Marshall, Tissue specific damage to the retinal pigment epithelium: mechanisms and therapeutic implications, *Lasers Light Ophthalmol.* 5 (1992) 17–28.
9. B. S. Gerstman, R. D. Glickman, Activated rate processes and a specific biochemical mechanism for explaining delayed laser induced thermal damage to the retina, *J. Biomed. Opt.* 4 (1999) 345–351.
10. H. Stringer, J. Parr, Shrinkage temperature of eye collagen, *Nature* 204 (1964) 1307.
11. R. Glickman, K.-W. Lam, Oxidation of ascorbic acid as an indicator of photooxidative stress in the eye, *Photochem. Photobiol.* 55 (1992) 191–196.

12. R. Glickman, R. D. Sowell, K.-W. Lam, Kinetic properties of light-dependent ascorbic acid oxidation by melanin, *Free Rad. Biol. Med.* 15 (1993) 513–547.

13. R. H. Burdon, C. Rice-Evans, Free radicals and the regulation of mammalian cell proliferation, *Free Radic. Res. Commun.* 6 (6) (1989) 345–358.

14. G. Murrell, M. Francis, L. Bromley, Modulation of fibroblast proliferation by oxygen free radicals, *Biochem. J.* 265 (1990) 659–665.

15. Macular Photocoagulation Study Group, Recurrent choroidal neovascularization after argon laser photocoagulation for neovascular maculopathy, *Arch. Opthalmol.* 104 (4) (1986) 503–512.

16. C. Lin, M. Kelly, Cavitation and emission around laser-heated microparticles, *Appl. Phys. Lett.* 72 (1998) 1–3.

17. J. Roegener, R. Brinkmann, C. Lin, Pump-probe detection of laser-induced microbubble formation in retinal pigment epithelium cells, *J. Biophys. Opt.* 9 (2004) 367–371.

18. A. Goldman, W. J. Ham, H. A. Mueller, Mechanisms of retinal damage resulting from the exposure of rhesus monkeys to ultrashort laser pulses, *Experimental Eye Research* 21 (1975) 457–469.

19. M. Niemz, *Laser-Tissue Interactions*, Springer, New York, 1996.

20. C. Sanghvi, R. McLauchlan, C. Delgado, L. Young, S. J. Charles, G. Marcellino, P. E. Stanga, Initial experience with the Pascal photocoagulator: a pilot study of 75 procedures, *British J. Ophthalmol.* 92 (2008) 1061–1064.

21. D. Modi, P. Chiranand, L. Akduman, Efficacy of patterned scan laser in treatment of macular edema and retinal neovascularization, *Clin. Ophthalmol.* 3 (2009) 465–470.

22. B. Lindblom, Effects of laser-induced retinal lesions on perimetric thresholds, *Documenta Ophthalmologica* 79 (3) (1992) 241–252.

23. S. Buckley, L. Jenkins, L. Benjamin, Field loss after pan retinal photocoagulation with diode and argon lasers, *Documenta Ophthalmologica* 82 (4) (1992) 317–322.

24. M. Lövestam-Adrian, C. D. Agardh, O. Torffvit, E. Agardh, Type 1 diabetes patients with severe non-proliferative retinopathy may benefit from panretinal photocoagulation, *Acta Ophthalmol. Scand.* 81 (3) (2003) 221–225.

25. M. Lövestam-Adrian, V. Andréasson, V. Ponjavic, Macular function assessed with mfERG before and after panretinal photocoagulation in patients with proliferative diabetic retinopathy, *Documenta Ophthalmologica* 109 (2) (2004) 115–121.

26. D. Palanker, A. Jain, Y. Paulus, D. Andersen, M. S. Blumenkranz, Patterned retinal coagulation with a scanning laser, in: *Proceedings of SPIE*, vol. 6426, ISSN 16057422, 2007.

27. L. Jixian, C. Yongbao, X. Jiehui, Laser treatment of diabetic retinopathy after cataract extraction combined with intraocular lens implantation, *Chinese J. Optometry Ophthalmol.* 11 (1) (2009) 73–75.

28. D. W. Goodwin, Lasers in surgery, *Phys. Technol.* 9 (1978) 248–253.

29. E. A. Boettner, J. R. Wolter, Transmission of the ocular media, *Invest. Ophthalmol. Vis. Sci.* 1 (1962) 776–783.

30. S. J. Till, J. Till, P. K. Milsom, G. Rowlands, A new model for laser-induced thermal damage in the retina, *Bull. Mathemat. Biol.* 65 (2003) 731–746.

31. L. Parver, C. Auker, D. Carpenter, Choroidal blood flow as a heat dissipating mechanism in the macula, *Am. J. Ophthalmol.* 89 (1980) 641–646.

32. Y. Barkana, M. Belkin, Laser eye injuries, *Survey Ophthalmol.* 44 (6) (2000) 459–478.

33. M. Whitachre, M. Mainster, Hazards of laser beam reflections in eyes containing gas, *Am. J. Ophthalmol.* 110 (1990) 33–38.

34. L. M. Jampol, M. F. Goldberg, N. Jednock, Retinal damage from a Q-switched YAG laser, *Am. J. Ophthalmol.* 62 (1983) 664–669.

35. C. J. Campbell, M. C. Rittler, C. J. Koester, The optical maser as a retinal coagulator: an evaluation, *Trans. Am. Acad. Ophthalmol. Otolaryngol.* 67 (1963) 58.

36. J. P. L'Huillier, G. Apiou-Sbirlea, Computational modeling of ocular fluid dynamics and thermodynamics, in *Medical Applications of Computer Modeling: Cardiovascular and Ocular Systems*, WIT Press, UK, 2000.
37. J. V. Forrester, A. D. Dick, P. McMenamin, W. Lee, *The Eye: Basic Sciences in Practice*, Elsevier Health Sciences, 2001.
38. A. F. Emery, P. Kramar, A. W. Guy, J. C. Lin, Microwave induced temperature rises in rabbit eyes in cataract research, *J. Heat Transfer* 97 (1975) 123–128.
39. P. S. Neelakantaswamy, K. P. Ramakrishnan, Microwave-induced hazardous nonlinear thermoelastic vibrations of the ocular lens in the human eye, *J. Biomechanics* 12 (3) (1979) 205–210.
40. J. J. W. Lagendijk, A mathematical model to calculate temperature distribution in human and rabbit eye during hyperthermic treatment, *Phys. Med. Biol.* 27 (1982) 1301–1311.
41. J. A. Scott, A finite element model of heat transport in the human eye, *Phys. Med. Biol.* 33 (1988) 227–241.
42. T. K. P. Chew, J. S. Wong, K. L. C. Chee, P. C. E. Tock, Corneal transmissibility of diode versus argon lasers and their photothermal effects on the cornea and iris, *Clin. Exper. Ophthalmol.* 28 (2000) 53–57.
43. V. M. M. Flyckt, B. W. Raaymakers, J. J. W. Lagendijk, Modelling the impact of blood flow on temperature distribution in the human eye and the orbit: fixed heat transfer coefficients versus the Pennes bioheat model versus discrete blood vessels, *Phys. Med. Biol.* 51 (2006) 5007–5021.
44. J. K. Luttrull, D. C. Musch, M. A. Mainster, Subthreshold diode micropulse photocoagulation for the treatment of clinically significant diabetic macular oedema, *Br. J. Ophthalmol.* 89 (2005) 74–80.
45. M. S. Blumenkranz, D. Yellachich, D. E. Andersen, M. W. Wiltberger, D. Mordaunt, G. Marcellino, D. Palanker, Semiautomated patterned scanning laser for retinal photocoagulation, *Retina, J. Retinal Vitreous Diseases* 26 (2006) 370–376.
46. E. A. Paysse, M. A. W. Hussein, A. M. Miller, K. M. B. McCreery, D. Coats, Pulsed mode versus near-continuous mode delivery of diode laser photocoagulation for high-risk retinopathy of prematurity, *J. AAPOS* 11 (2007) 388–392.
47. H. H. Pennes, Analysis of tissue and arterial blood temperature in the resting human forearm, *J. Appl. Physiol.* 1 (2) (1948) 93–122.
48. A. Narasimhan, K. K. Jha, Transient simulation of multi-spot retinal laser irradiation using a bio-heat transfer model, *Numerical Heat Transfer*, Part A; 57 (7) (2010) 520–536.
49. A. Narasimhan, K. K. Jha, L. Gopal, Transient simulations of heat transfer in human eye undergoing laser surgery, *Int. J. Heat Mass Transfer* 53 (1-3) (2010) 482–490.
50. E. Y. K. Ng, E. H. Ooi, FEM simulation of the eye structure with bioheat analysis, *Computer Methods and Programs in Biomedicine* 82 (3) (2006) 268–276.
51. E. Y. K. Ng, E. H. Ooi, Ocular surface temperature: A 3D FEM prediction using bioheat equation, *Computers in Biology and Medicine* 37 (6) (2007) 829–835.
52. C. P. Cain, A. J. Welch, Measured and predicted laser-induced temperature rises in the rabbit fundus, *Invest. Ophthalmol. Vis. Sci.* 13 (1974) 60–70.
53. A. Taflove, M. Brodwin, Computation of the electromagnetic fields and induced temperatures within a model of the microwave irradiated human eye, *IEEE Trans. Microwave Theory Tech.* 23 (1975) 888–896.
54. K. A. Al-Badwaihy, A. B. A. Youssef, Biological thermal effect of microwave radiation on human eye, in: C. C. Johnson, M. L. Shore (Eds.), *Biological Effects of Electromagnetic Waves,* vol. 1, DHEW Publication, Washington, DC, 61–78, 1976.
55. J. A. Scott, The computation of temperature rises in the human eye induced by infrared radiation, *Phys. Med. Biol.* 33 (1988) 243–257.
56. E. H. Amara, Numerical investigations on thermal effects of laser-ocular media interaction, *Int. J. Heat Mass Transfer* 38 (13) (1995) 2479–2488.

57. C. R. Thompson, B. S. Gerstman, S. L. Jacques, M. E. Rogers, Melanin granule model for laser-induced damage in the retina, *Bull. Math. Biol.* 58 (1996) 513–553.

58. M. Cvetkovic, D. Poljak, A. Peratta, Thermal modelling of the human eye exposed to laser radiation, *Software, Telecommunications and Computer Networks, SoftCOM.* (2008) 16–20.

59. K. J. Chua, J. C. Ho, S. K. Chou, M. R. Islam, On the study of the temperature distribution within a human eye subjected to a laser source, *Int. Comm. Heat Mass Transfer* 32 (2005) 1057–1065.

60. J. Kandulla, H. Elsner, R. Birngruber, R. Brinkmann, Noninvasive optoacoustic online retinal temperature determination during continuous-wave laser irradiation, *J. Biomed. Optics* 11 (4) 041111.

61. J. Sandeau, J. Kandulla, H. Elsner, R. Brinkmann, G. Apiou-Sbirlea, R. Birngruber, Numerical modelling of conductive and convective heat transfers in retinal laser applications, *J. Biophotonics* 1 (1) (2008) 43–52.

62. A. Hirata, Improved heat transfer modeling of the eye for electromagnetic wave exposures, *IEEE Trans. Biomed. Eng.* 54 (5) (2007) 959–961.

63. E. H. Ooi, W. T. Ang, E. Y. K. Ng, Bioheat transfer in the human eye: a boundary element approach, *Eng. Anal. Boundary Elements* 31 (6) (2007) 494–500.

64. K. K. Jha, A. Narasimhan, Numerical simulations of heat transport in human eye undergoing laser surgery, in: *Proceedings of the 20th National and 9th International ISHMT-ASME Heat and Mass Transfer Conference*, 10HMTC430, Mumbai, India, 2010.

65. A. Kohtiao, I. Resnick, J. Newton, H. Schwell, Threshold lesions in rabbit retinas exposed to pulsed laser radiation, *Am. J. Ophthalmol.* 62 (1966) 664–669.

66. C. Ren-yuan, L. Jia-hua, L. Meng-chang, Pulsed ND:YAG laser irradiation threshold of Chinese retinas, *Chinese Med. J.* 100 (1987) 855–858.

67. A. Vassiliadis, H. C. Zweng, N. A. Peppers, Thresholds of laser eye hazards, *Arch. Environ. Health* 20 (1970) 161–170.

68. C. P. Cain, C. A. Toth, C. D. DiCarlo, Visible retinal lesions from ultrashort laser pulses in the primate eye, *Invest. Ophthalmol. Vis. Sci.* 36 (1995) 879–888.

69. M. F. Blankenstein, J. Zuclich, R. G. Allen, Retinal hemorrhage thresholds for Q-switched neodymium-YAG laser exposures, *Invest. Ophthalmol. Vis. Sci.* 27 (1986) 1176–1179.

70. W. D. Gibbons, R. G. Allen, Retinal damage from suprathreshold Q-switch laser exposure, *Health Phys.* 35 (1978) 461–469.

12 A Geometric Model of the 3D Human Eye and Its Optical Simulation

Leandro Paganotti Brazil and
Odemir Martinez Bruno

CONTENTS

12.1   INTRODUCTION

The interest in understanding quality of vision, the optical properties of the human eye, and its relation to physical and physiological properties of its components, is ancient [7]. Helmholtz, in the nineteenth century, was one of the pioneers in this study, which was compiled in the famous collection *Helmholtz Treatise on Physiological Optics* [8]. Since then, a great number of techniques and instruments for visual quality measurements have been implemented.

The technical and scientific development of medical instrumentation achieved its maximum in the last three decades with the development of medical image techniques. The great advantage of these image techniques is that they extract more information, often with very high quality and accuracy.

Modern medicine is dependent on the image information based on magnetic resonance, x-ray, and ultrasonic techniques. These images have allowed great advances in medical science (i.e., with regard to understanding and explaining details of how the organs and human systems work), diagnostics, and surgical techniques.

On the other hand, development of image-based techniques for ophthalmology found a great barrier: the nature of the eye. The human eye is mostly composed of liquids or soft cells, which are substances not differentiable by x-ray or resonance magnetic, making these techniques impractical for human eye analysis. Although ultrasonic techniques can distinguish the parts of the eye, they do not have enough resolution to analyze most of the eye's physiology, for instance the accommodation process.

These deficiencies of measure and analysis techniques have made computer modeling the most important tool to investigate the optical and physiological phenomena of the human eye.

Eye modeling and simulation is a challenging task, especially when realistic models are required. Even basic questions such as the computational modeling of the structures comprising the human eye system and how to simulate the projection of an image onto the retina for a specific eye have not been addressed suitably. Few works devoted to the simulation of optimal correction for aberrations and lens accommodation process have been proposed.

This chapter presents one of the first steps toward tackling some of the questions above, proposing a framework for computational modeling and simulation of the human eye system. Making use of geometric modeling and computer graphics techniques, the proposed approach is able to handle both synthetic and *in vivo* corneal topography data from which it is possible to visualize and analyze retinal images of a specific eye.

The system, called *Virtual Eye (VEye)* [28], was created by a Brazilian group from the University of São Paulo at the Institute of Mathematics and Computer Science [27] in São Carlos. The group has been showing great progress in this research with significant results such as a modeler and viewer of the human visual system [20,28], optical simulations and physiological phenomena of the eye [21,23], and also modeling and simulation of phenomena regarding the retina of the eye [22].

The Virtual Eye presents some special characteristics compared with other approaches described in the literature. For example, the eye model is comprised of cornea, crystalline, and spherical retina. All of them are modeled by triangular meshes in a 3D environment, facilitating computational simulation with such structures and allowing a wide flexibility in simulation as an optical system. It is a realistic anatomical model of a human eye in a virtual environment that reproduces its structures to simulate the human vision process and some optical properties concerned with it. The technique presented here can lead to further contributions to the understanding and planning process for customized refractive surgeries.

Not limited to optical simulations, the Virtual Eye can also reproduce an interpretation of retinal images, highlighting their different resolutions and also psychophysical phenomena involved in them.

12.2   GEOMETRIC SIMULATION OF THE HUMAN EYE

Different approaches for computational modeling of the human visual system exist, the schematical and reduced models being the most commonly used. In schematical modeling the goal is to create precise models for the ocular system, respecting, at least to a certain degree, certain anatomical parameters of the biological eye. Although schematical models can precisely represent certain properties and functionalities of the biological eye, their complexity may impair computational simulation, which demands a more simplified modeling.

The objective of the reduced models is to reproduce the optic characteristics of the human ocular system through a simplified set of anatomical structures of the human eye. The simplifications introduced by the reduced models, which sometimes arrive to consist of only one refractory structure, help enormously in the calculation of simple parameters. For problems whose goal is to reach the real performance of the human visual system such models can be incomplete.

One of the first works related to the modeling of the human eye was written by Helmholtz [8]. This schematical model, said to be almost accurate, intends to represent an eye with correct biological functioning, including the majority of the anatomical structures; even so, the values of the refractive indices as well as some values of radius of curvature are not biologically consistent. Although all schematical eye models have different degrees of discrepancy with the biological model, the Helmholtz model is considered one of the most faithful to the biological eye in terms of optic properties.

Gullstrand [11] proposes simplifications in the Helmholtz's schematical model, considering the cornea as being constituted of only one refractive surface. The reduced model of Emsley [9], derivative from Gullstrand's schematical model, is one of the most spread out, mainly due to its simplicity. This model has only retina and cornea, both represented as a single surface, with refraction power of 60 diopters, and an internal medium with refractive index of 1.333.

The previously described models use spherical surfaces to model the components of the eye, making it difficult to accomplish realistic simulations due to spherical aberration present in these models. To overcome such a problem, Lotmar [10] considers a model where parabolic surfaces replace the spherical models. Although the proposed surfaces do not agree with the anatomical structures, the results obtained are in accordance with experimental tests. More general approaches have also been proposed, such as the elliptical, parabolic, and hyperbolic models proposed by Kooijman [12], whose results are quite similar to the Lotmar model.

With the objective of improving the simulation of chromatic aberrations, Thibos [13] proposes a new reduced model, called *Chromatic Eye*. The chromatic eye introduces a pupil to the model and uses elliptical surfaces to model the corneal lens, ensuring a null spherical aberration. Changing the elliptical surface by a family of models with rotational symmetry, Thibos [14] introduces a degree of freedom to the model, making it possible to simulate spherical aberration. This new model has been called *Indiana Eye*.

Doshi [15] has compared the effectiveness of Kooijman's model, Chromatic Eye, and Indiana Eye in computer simulation. Although all models have presented satisfactory results, Chromatic Eye has obtained the best behavior in experiments. Some of the above-mentioned eyes are discussed in greater detail in Smith [1].

A different approach for computer simulation of the human eye has been proposed by Camp et al. [16]. Camp's approach makes use of real data to model the cornea and a plane to model the retina. Using ray-tracing to simulate light rays through the eye, this strategy can compute a spot diagram on the plane defining the retina. By convolving the spot diagram with Snellen's letters the system is able to infer how a person sees. Aspherical algebraic surfaces have been employed by Langenbucher [17]. Although such an approach enables one to compute normals and ray intersections analytically, handling a real corneal data set becomes difficult, therefore limiting the technique to general surfaces. Carvalho et al. [18] propose a framework to deal with a real corneal data set, using the Emsley Eye as base to accomplish the simulation.

In this chapter is presented the Virtual Eye proposal, which is also able to deal with real data to model the cornea while including additional structures as crystalline lens and spherical retina, making it more complete than others. Furthermore, the Virtual Eye simulation scheme is based on triangular mesh to model the anatomical structures, an original approach in the context of eye simulation. This framework makes the basic operations involved in human eye simulation, such as the ray-tracing process, more robust and efficient.

12.3 THE VIRTUAL EYE SYSTEM

The Virtual Eye system is divided into three main modules: *modeling* (in the computational sense), *simulation*, and *visualization*. Modeling has the objective of structuring the components of the eye, such as cornea, retina, and crystalline lens. Simulation is responsible for the optical system, casting rays, and computing the intersections and refraction of the rays. Outputs from the simulation are handled by the visualization module. The following subsections describe in more details the functionalities of each module.

12.3.1 Modeling

As the name suggests, this module is responsible for modeling the three main components of the eye: cornea, retina, and crystalline lens. Models based on the quadric

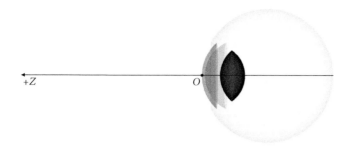

FIGURE 12.1 Position of the Virtual Eye in the Cartesian coordinate system. The x-axis is going out from the paper and the origin is the apex of the anterior cornea. (Please see color insert.)

equation (Section 3.1.1) and triangular superficial meshes (Section 3.1.2) have been created to represent all the components of the human eye. Figure 12.1 shows the position of the Virtual Eye in the Cartesian coordinate system where the apex on the center of anterior cornea is placed at the origin of the coordinate system.

12.3.1.1 Modeling by Quadrics

In general, schematic models of artificial eyes are constructed with quadric surfaces [1]. At first, each surface is generated at the system origin and after this it is moved to the correct position. Equation 12.1 is used to express such surfaces.

$$h^2 + (1+Q)z^2 - 2zr = 0 \qquad (12.1)$$

where z is the optical axis, $h^2 = x^2 + y^2$, r is the radius of curvature, and Q is the surface asphericity:

- $Q < -1$: specifies a hyperboloid
- $Q = -1$: specifies a paraboloid
- $-1 < Q < 0$: specifies an ellipsoid, with the z-axis being the major axis
- $Q = 0$: specifies a sphere
- $Q > 0$: specifies an ellipsoid, with the major axis in the x-y plane

One example of a mesh generated by quadrics is shown in Figure 12.5(a).

12.3.1.2 Modeling by Meshes

The mesh generation for modeling surfaces is based on Equation 12.1. Cornea, crystalline, and retina are all created with different quadrics. At first, one layer is defined that will pass through successive processes of refinement until the mesh reaches the satisfactory level, resulting in the desired surface.

Five vertices are initially defined: v_0, the apex of surface, v_1, v_2, v_3, and v_4. All of them are placed to form a prism M, as shown in Figure 12.2. The v_0 vertex is the top

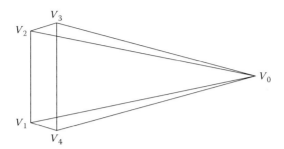

FIGURE 12.2   Initial mesh composed of prism with five vertices.

of the prism and the intersection between the optical axis and the surface. The last four vertices define the base of the prism and the plane that limits the surface. This prism is the initial step of mesh generation.

Then, new layers are added to the prism. If the model is composed of one layer, four vertices are added to it, forming a plane that divides the prism into two areas or two layers. If three layers are desired, eight new vertices, forming two parallel planes, are added to the initial model, dividing the prism into three areas or layers, and so on for larger models. Figure 12.3 illustrates the initial layers in the mesh generation process of Virtual Eye.

The next step is the refinement. The triangles created in the layers step are divided into smaller triangles, making the geometrical surface more similar to the theoretical quadric. The refinement step is described as follows: Let t be any triangle in the mesh M, where $t = \Delta v_i v_{i+1} v_{i+2}$. Find out the three middle points of the three edges that compose the triangle t and make them the three new vertices $v_k v_{k+1} v_{k+2}$ to form new smaller triangles in the mesh. These new triangles are added to M and the older triangle t is removed from it.

Figure 12.4 shows a model of mesh for a retina created by Virtual Eye. There is a difference of refinement between the last layer (the rightmost one) and the others. The last layer defines the place where the fovea stay on the retina and there must be many more photoreceptor cells in this place than others.

12.3.1.3   Modeling *in Vivo*

Besides the theoretical cornea generated by computer, there is also a set of real corneal data *in vivo*, obtained by a corneal topographer from the Group of Optical Ophthalmologic at the University of São Paulo in São Carlos. The topographer measures the relative elevations by center of cornea, where it is the coordinate system origin O and the elevation point is null. Each point is represented by the triple (r, θ, h), where r is the distance from the point until the origin O, θ is the angle measured from the x-axis, and h is the relative elevation from orthogonal plane to z tangent to the corneal vertex. The elevations are caught by degree at different circumferences with center O.

Then, the surface is approximated by a triangular surface mesh generated by the triangulation of the set of points and their elevations obtained by the topographer. As result, there will be a mesh similar to Figure 12.5(b).

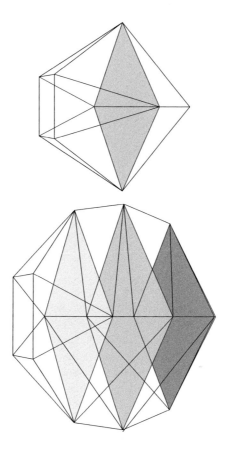

FIGURE 12.3   Initial mesh (a) with two layers and (b) with four layers.

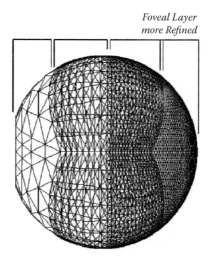

FIGURE 12.4   Retina model with four layers. The last one is the fovea layer.

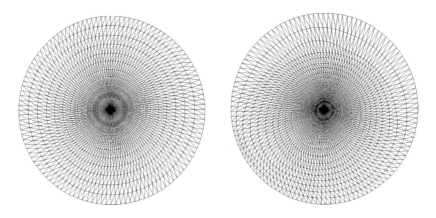

FIGURE 12.5 Mesh generated by (a) simulated data and (b) real data from topographer.

12.3.2 SIMULATION

To make the simulations of the Virtual Eye, two schematic models of eyes found in the literature were implemented for this chapter: *Le Grand* and *Liou-Brennan*. The Le Grand model was chosen because it is simple and flexible, and the Liou-Brennan was chosen because it is an eye model that uses the refractive index distribution for each part of the lens, such as the posterior and anterior part.

The Le Grand model is presented in its unaccommodated *(lgr_u)* and accommodated *(lgr_a)* state, and Liou-Brennan only in its unaccommodated *(lbr_u)* state. Table 12.1 shows specified values for the *(lgr_u)* model and Table 12.2 for *(lgr_a)* [5].

The Liou-Brennan model, shown in Table 12.3, is based on data obtained experimentally from the human eye [6]. Both the anterior n_A and the posterior n_P distribution are given by Equation 12.2.

$$n(\rho',z') = n_{00} + n_{01}z' + n_{02}z'^2 + n_{10}\rho'^2 \qquad (12.2)$$

where $\rho'^2 = x'^2 + y'^2$ and (x',y',z') are a centered coordinate system at z_0 on the optical axis z and n_{00}, n_{01}, n_{02}, and n_{10} are constants that are explained in Table 12.4.

TABLE 12.1
Le Grand Unaccommodated Full Theoretical Eye

	Radius (mm)	n (Index mm)	d (Thick mm)
Anterior Cornea	7.8	1.377	0.55
Posterior Cornea	6.5	1.377	3.05
Anterior Lens	10.2	1.420	4.0
Posterior Lens	−6.0	1.336	16.59

Note: Power = 59.940.

TABLE 12.2

Le Grand Accommodated Full Theoretical Eye

	Radius (mm)	n (Index mm)	d (Thick mm)
Anterior Cornea	7.8	1.377	0.55
Posterior Cornea	6.5	1.377	2.65
Anterior Lens	6.0	1.427	4.5
Posterior Lens	−5.5	1.336	16.49

Note: Power = 59.940, A = 7.053D.

TABLE 12.3

Liou-Brennan Accommodated Eye

	Radius (mm)	n (Index mm)	d (Thick mm)
Anterior Cornea	7.77	1.376	0.55
Posterior Cornea	6.40	1.336	3.16
Lens	12.40	n_A	1.59
Lens	∞	n_P	2.43
Lens	−8.10	1.336	16.27

Note: Power = 60.314.

TABLE 12.4

Constants of Equation 12.1 Which Show the Refractive Index Distribution in the Anterior n_A and Posterior n_P Part of Crystalline

	n_A	n_P
n_{00}	1.386	1.407
n_{01}	0.049057	0.0
n_{02}	−0.015427	−0.0006605
n_{10}	−0.001978	−0.001978
z_0	−3.71	−5.30

The simulation consists of casting rays toward the eye, computing the refractions on the cornea and crystalline lens, and finally obtaining the intersection points among rays and retina (ray-tracing process). The next two sections show how this process is done. Section 12.3.2.1, "The Ray-Tracing Process," explains how one ray is simulated from the origin point until it gets to the surface of the retina. Then Section 12.3.2.2, "Projection of Cones," shows how a set of these rays is grouped in cones to be shot forward in the eye and transformed into an image.

12.3.2.1 The Ray-Tracing Process

The calculation of refractions involves two geometrical estimates: the intersection points between each ray and the refractive surfaces (cornea and crystalline) and the normal vectors in these intersection points.

The Virtual Eye system implements two ways to calculate the intersection between the ray and surface and the normal at this point. The first one is used when the surface is generated by simulated data with Equation 12.1. The second one is used when the surface is based on real data *in vivo* from the topographer; in this case, three-dimensional surface meshes are used.

In the first case, the intersection is obtained by replacing Equation 12.3 in Equation 12.1, solving the second-degree system. There will be two solutions α_1 and α_2 from the system. It must pick out the one that produces the less positive value β_1, β_2 in Equation 12.4.

$$R_i = R_0 + \alpha L \tag{12.3}$$

$$\beta_i = a \cos\left[\frac{L*(R_i - R_0)}{\|R_i - R_0\|}\right] \tag{12.4}$$

$$R_i = R_i + \alpha_i L \tag{12.5}$$

So the intersection W is given by

$$W = R_0 + \alpha_k L \tag{12.6}$$

where α_k is the square root. The normal at W is calculated by the gradient operator:

$$N_W = \nabla S(W) \tag{12.7}$$

where

$$\nabla S(x, y, z) = \begin{bmatrix} \dfrac{\partial S}{\partial x} \\[2ex] \dfrac{\partial S}{\partial y} \\[2ex] \dfrac{\partial S}{\partial z} \end{bmatrix} \tag{12.8}$$

with

$$\frac{\partial S}{\partial x} = 2x, \frac{\partial S}{\partial y} = 2y \quad and \quad \frac{\partial S}{\partial z} = 2[(1+Q)z - R] \tag{12.9}$$

The second case, in which the intersection is between the ray and the mesh, uses the *door-in–door-out* principle, explained as follows.

Let v_1, v_2, and v_3 be three vertices defining a triangle t in a mesh. Suppose that a ray l is cast from point x in direction u (Figure 12.6). The ray l intersects the plane defined by t at one point w, in mathematical terms $w = x + \alpha u$. The point w can also be written as $w = \lambda_1 v_1 + \lambda_2 v_2 + \lambda_3 v_3$. From these two expressions for w we derive the following linear system:

$$\begin{pmatrix} 1 & 1 & 1 & 0 \\ v_1 & v_2 & v_3 & u \end{pmatrix} \begin{pmatrix} \lambda_1 \\ \lambda_2 \\ \lambda_3 \\ \alpha \end{pmatrix} = \begin{pmatrix} 1 \\ x \end{pmatrix} \qquad (12.10)$$

The system in Equation 12.10 gives values to $\lambda_1, \lambda_2, \lambda_3$, and α. If $\lambda_i \geq 0$ for all $i = 1,2,3$, then w is within the triangle t; otherwise at least one λ_i is negative. A negative λ_i indicates that w is opposite to v_i; for example, in Figure 12.6 w is opposite to v_2 regarding the edge $v_1 v_3$, so $\lambda_2 < 0$. Notice that if we "jump" from t to the adjacent triangle opposite to v_i we go toward w. Following this principle we shall reach a triangle containing w where $\lambda_i \geq 0$, with, $i = 1,2,3$. It is worth noting that the door-in–door-out principle does not work if the mesh presents "strong" concavities (high-intensity curvatures), but this is not the case in our context.

Besides revealing the intersection points, the values of λ can also be employed to interpolate normals on the mesh. Let v_1 v_2, and v_3 be the vertices of a triangle t containing w and n_1, n_2, and n_3 be the normals in these vertices (the normals n_i can be estimated by averaging the normals of the triangles surrounding the vertex v_i). As $\lambda_i \geq 0$, $i = 1,2,3$ in t, the normal n_w in w can be estimated as

$$n_w = \lambda_1 n_1 + \lambda_2 n_2 + \lambda_3 n_3 \qquad (12.11)$$

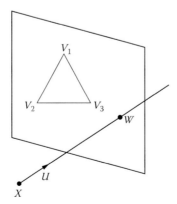

FIGURE 12.6   Door-in–door-out principle.

In that way, the door-in–door-out principle allows the computation of intersection points and normals in a very efficient way, as it avoids the necessity of testing each ray against all triangles in the mesh. Since all eye structures are modeled as triangular meshes, the door-in–door-out technique can be employed in all geometrical calculations present in the ray-tracing.

Refractions are computed from Snell's law, $n_i \sin(\theta_i) = n_r \sin(\theta_r)$, where n_i, θ_i are the index of refraction and angle of incidence of the incident medium and n_r, θ_r are the index and angle of refraction of the refractive medium.

12.3.2.2 Projection of Cones

With the ray-tracing described in the previous section the Virtual Eye can simulate the image formation on the retinal surface. A lot of light rays leave any point (pixel) in the image I toward the eye. However, in the real world, only some of them enter the human eye, forming a light ray cone, as shown in Figure 12.7. Thus, many light ray cones are shot from each pixel in the image I computing the refractions on the cornea and crystalline lens, finally obtaining the intersection points among rays and retina (ray-tracing process). This set of final points is called the cloud of point. It is necessary to transform each pixel in the image I into Cartesian coordinates to simulate the ray-tracing process. Equation 12.12 changes any pixel (i,j) from I into (x,y) real coordinate.

$$
\begin{aligned}
x_i &= x_0 + i\Delta x \\
y_j &= y_0 + j\Delta y \\
color_{i,j} &= I[i,j]
\end{aligned}
\tag{12.12}
$$

with $i = 0, 1, 2, ..., r_x - 1$, and $j = 0, 1, 2, ..., r_y - 1$, where z_0 is the object plane position on the optical axis, x_0 and y_0 are the image positions on the object plane, r_x and r_y are the image I resolutions, and $\Delta x = h/r_x$ and $\Delta y = h/r_y$, where h is the height and width in image I.

Then, the inverse process is done to get the final image I'. All cloud of points Ω (x',y') are changed into integer coordinates (i',j') in I' by Equation 12.13.

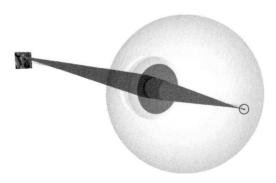

FIGURE 12.7 Projection of cones and set of points Ω on the retina. (Please see color insert.)

$$i' = round\left[\frac{h'-y'_i}{h'}\right](r'_y-1)$$

$$j' = round\left[\frac{h'-x'_j}{h'}\right](r'_x-1) \qquad (12.13)$$

$$I'[i',j'] = color_{i,j}$$

where h' is the height and width of the image I', r'_x and r'_y are the resolutions.

12.3.3 VISUALIZATION

The visualization module is composed of a set of graphical tools devoted to visualize the mesh models and the output of the simulation module. They are built tools using libraries such as *GLUT* [24] and *OpenGL* [25] under Gnu/Linux systems. The *ParaView* [26] application can be used to provide visualization of results.

The meshes can be visualized either in *wire-frame* or *shading*. Examples of wireframe visualization have been presented in Figures 12.4 and 12.5(a). Figure 12.7 shows a view of all eye components in shading and the ray-tracing process.

12.4 OPTIC SIMULATION

Optic simulation consists of the generation of environments, which can guide the decision process, make analysis and evaluations of systems, and propose solutions to improve performance and understanding of the simulated process.

In this case, optical simulation intends to reproduce the behavior of the human eye as an entire optical system. This process allows the acquisition of certain measures such as Gaussian properties, spot diagram, and circle of confusion that are widely used for validating models of eyes. This section is dedicated to validate and verify the accuracy of the optical behavior in the Virtual Eye. The results are compared with those found in literature and are presented as follows.

12.4.1 GAUSSIAN PROPERTIES

Every centered optical system that has some equivalent power has six cardinal points that lie on the optical axis. These are in three pairs. Two are focal points, which we denote by the symbols F and F'; two are principal points, denoted by the symbols H and H'; and two are nodal points, denoted by the symbols N and N'. The positions of these cardinal points in an eye depend upon its structure and the level of accommodation.

One of the main applications of paraxial schematic eyes is predicting the Gaussian properties of real eyes. Of these, probably the most important are the equivalent power F, positions of the six cardinal points, and the positions and magnifications of the pupil.

To validate and check the accuracy of algorithms and models employed in Virtual Eye, we computed the Gaussian properties for the Le Grand model by the finite ray-tracing method [1]. The paraxial ray-tracing is emulated, shooting some rays next to the optical axis and making a less possible paraxial ray with $h = 1.0$ mm high of optical axis.

The focal points F and F' are computed, shooting a light ray parallel to the optical axis of the eye and getting the intersection between the refracted ray and optical axis. The principal points H and H' are $H = F + HF$ and the same to $H' = F' + H'F'$. The measures $HF = f$ and $H'F' = f$ are $f = -h/\varphi'$ and $f = -h/\varphi$, where φ' and φ are the angles formed by intersection of the incident and refracted rays, respectively with the optical axis of surface and h is the distance of optical axis with the intersection between incident ray and surface.

The nodal points N and N' are $N = H + HN$ and $N' = H' + H'N'$ and $H'\,N' = HN = (n'-n) / D$, where n' and n are the refractive indices and D is the diopter of the lens.

Based on this theory the Virtual Eye simulates the Gaussian properties of the following models of eyes described in Section 12.3.2: unaccommodated Le Grande (lgr_u), accommodated Le Grand (lgr_a), and unaccommodated Liou-Brennan (lbr_u). In tables in this section the distances are measured in millimeters (mm) and the power and the accommodation in diopters D.

Table 12.5 shows a comparison of the Gaussian properties between the results computed by Virtual Eye and Smith [1] for a paraxial accommodated Le Grand model (lgr_a). It can be noticed that the diopter in Virtual Eye is $D = 67.1511D$, almost the same value in Smith of $D = 67,6780D$, and there is not much difference between other Gaussian properties values shown in the table.

Table 12.6 shows the Gaussian properties for an unaccommodated Le Grand model (lgr_u). The diopter of (lgr_u) model is $D = 59.941D$, which is slightly lower than the more accepted mean value $<D> = 60.00D$ for adults. It can be noticed again that there is not much difference between the values obtained from Virtual Eye and Smith.

The last model is based on *in vivo* data collected from the literature and developed as described in Section 12.3.1.3. The Gaussian properties in an unaccommodated

---

TABLE 12.5

Gaussian Properties of Le Grand Accommodated (lgr_a)

	Virtual Eye	Smith	Deviation
Power	67.1511	67.678	0.5269
VF	−12.8638	−12.957	0.0932
VF′	22.1482	21.932	0.2162
VH	1.9057	1.819	0.0867
VH′	2.2528	2.192	0.0608
VN	6.7947	6.784	0.0107
VN′	7.2564	7.156	0.1004
H′N′=HN	5.00364	4.965	0.03864
F	14.7694	14.776	0.0066
f′	19.8954	19.741	0.15554

Note: A = 6.96D.

TABLE 12.6

Gaussian Properties of Le Grand Unaccommodated (lgr$_u$)

	Virtual Eye	Smith	Deviation
Power	59.941	59.940	0.001
VF	−15.0881	−15.089	0.0009
VF′	24.197	24.197	0.0
VH	1.595	1.595	0.0
VH′	1.908	1.908	0.0
VN	7.200	7.200	0.0
VN′	7.513	7.513	0.0
H′N′=HN	5.6055	5.606	0.0005
F	16.6832	16.683	0.0002
f′	22.2887	22.289	0.0003

Liou-Brennan model were calculated, shooting rays at $h = 0.01$ mm high from the z optical axis. This model presents power of $D = 60.3217D$, which is higher than the value $<D>$. The results shown in Table 12.7 present consistent values with those reported in Smith.

12.4.2 SPOT DIAGRAM

Spot diagram SD is a set of intersections $P'_i=(x'_i,y'_i,z'_i)\in S$, with $i=1,2,3,...,N$, between the rays $l \in C$ and $S \subset R^3$, where C is a light cone shot from point P in object space and S is the retinal surface.

Light passing through a small circular opening forms a pattern of diffraction called the *Airy disc*. This pattern consists of a bright central circle, or *blot*, composed of concentric rings with low contrast in the periphery. At the moment the eye focuses on an object point, a circular image with the same size as the Airy disc forms on the retina. This even happens for ideal cases in which there is no aberration in the lens because, in this context, the effects of diffraction are more influential than the aberrations in the image formation process. The Airy disc diameter is given by

$$D_a = 1,22\lambda\frac{f}{d} \tag{12.14}$$

where f is the focal length and d the pupil diameter.

The root mean square value (RMS) in Equation 12.15 is one quantitative measure associated with the spot diagram SD.

$$RMS = \sum_i \frac{\sqrt{(x'_i-x'_0)^2 + (y'_i-y'_0)^2}}{N} \tag{12.15}$$

Another usual measure is the circle of confusion or geometrical radius ρ'. Let C be the set of light rays l in the light cone shot from point P. Let $\Omega' \subset S$ be the set of

TABLE 12.7

Gaussian Properties of Liu-Brennan Unaccommodated (lbr$_u$)

	Virtual Eye	Smith	Deviation
Power	60.3217	60.343	0.0213
VF	−15.0352	−15.040	0.0048
VF′	23.9665	23.950	0.0165
VH	1.5436	1.532	0.0116
VH′	1.8190	1.810	0.009
VN	7.1136	7.100	0.0136
VN′	7.3890	7.378	0.011
H′N′=HN	5.570	5.568	0.002
F	16.5788	16.572	0.0068
f′	22.140	22.140	0.0

n points $P'_k=(x'_k,y'_k,z'_k)\in S$ generated by intersections between l and S, where $S\subset R^3$ is the retinal surface. The circle of confusion or geometrical ray ρ' is given by

$$\rho'^2_k = x'^2_k + y'^2_k$$

$$\rho' = \max\{\rho'_k\}$$

(12.16)

The spot diagram can be considered in two cases. In the first one, C associated with SD was shot from a point P on the optical axis, and in the second case, C was shot from a point P which forms a visual angle $\alpha = 5$ with the optical axis. Figures 12.8 and 12.9 show the spot diagrams with their Airy discs in unaccommodated and accommodated Le Grand model, respectively.

It is possible to notice that the spot diagrams are not equivalent to the ideal diagram, which consists of only one point in S. In both levels of accommodation the Airy disc is smaller than the blot produced by aberration, suggesting that these models do not reflect the aberrations of the human eye. It is also possible to check the RMS and ρ' increase with the pupil size.

12.4.3 RETINAL IMAGE FORMATION

To investigate the retinal images formed by a theoretical eye model, a simulation of an actual object (a bitmap image) was implemented. Each pixel on the object corresponds to a light ray launched in direction of the eye.

Figure 12.10(a) has dimension $h = 11.6$ mm and is used as input I, being placed at plane $z = 141,787$ mm in the object space for the accommodated Le Grand model. In this situation, the circle of confusion ρ' of the light cone shot from z has also been computed. The radius R of pupil of the Le Grand model was changed to check what happens in the image formation of I.

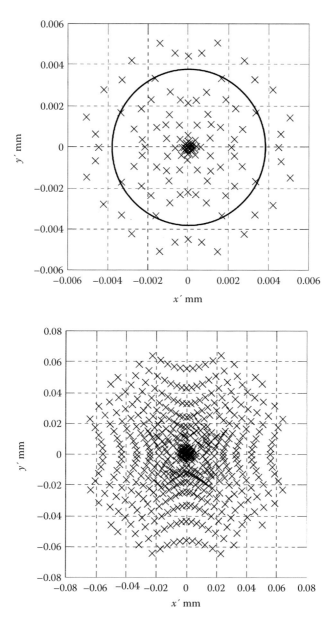

FIGURE 12.8 Spot diagram in unaccommodated Le Grand model (lgr_u) and Airy disc. (a) $R = 1$ mm, $RMS = 0.0019$ mm, $\rho' = 0.0053$ mm, and $D_a = 0.0037$ mm; (b) $R = 2.0$ mm, $RMS = 0.0250$ mm, $\rho' = 0.0680$ mm, and $D_a = 0.0019$ mm.

(*Continued*)

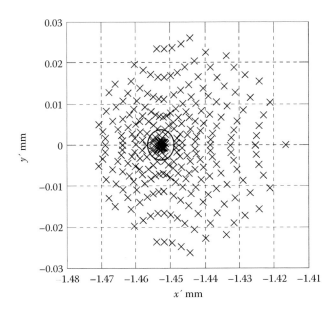

FIGURE 12.8 (Continued)   Spot diagram in unaccommodated Le Grand model (lgr_u) and Airy disc. (c) $R = 1.0$ mm, $\alpha = 5$, RMS = 0.0023 mm, $\rho' = 0.0010$ mm, and $D_a = 0.0037$ mm.

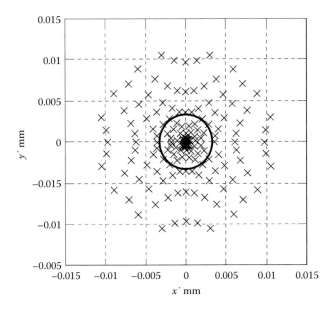

FIGURE 12.9   Spot diagram in accommodated Le Grand model (lgr_a) and Airy disc. (a) $R = 1$ mm, $RMS = 0.0048$ mm, $\rho' = 0.0110$ mm, and $D_a = 0.0066$ mm.

(Continued)

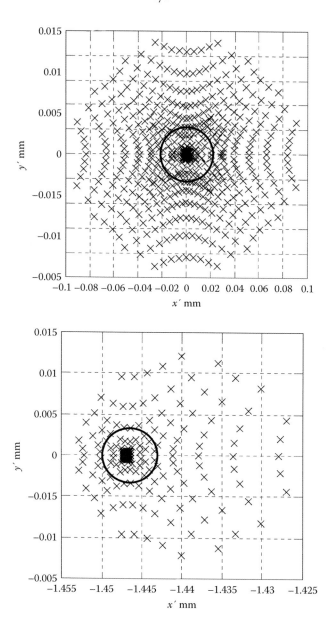

FIGURE 12.9 (Continued) Spot diagram in accommodated Le Grand model (lgr$_a$) and Airy disc. (b) R = 2.0 mm, RMS = 0.0373 mm, ρ' = 0.0943 mm, and D_a = 0.0033 mm; (c) R = 1.0 mm, α = 5, RMS = 0.0058 mm, ρ' = 0.0200 mm, and D_a = 0.0066 mm.

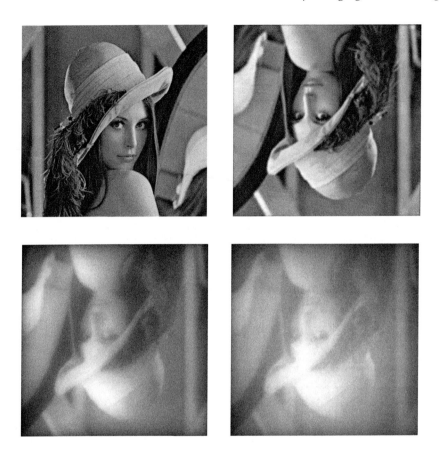

FIGURE 12.10   Original image and images formed by the accommodated Le Grand model in Virtual Eye. (a) Original image. (b) Radius of the pupil $R = 1.0$ mm and circle of confusion is $\rho' = 0.032$ mm. (c) Radius of the pupil $R = 2.5$ mm and circle of confusion is $\rho' = 0.198$ mm. (d) Radius of the pupil $R = 4.0$ mm and circle of confusion is $\rho' = 1.125$ mm.

Light cones were projected from each pixel of I. The radiuses of pupil are $R = 1.0$ mm, $R = 2.5$ mm and $R = 4.0$ mm. The results are shown in Figure 12.10(b), Figure 12.10(c), and Figure 12.10(d). They are real inverted images with some blur for radius 2.5 mm and 4.0 mm.

When examining the results, we realized that the flow of light rays incident in the retina increases with the size of the pupil, focusing their gray levels at the white regions and indicating the increase in brightness of the image in its center. The circle of confusion shows the increase in the blur of image I because of the aberrations present in Le Grand. In all cases, the size of image is $h' = 1.3288$ mm, which results in increasing lateral of M, where:

$$M = \frac{-1.3288mm}{11.6mm} = -0.1145.$$

12.5   THE RETINAL MODEL IN THE VIRTUAL EYE

To simulate the natural behavior of the human retina, one must first understand its basic functionality. The next section is dedicated to explaining the theoretical basis for simulations that are made in the retinal Virtual Eye.

12.5.1   BIOLOGICAL RETINA

Approximately 0.05 mm thick, the retina is the layer of tissue lining the eye chamber. It has a high concentration of nerve endings essential for the inflow of light; these nerve endings are the photoreceptors (rods and cones). The retina is responsible primarily for the formation of images, acting as a "projection screen" on which the images are projected. It retains the light rays that enter the eye and translates them into electrical impulses that are sent to the brain by the optic nerve.

The cells of the retina are organized in a layered architecture in sequence, from the receptors responsible for the acquisition of light received to the ganglion cells that send visual information to the brain as electrical signals. There are five different types of cells within the retina: light receptors, horizontal cells, bipolar cells, amacrine cells, and ganglion cells. The light passes through all the retina layers and is detected by the last layer, which is made by the receptor cells. The receptor cells, composed of rods and cones, convert the light into neuronal electric signals and then transmit the information to the horizontal cells, bipolar and amacrine, finally arriving in the ganglion cells. The ganglion cells send the information to the brain.

There are two types of photoreceptors in the human eye: rods and cones. Cones are responsible for the visual acuity and color perception. They are smaller and thicker than rods. There are three types of cones in humans; each is intended to perceive a certain light wavelength (long, medium, and short). Each wavelength and its combination is perceived as color by the brain. The long wavelength is related to the red color, the medium to the green, and short to the blue. The cones are able to perceive thinner spatial details and they are present in a high density in the central region of the retina that is called the fovea. Thus the image formed on this area is sharper than others.

The rods, on the other hand, are more sensitive to movement but are not capable of distinguishing the colors. They are the luminance senses, being able to perceive low-intensity light, covering mostly the peripheral retina and almost absent in the fovea region. The rods are also responsible for night vision and peripheral vision. They are most useful in darker environments, being more sensitive to light than cones, but only detect shades of gray. The distribution of retinal receptor cells is shown in Figure 12.11.

The signal captured by the receptors travels through cells horizontal, bipolar, and amacrine to finally reach the ganglions and then goes to the brain via the optic nerve. One important property of this network of neurons is that the signals from many receptors converge on a single ganglion. In the field of vision, the receptive field of a ganglion cell G is defined as the area in the retina which, when stimulated by light, influences the neuron's response rate of G; in other words, it is the corresponding area on the retina formed by cell receptors (rods and cones) that converge to the ganglion G.

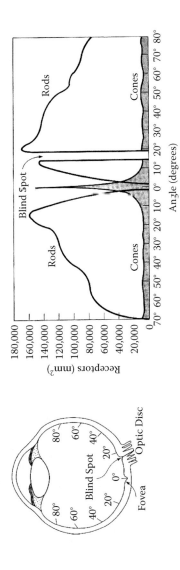

FIGURE 12.11 Distribution of receptor cells in the retina produced by Osterberg (1935) and adapted by Lindsay and Norman (1977) [2].

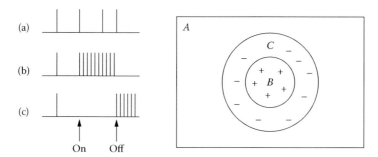

FIGURE 12.12 Response of a stimulus in the receptive field in different regions. (a) Outside the receptive field (area *A*). (b) Within the area of the excitatory receptive field (area *B*). (c) Within the area of the inhibitory receptive field (area *C*).

Figure 12.12 shows a receptive field with different areas labeled *A*, *B*, and *C*. The left side of the figure presents the response rate of the field in three different situations. If any region within the area *A* is stimulated by light rays, there will be no effect on the activity of the neuron; see Figure 12.12(a). If the region *B* is stimulated, there will be an increase in response rate of the neuron; see Figure 12.12(b). To represent this phenomenon, region *B* is marked with a plus sign (+) to indicate that the response to a stimulus in this area is excitatory. On the other hand, if the stimulus is on the area *C*, there will be an inhibitory response causing a decrement in the response rate of the neuron; see Figure 12.12(c). This area is marked with a minus sign (–) to indicate that the response on this place is inhibitory. Thus, areas *B* and *C* together form a receptive field of a neuron.

The receptive field in Figure 12.12 is called center-surround because the excitatory and inhibitory areas are arranged in a circular area, responding in a particular way in its central region and the opposite way on the periphery. The receptive field in this case is called *ON-Center OFF-Surround*, but there are also receptive fields *OFF-Center ON-Surround*.

12.5.2 Modeling of the Retina

12.5.2.1 Receptors

The Virtual Eye simulation process carries out a set of points Ω (coordinates and colors) that belong to the quadric model, as described in Section 12.3.2.2. To visualize the image formed in the eye, these points are projected onto a projection plane π, where an image is defined in coordinates *(i,j)* in PMG type. It is on this plane that receptors are also mapped.

The distribution of receptor cells is based on the eccentricity of the retina in angle relative to the fovea (Figure 12.11); the retina is divided into several subregions called concentric rings. Each ring is defined on quadric surface model as $A_i = (R_i, r_i, \alpha_i)$, where R is a larger radius, r is a smaller radius, and α_i is the angle between A_i and fovea. Figure 12.13(a) shows how the rings are defined; the red part is one ring A_i.

The program calculates the set of points $S = S_0, S_1, S_2, ..., S_n$, where S_i is a point *(x, y, z)* belonging to a circle that separates rings A_i and A_{i+1}. Then the set S is projected and mapped onto a projection plane (PGM image (mxn)) becoming the set $P = P_0, P_1, P_2, ..., P_n$, where P_i is a point (i,j) in the circle that separates rings A_i and A_{i+1} in PGM image (mxn). At this stage the angle α_i of each ring is stored to calculate the density of receptors on the component. Figure 12.13 helps clarify the process.

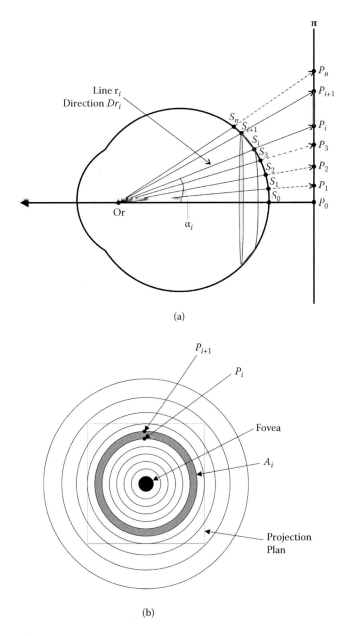

(a)

(b)

FIGURE 12.13 (a) Concentric rings on the surface of the retina. (b) Concentric rings in the projection plane image PGM image (mxn). (Please see color insert.)

The points of S are obtained by intersections between quadric surface and rays r_i, which originate in Or and have directions Dr_i defined in relation to the angle α_i. Equation 12.17 shows how to calculate each Dr_i.

$$Dr_i.x = sen(\alpha_i)$$

$$Dr_i.y = 0.0 \qquad\qquad (12.17)$$

$$Dr_i.z = -\cos(\alpha_i)$$

After finding out all the rings on the image, the next step is to map receptor cells. The graph in Figure 12.14 is a discretization (for angles) of the graph of Figure 12.11 with values normalized between 0 and 1 (for density).

In Figure 12.12, each angle α_i corresponds to one ring A_i and the density of receptors in one ring is given by $D(A_i) = NR(A_i) / P(A_i)$, where $D(A_i)$ is the density of receptors. $NR(A_i)$ is the number of receptors and $P(A_i)$ is the number of pixels in the ring A_i on PGM image. In this case, the area of a ring maps as the number of pixels that belongs to that region. Therefore, the number of receptors in any ring A_i is given by Equation 12.18:

$$NR(A_i) = D(A_i) \cdot P(A_i) \qquad\qquad (12.18)$$

Consequently, as the values for density are normalized between 0 and 1, a ring with a maximum density (equal to 1 in the fovea, where the cones are) will have as many cells as there are pixels. In this case, all the pixels belonging to the ring will be selected as a receiver and there will be no loss of information in this region, because the light incident on all the pixels will be detected (Figure 12.15a). If the density is lower than 1, the number of cells will be less than the total number of pixels, causing

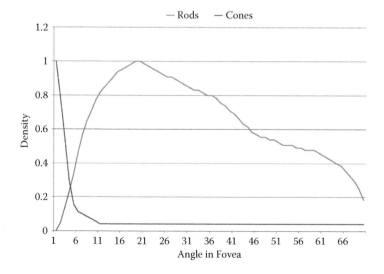

FIGURE 12.14 Discrete values for density of receptor cells in the retinal eccentricity. (Please see color insert.)

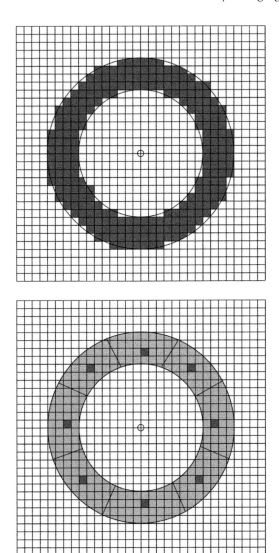

FIGURE 12.15   (a) Ring with maximum density; all the incident light will be detected in this ring. (b) Ring with lower density; much of the incident light in this ring is lost, because there is no receptor to detect it. (Please see color insert.)

a loss of information because part of the incident light will not be detected in this region (gray region in Figure 12.15b).

12.5.2.2   Receptive Fields

In the Virtual Eye, a receptive field is modeled by a simplification of the Marr-Hildreth filter [3], CR_{hxh} as a mask, with a smaller radius (r) that defines the central area and a larger radius (R) that defines the periphery. Therefore, the mask CR is defined by Equation 12.19:

$$CR_{i,j}^+ = \begin{cases} +1/N_r \Rightarrow d \le r \\ -1/N_R \Rightarrow r < d \le R \\ 0 \Rightarrow d > R \end{cases} \qquad (12.19)$$

N_r is the number of elements within the central area and N_R is the number of elements within the peripheral area and $d = \sqrt{i^2 + j^2}$. Thus the receptive field in Equation 12.19 defines an *On-Center Off-Surround* receptive filed. To define receptive field *Off-Center On-Surround* the signal should be inverted:

$$CR_{i,j}^- = \begin{cases} -1/N_r \Rightarrow d \le r \\ +1/N_R \Rightarrow r < d \le R \\ 0 \Rightarrow d > R \end{cases} \qquad (12.20)$$

If an image *I (mxn)* features a ganglion cell at pixel *(k, l)*, the response of the receptive field of this cell is given by the convolution operation *I (k, l)* * *CR*, matching the center point of *CR* mask with point *(k, l)* in *I*.

The human retina performs several image-processing filters using and combining the receptive fields; for instance, the combination of the two types of receptive field *(On-Center* and *Off-Center)* can be used to model edge detectors. In this case, the gradient operator between the two of them, CR^+ CR^-, defines an edge detector, *ED*, and it is given by Equation 12.21:

$$ED_{i,j} = \sqrt{CR_{i,j}^{+2} + CR_{i,j}^{-2}} \qquad (12.21)$$

12.5.3 SIMULATIONS

12.5.3.1 Fovea and Periphery

Simulations of the process of image formation in fovea and periphery area are made to show the difference in resolution between images in these two regions. The first row in Figure 12.16 contains a graphical representation of three (D_1, D_2, D_3) different cell distributions (cones, in this case). The other rows are shown to their resulting images of retinal simulation. Then, D_1 represents a distribution of cones for an image formed totally in the region of fovea, the distribution of D_2 is for an image formed in the fovea and also in the periphery (0 to 16 degrees of eccentricity), and the last one is D_3 for a distribution of cones to an image formed in the fovea and periphery, but for 0 to 56 degrees of eccentricity.

The results in Figure 12.16 show that the image resolution decreases with distance from the center. It may be noted that in the fovea there are many more cells than in the periphery. Because of that this place has a highest quality of vision and perception of details. The graph in Figure 12.17 shows the density of cone cells in the eccentricities for the D_3 distribution given in Figure 12.16. The density is given by $D = N^oCell/Area$, where area is given in mm^2 corresponding to the area

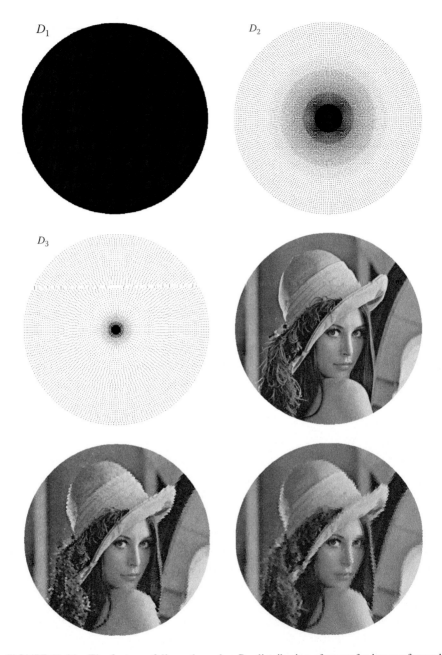

FIGURE 12.16 The first row follows the order: D_1, distribution of cones for images formed only in the fovea; D_2, distribution of cones to images formed in the regions of the fovea and periphery with eccentricities of 0° to 16°; D_3, distribution of cones to images formed in the regions of the fovea and periphery with eccentricities of 0° to 50°.

(Continued)

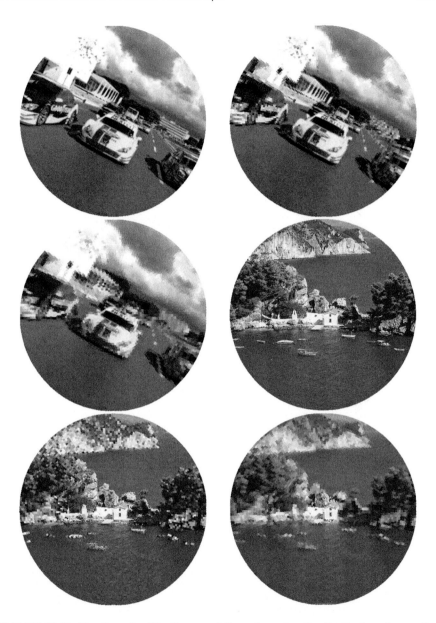

FIGURE 12.16 (*Continued*) The first row follows the order: D_1, distribution of cones for images formed only in the fovea; D_2, distribution of cones to images formed in the regions of the fovea and periphery with eccentricities of $0°$ to $16°$; D_3, distribution of cones to images formed in the regions of the fovea and periphery with eccentricities of $0°$ to $50°$.

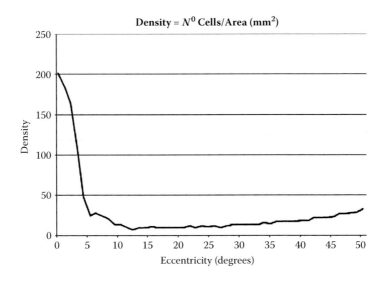

FIGURE 12.17   Density of cones in D_3, with area in mm^2.

that occupies a ring on the quadric surface of the retina. It can be seen that the curve of cell distribution in Virtual Eye is consistent with the distribution proposed by Osterberg in Figure 12.11.

12.5.3.2   Receptive Field

Figure 12.18 shows the result of a receptive field simulation of cone cells for an image completely formed in the fovea. The fields in this region have smaller sizes than others, allowing capture of details in the scene. In the figure is shown the signal produced by fields in *On-Center Off-Surround*, *Off-Center On-Surround* and a combination of fields to act as edge detector in the retina.

12.5.3.3   Experiment Simulation: Hermann Grid

Looking at Figure 12.19, it is possible to see spots or dark "ghosts" in almost all intersections between the white bars. It can be proved that these dark spots are not physically present. Note that they disappear when the gaze shifts to any point of intersection of the bars. Described by Ludimar Hermann in 1870 [4], this phenomenon is due to center-surround neurophysiologic mechanism of the receptive fields of retinal ganglion cells.

We can make use of the receptive fields *On-Center Off-Surround* to explain how those spots are seen by the eye. Two questions must be answered:

- Why do the spots appear only at the intersections of white bars?
- Why do the spots disappear when you stare at the intersection?

To answer the first question, take a look at Figure 12.20. It lets you compare how the image of Hermann Grid affects the retinal receptive fields in two different

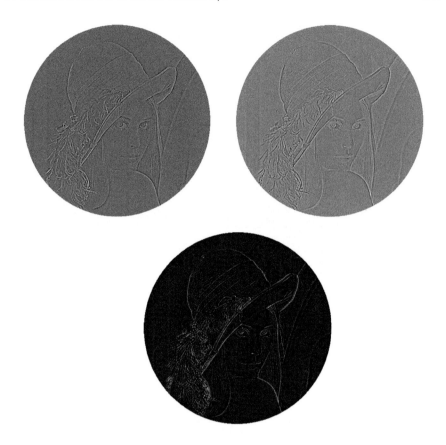

FIGURE 12.18 Receptive fields On-Center Off-Surround, Off-Center On-Surround, and edge detector, respectively.

positions: one centered at the intersection of two bars and the other centered between two intersections. Note that the centers of both receptive fields receive the same amount of light, but the outlying areas receive different amounts. Therefore, the field on the right side receives much more light on its OFF part, which causes a reduction in its response rate. Meanwhile, the other field gets a little light on its OFF part, causing it to have a higher response rate.

To answer the second question, we must think about the size of the receptive fields stimulated. The smallest are present in the fovea of the retina. When one looks directly at an intersection point of two bars, the receptive fields are stimulated in the fovea, in which the center and periphery are so small that both regions are formed within a white bar. It can be seen in Figure 12.21 that these smaller receptive fields receive the same amount of light in their entire region, which generates a low response rate.

Figure 12.22(a) shows a simulation of the receptive fields *On-Center Off-Surround* at the fixation point and Figure 12.22(b) a simulation in the peripheral region. These

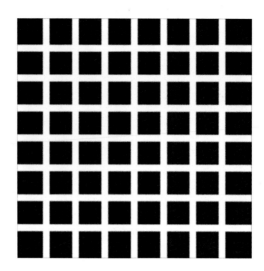

FIGURE 12.19 Hermann Grid illusion. Dark spots appear at the intersections of white bars and disappear when you stare at them.

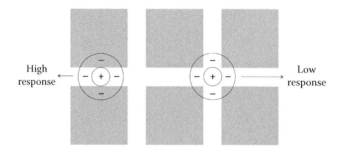

FIGURE 12.20 Possible explanation for Hermann Grid.

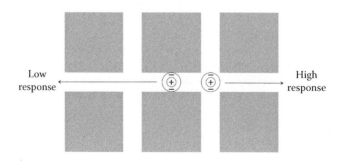

FIGURE 12.21 Possible explanation for Hermann Grid at the point of fixation.

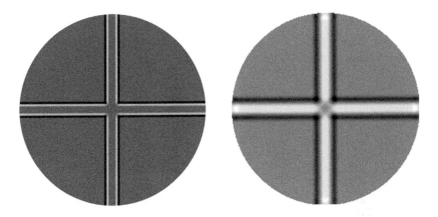

FIGURE 12.22 Simulation of the receptive fields for the Hermann Grid illusion: (a) peripheral region; (b) focal point.

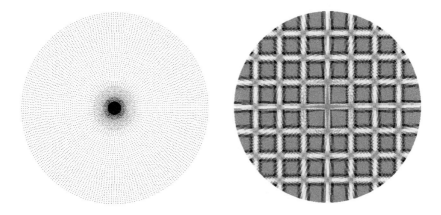

FIGURE 12.23 Simulation of the receptive fields for the Hermann Grid illusion of the fixation point and peripheral regions.

results demonstrate that the receptive fields of retinal Virtual Eye behave according to the model suggested in Figures 12.20 and 12.21.

Figure 12.23 presents a simulation with the image of the Hermann Grid being formed in various retinal eccentricities. For this experiment, the model of accommodated Le Grand (lgr_a) was used with 1.0 mm of radius of pupil. The image was placed at a distance of 147,747 mm in front of the eye with 20 cm in diameter. The result is an image formed in the eccentricities of 0° (fovea) to 32° (periphery).

This experiment lets you compare the difference in performance of the receptive fields in different retinal eccentricities. This difference is caused by varying the diameter of the fields where the largest are located in the periphery and the lowest in the center.

12.6   CONCLUSION

Medical image techniques have become an important tool for both research and medicine in recent decades. Due to medical images, our knowledge about human physiology and anatomy has increased substantially, which has allowed discovery and understanding of how many human organs work and the phenomena behind their functionality.

Although medical images and instrumentation have led to advances in ophthalmology, the nature of the human eye (composed mostly of liquids and soft cells which are not differentiable by x-ray or magnetic resonance) is a barrier to the detailed understanding of its optics and physiology. Many basic human eye phenomena are not well understood yet. This is highlighted when the lens accommodation process is taken into account. Although studied since Helmholtz in the nineteenth century, the accommodation process is still under research. There are contradictory theories now, which explain the phenomena in completely opposite ways [19]. Another example related to this subject is the presbyopia. The lack of a detailed understanding of the eye's optics and physiology make presbyopia surgical correction unsatisfactory.

The solution to a better understanding of the eye's optical and physiological phenomena arise from eye computer simulations. There are a lot of studies in this field, and eye simulation has demonstrated that it is the best solution to show details about how the human eye works and bring ophthalmology to the next stage.

Another challenge in human eye research is the understanding of how the retina works. Understanding retina behavior is a complex task. The retina could be considered as a part of the brain that is outside. It is a cortical layer, which converts the light into neuron signal, processes the visual information, and sends the processed signals to the brain. The study of retina behavior is one of the keys to understanding vision. Although the understanding of how the retina works and processes visual information is in the field of neuroscience, the optical aspects of the retina are in the domain of ophthalmology. As with the eye's optics and physiology, the simulation and modeling arises as a solution to study of the retina. Due to its importance, it is fundamental that realistic models of the retina be contemplated in computer eye modeling and simulation.

This chapter showed the advances of the 3D geometric eye simulation with the retina, presenting the Virtual Eye system. Although Virtual Eye, in actual stage, does not reproduce all optical effects, such as blur, dispersion, contrast, and interference, it allows the analysis of the geometric distortions of retinal images. The system is in the early stage and it is a first step toward a realistic 3D geometric eye and retina computer simulation.

REFERENCES

1. Atchison D.A., Smith G. *Optics of the human eye*, London: Reed Educational and Professional Publishing, 2000.
2. Goldstain E.B. *Sensation and perception*. Belmont: Wadsworth, 6th ed., 2002.
3. Mar, D. *Vision*, Cambridge, MA: MIT Press, 2010.
4. Sekuler R. and Blake R. *Perception*. NY: McGraw-Hill, 1990.
5. Le Grand, Y., El Hage, S.G. *Physiological optics*. Berlin: Springer-Verlag, 1980.

6. Brennan N.A. and Liou H. Anatomically accurate, finite model eye for optical modeling. *Opt. Soc. Am.*, A 14:1684–1695, 1997.

7. Scheiner C. *Sive fundamentum opticum*, Germany: Innspruk, 1619.

8. Helmholtz von H.H. *Handbuch der Physiologishen Optik*. In Southall J.P.C. (Translator), *Helmholtz's treatise on physiological optics*. New York: Dover, 1962.

9. Emsley H. *Visual Optics*. London: Hatton Press, 5th ed, 1952.

10. Lotmar W. Theoretical eye model with aspherics surfaces. *Opt. Soc. Amer.*, 61:1522–1529, 1971.

11. Gullstrand A. *Helmholtz's Handbuch der Physiologischen Optik*, Hamburg: Voss 1909.

12. Kooijman A.C. Light distribution on the retina of a wide-angle theoretical eye. *J. Opt. Soc. Amer.*, 73:1544–1550, 1983.

13. Thibos N., Zhang X., and Bradley A. The chromatic eye: A new reduced-eye model of ocular chromatic aberration in humans. *Appl. Opt.*, 31(19):3594–3600, 1992.

14. Thibos N., Zhang X., and Bradley A. *Spherical aberration of the reduced schematic eye with elliptical refracting surface*, Indiana School of Optometry, 1997.

15. Doshi J., Sarver J., and Applegate B. Schematic eye models for simulation of patient visual performance. *Journal of Refractive Surgery*, 17:414–419, 2001.

16. Camp J., Maguire, J., et al. A computer model for the evaluation of the effect of corneal topography on optical performance. *Am. J. Ophthalmol.*, 109(4):379–385, 1990.

17. Langenbucher A., Viestenz A., Viestenz A., Brunner H., and Seitz B. Ray tracing through a schematic eye containing second-order (quadric) surfaces using 4 × 4 matrix notation. *Ophthalmic Physiol. Opt.*, (2):180–8, 2006.

18. Carvalho L.A. Simple mathematical model for simulation of the human optical system based on in vivo corneal data. *Revista Brasileira de Engenharia Biomdica*, 19(1):29–38, 2003.

19. Agarwal A. MS. FRCOphth. *Presbyopia: A Surgical Textbook*, University of Michigan: Slack; 2002.

20. Duran R.S. Modeler and viewer of the human visual system. Master's thesis, University of São Paulo–São Carlos, 2005.

21. Henrique L., Fernandes O. Simulation of optical phenomena and physiology of human vision system. Master's thesis, University of São Paulo–São Carlos, 2008.

22. Brazil L.P. Simulation and modeling of the sensory retina. Master's thesis, University of São Paulo–São Carlos, 2009.

23. Brazil L.P., Fernandes L.H.O., Nonato L.G., Carvalho L.A.V., and Bruno O.M. Modeling and simulation of the human eye. *International Symposium on Mathematical and Computational Biology*. Campos do Jordão–São Paulo/Brasil, 2008.

24. OpenGL. Glut and OpenGL utility libraries. http://www.opengl.org/resources/libraries/, 2011. [Accessed at 2011 29 January.]

25. OpenGL. Open graphics library. http://www.opengl.org, 2011. [Accessed at 2011 29 January.]

26. ParaView—Open Source Scientific Visualization. http://www.paraview.org/, 2011. [Accessed at 2011 29 January.]

27. Institute of Mathematics and Computer science. http://www.icmc.usp.br, 2001. [Accessed at 2011 30 January.]

28. Bruno O.M. and Carvalho L.A. *Óptica e Fisiologia da Visão: Uma Abordagem Multidisciplinar*, Roca, 2008.

13 Human Eye Heat Distribution Using 3D Web-Splines Solution

Fulya Callialp Kunter and S. Selim Seker

CONTENTS

13.1 INTRODUCTION

This study presents on the use of web-splines in the finite element method (FEM). The spline functions are often used in approximation, data fitting, computer-aided design (CAD), and many other applications [1,2]. The contributions of de Boor, de Casteljau, and Bezier have played an important role for splines. The b-splines can be used as basis functions for their flexibility and continuity between points. Many studies have been done on spline finite element solutions [3–5]. Despite the fact that boundary conditions and stability requirements prevent b-splines from being used on uniform grids, these difficulties can be overcome with the new method called web-spline. Hollig [6] constructed the web-spline method and used it with the FEM. Thus the combined advantages of standard finite elements and web-spline representations inspired many authors to work on this new subject [7–15].

This study illustrates the web-splines as basis functions for FEM in bioheat transfer problems for analyzing the temperature distribution in 2D and 3D models of the human eye with and without external sources. The benefits of using web-splines in solving axisymmetrical problems and approximating the heat distribution in the eye are that no mesh generation is required and uniform grids are used instead of irregular partitions of domain, thus eliminating the difficult and time-consuming preprocessing step. As reported here, high accuracy can be obtained with relatively few parameters.

13.2 FEM WITH B-SPLINES

The use of b-splines as finite element basis functions is very functional with geometric modeling and numerical simulation closely linked in engineering applications. However, at first sight this seems infeasible for two reasons. Firstly, there are some difficulties in modeling essential boundary conditions. For instance, if a linear combination of b-splines is required to vanish on the boundary of the domain, then all coefficients of b-splines with support intersecting the boundary must be zero. Hence this results in very poor approximation order for solutions of differential equations with Dirichlet boundary conditions. This difficulty can be overcome by modeling homogeneous essential boundary conditions via weight functions. Thus, solutions that vanish on the boundary are approximated with linear combinations of weighted b-splines. Secondly, the restricted b-spline is not uniformly stable because the outer b-splines have very small support in the domain. This leads to excessively large condition numbers of finite element systems and can cause extremely slow convergence of iterative methods. The stability problem is resolved by adjoining the outer b-splines to the inner b-splines to form the extended b-splines having stable basis.

Combining the above ideas gives rise to the definition of weighted extended b-splines. These basis functions possess the usual properties of standard finite elements. FEM applications use basis functions and meshes. But mesh generation causes consumption in computation duration for higher dimensions. Given the difficulty of constructing finite element meshes [16,17,18], not being required to generate meshes is the most important advantage of using the b-splines. In addition, the use of web-splines reduces the dimension of finite element systems, in particular, when high accuracy is required [6,19–24].

13.2.1 FLOW CHART

The flow chart of FEM using web-spline method is focused. Figure 13.1 shows the flow diagram. First of all, the simulation region and the problem are defined by the storage of inputs for the region, PDE, and boundary conditions. Then the generation of the grid cells and classification of b-splines are done for the simulation region. The next step is to compute the extension coefficients. If there is homogeneous Dirichlet boundary condition, the weight function for the region is determined. After assembling the system of equations, the approximate solution is computed. At the end, the results are shown as an output.

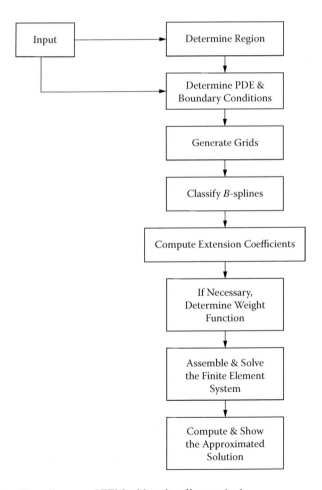

FIGURE 13.1   Flow diagram of FEM with web-spline method.

13.2.2 CLASSIFICATION OF B-SPLINES

There are two types of b-splines: the inner and outer b-splines, which depend on the size of their support in the domain. The outer b-splines are adjoined to the inner b-splines to eliminate instability.

For the domain Ω, firstly grid generation is completed. Figure 13.2 shows the grid generation for the given region. The grid width is taken as 0.5. The next step is to classify b-splines. The relevant b-splines, which are supporting in the domain, are determined. According to the size of their support, they are classified as inner and outer b-splines. The inner b-splines have at least one complete grid cell of their support in the domain. The other ones supporting the domain are called outer b-splines [6,19–24]. For the outer b-splines, the grid cells of their supports are not completely contained in the boundary. Figure 13.2 shows all the relevant inner and outer b-splines. According to their center of supports, the inner and outer b-splines are marked by (•) and (o), respectively.

13.2.3 EXTENSION COEFFICIENTS

The relevant b-splines supporting in the domain are classified as inner and outer b-splines. The inner b-splines (b_k, $k \in I$) have at least one complete grid cell of their support in the domain. The others are outer b-splines ($b_i \in J(k)$). For the outer b-splines, the grid cells of their supports are not entirely contained in the domain. Although the outer b-splines have small effect, they must be taken into consideration for stability. So they are adjoined to the closest inner b-splines to form the extended b-splines B_k.

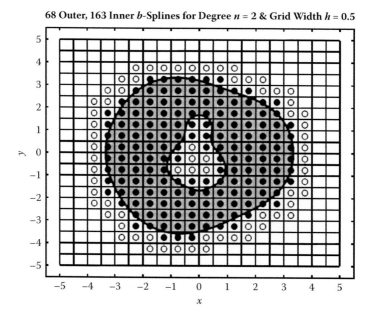

FIGURE 13.2   All relevant b-splines for the given domain.

$$B_k = b_k + \sum_i e_{k,i} b_i \qquad \text{for } k \in I, i \in J(k) \qquad (13.1)$$

where e_k, i are the extension coefficients. These extended b-splines inherit all basic features of the standard b-splines b_k. The extension coefficients are computed by using Lagrange polynomials as

$$e_{k,i} = \begin{cases} \displaystyle\prod_{d=1}^{m} \prod_{\mu=0}^{n} \frac{i_d - l_d - \mu}{k_d - l_d - \mu}, & \text{for } i = j \in J, k \in I(i), l_d + \mu \neq i_d \\ 1, & \text{for } i = k \in I \\ 0, & \text{otherwise} \end{cases} \qquad (13.2)$$

where $l = [l_1, l_2, \ldots] \in Z_m$ is the index for the lower left position of $I(j)$.

13.2.4 THE WEIGHT FUNCTION

The weight function is a continuous positive function in the domain and zero on the boundary. It can be constructed by using smooth distance function as [25,26,27]

$$w(x) = \begin{cases} 1 - (1 - \frac{\text{dist}(x,\partial\Omega)}{\delta})^\gamma & \text{dist}(x) < \delta \\ 1 & \text{otherwise} \end{cases} \qquad (13.3)$$

where δ is the boundary strip, γ is the smoothing parameter, and *dist* is the function that determines the minimum distance to the boundary.

If analytical equations are used for the boundaries, the weight function can be constructed by using Rvachev's R-functions. The intersection, union, or complement of R-functions can be considered as [25,26,27]

$$w_\cap(w_1, w_2) = \frac{1}{1+\tau}\left(w_1 + w_2 - \sqrt{w_1^2 + w_2^2 - 2\tau w_1 w_2}\right) \qquad (13.4)$$

$$w_\cup(w_1, w_2) = \frac{1}{1+\tau}\left(w_1 + w_2 + \sqrt{w_1^2 + w_2^2 - 2\tau w_1 w_2}\right) \qquad (13.5)$$

$$w^c = -w \qquad (13.6)$$

respectively where τ is a constant ($-1 < \tau \leq 1$). Taking $\tau = 0$ provides good results in simulations.

13.2.5 WEIGHTED EXTENDED B-SPLINES

The extended b-splines are multiplied by the weight function $w(x)$ if the Dirichlet boundary conditions are taken into consideration. The weight function is a continuous positive function in the domain, and zero on the boundary. It can be constructed by using analytical function, distance function, or Rvachev's R-function. As a result, the web-splines are obtained as

$$B_k = \frac{w(x)}{w(x_k)} \left(b_k + \sum_i e_{k,i} b_i \right) \qquad \text{for } k \in I, i \in J(k) \qquad (13.7)$$

where x_k is in the center of a grid cell that intersects the support of b-spline and the domain completely for normalization, $w(x)$ is the weight function for $x \in R^m$, and $w(x_k)$ is the value of weight function at the center of the grid cell.

The significance of web-splines is that the contribution of basis functions that are near the boundary is added to the inner basis functions. So the number of nodes and computing time are reduced. Secondly, the instability problem can be solved by coupling the outer b-splines with the inner b-splines. If we have a boundary value problem with homogeneous Dirichlet boundary conditions, Equation (13.7) is constructed as a basis function. The other boundary conditions use Equation (13.1) as a basis function.

Figure 13.3 shows the outer b-splines (○), extended inner b-splines (▲), and standard inner b-splines (•) for linear b-splines with the grid width $h = 0.5$. The outer b-splines are adjoined to the inner b-splines, which are called extended b-splines. These extended b-splines form a stable basis with the properties of standard finite elements [6,19–24].

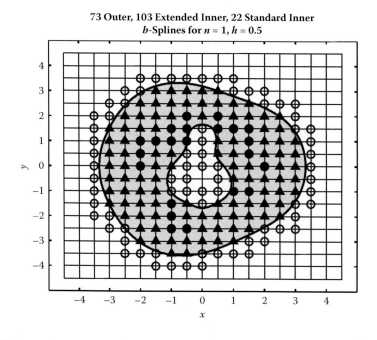

FIGURE 13.3   Outer, extended, and standard linear b-splines for h = 0.5.

13.3   WEB-SPLINE APPLICATIONS FOR UNEXPOSED HUMAN EYE HEAT DISTRIBUTION

Modeling of the heat distribution in the human eye has been popular for the last century with different kinds of techniques taking advantage of the advancements in computational technology. In earlier studies, the finite difference time domain method (FDTD) was used to solve Pennes bioheat equations numerically. One of the first eye models in the literature was developed by [28]. They used the FDTD to calculate the transient solutions of the temperature distribution in a microwave-irradiated human eye. [29] also examined the thermal effects of microwave radiation on the human eye for the steady-state temperature distribution. [30] then developed a mathematical model based on the FDTD method to calculate the transient and steady state temperature distributions in the normal unexposed human eye using the data he observed from the measurements on rabbit eyes. More recently, [31] applied FDTD method to study the temperature rise in the human eye exposed to electromagnetic waves. The drawback of these models was that they assumed the structure of the eye to be homogeneous in the sense that it is composed of a single uniform tissue. Thus this model, by not taking into account the presence of the cornea and the iris and simplifying the blood flow inside the eye, caused significant error.

Although it is observed that the FDTD mathematical model cannot represent the human eye perfectly, as the grids are rigid, the FEM allows precise representation of the ocular surface. The earliest reported model for temperature distribution in the eye using FEM was by [32] and [33]. Their numerical results, which were for rabbit eyes subject to electromagnetic waves, were reported to be in good agreement with data from experimental measurements. [34] and [35] constructed a 2D FEM of the human eye to analyze the temperature profile during steady state. Later [36] used her model to compute the temperature rise in the eye when exposed to infrared radiation. The studies of [35,36] were improved by [37,38], and [39], respectively. They presented a 2D and 3D finite element and 2D boundary element human eye models, which were developed to simulate thermal steady state conditions of the eye based on the properties and parameters reported in the open literature. In addition, a 3D axisymmetric human eye model was developed using boundary element method (BEM) during treatment of laser thermokeratoplasty [40]. The specific regions such as tumor and anterior chamber of the human eye's effects on the ocular heat transfer were also examined using BEM, respectively [41,42]. A brief summary of the various mathematical models of the human eye developed to date were reviewed in [43].

This section proceeds as follows. The mathematical model of the human eye with its properties for different domains is introduced in Section 13.3.1. Section 13.3.2 is dedicated to the method of analysis. The FEM formulation of the Pennes bioheat equation with the governing boundary equations is presented along with the web-spline method where grid cell classification on the domain, weight functions, and numerical integrations are given in detail. Section 13.3.3 presents the results of comparing the 2D and 3D web-spline human eye model simulations with the other available FEM and experimental data, which are followed by the conclusion.

13.3.1 MATHEMATICAL MODEL OF THE HUMAN EYE

The 2D and 3D models of the human eye are developed in this section. A 2D schematic cross-section of the eye with the assumption that it is symmetric about the pupillary axis is given in Figure 13.4, whereas the 3D model is formed by revolving this 2D model 360° around its horizontal pupillary axis. Simplifying assumptions concerning the geometry and structure of the eye are made to validate our web-spline model of the human eye using the latest studies done with FEM. First, the optic nerve is not simulated due to its minimal effect on the temperature distribution in the eye. Next, the eye is divided into six regions comprising the cornea, the aqueous humor, the lens, the iris, the vitreous humor, and the sclera. Each region is assumed to be homogeneous and isotropic. The thermal properties for each region are obtained based on [37] and the value for each is tabulated in Table 13.1. In addition, the coordinates of each region are modeled as in [37]. The properties and parameters used for the 3D model are similar to those of the 2D model.

The governing differential equation for temperature distribution is the Pennes bioheat transfer equation:

$$\rho c \frac{\partial T}{\partial t} = \nabla(k \nabla T) + H \quad \text{in } \Omega \quad \text{(inside the eye)} \tag{13.8}$$

where Ω is the domain studied and Γ_1, Γ_2, Γ_3 are its boundaries, as indicated in Figure 13.4. The boundary conditions are specified on the pupillary axis, the sclera, and the cornea, given in (13.9), (13.10), and (13.11), respectively.

$$k \frac{\partial T}{\partial n} = 0 \quad \text{on } \Gamma_1 \text{(the pupillary axis)} \tag{13.9}$$

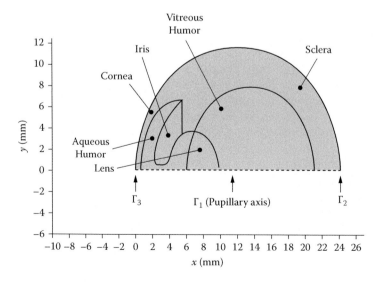

FIGURE 13.4 The 2D human eye model.

TABLE 13.1

Properties of the Human Eye for Different Domains

Domains	Thermal Conductivity (Whm^{-1}C^{-1})	Density (kgm^{-3})	Specific Heat Capacity (Jkg^{-1}C^{-1})
Cornea	0.58	4178	1050
Aqueous humor	0.58	3997	996
Lens	0.40	3000	1050
Iris	1.0042	3180	1100
Vitreous humor	0.603	4178	1000
Sclera	1.0042	3180	1100

Source: From Ng, E. Y. K., E. H. Ooi: FEM Simulation of the Eye Structure with Bioheat Analysis, *Comput. Methods Programs Biomed.*, **82**, 3, 268–276 (2006).

$$-k\frac{\partial T}{\partial n} = h_s(T - T_b) \quad on \; \Gamma_2 \text{(the sclera)} \tag{13.10}$$

$$-k\frac{\partial T}{\partial n} = E + h_c(T - T_{amp}) + \sigma\varepsilon(T^4 - T_{amp}^4) \quad on \; \Gamma_3 \text{(the anterior cornea surface)}$$

$$\tag{13.11}$$

The parameters k, ρ, and c, which refer to thermal conductivity, specific heat capacity, and density, respectively, are assumed constant within each region and with temperature variations. The coefficients h_s (65 Wm^{-2}C^{-1}) and h_c (10 Wm^{-2}C^{-1}) describe the thermal exchanges by convection on the eye's surface, respectively, from sclera to body core and from cornea to the surroundings. The other terms describing the radiative heat transfer are represented by T, unknown temperature (°C); t, time (s); E, evaporation rate (40 Wm^{-2}); T_{amb}, ambient temperature (25°C); T_b, blood temperature (37°C); n, the unit vector outward normal (m); σ, Stefan constant (5.67 × 10^{-8}Wm^{-2}K^{-4}); ε, emissivity of corneal surface (0.975); and H, heat source (Wm^{-3}).

The initial temperature distribution ($t = 0$) is found by solving the steady state heat transfer equation with no external heat sources as in

$$\nabla(k\nabla T) = 0 \tag{13.12}$$

13.3.2 METHOD OF ANALYSIS

In this section, first procedures for applying the FEM to the bioheat equation are described. The b-splines and web-splines will be outlined only in 3D, since the detailed account of the method can be found in the literature [6].

13.3.2.1 The Weak Formulation of the Bioheat Equation

The bioheat transfer equation is used in calculating the temperature distribution in the human eye wherein the domain Ω has smooth subdomains Γ_{1-3}. To calculate the approximate temperature T_h, a variational statement of the steady state problem is obtained by multiplying (13.8) by an arbitrary test function B_k and integrating the equality. The weak formulation becomes

$$\int_\Omega \left(-\nabla(k\nabla T_h) + \rho c \frac{\partial T_h}{\partial t} - H \right) B_k d\Omega \tag{13.13}$$

Employing Green's theorem, (13.13) can be expressed as the sum of the functions T_1, T_2, and T_3, which yield the differential equations

$$T_1 = -k \int_\Omega (\nabla T_h . \nabla B_k^t) d\Omega - \rho c \int_\Omega B_k \frac{\partial T_h}{\partial t} d\Omega + H \int_\Omega B_k d\Omega \quad \text{volume term} \tag{13.14}$$

$$T_2 = -\int_{\Gamma_2} h_s B_k (T_h - T_b) d\Gamma_2 \quad \text{sclera term} \tag{13.15}$$

$$T_3 = -\int_{\Gamma_3} [h_c B_k (T_h - T_{amp}) + \sigma \varepsilon B_k (T^4 - T_{amp}^4)] d\Gamma_3 \quad \text{cornea term} \tag{13.16}$$

where B_k^t denotes the transposed matrix of B_k. The approximate temperature T_h is replaced with the solution which consists of e nodes:

$$T_h = \sum_{i=1}^e \alpha_i B_i \tag{13.17}$$

where α_i indicates the coefficient of the basis functions B_i. Following the derivation for $\partial(T_1, T_2, T_3) / \partial T$, the matrix formulation below is obtained:

$$\left\{ \frac{\partial \Sigma T}{\partial T} \right\}^e = [K]^e \{T_h\}^e + [M]^e \left\{ \frac{\partial \Sigma T_h}{\partial t} \right\}^e - \{G\}^e \tag{13.18}$$

where $i,k = 1 \ldots e$,

$$[K]^e = k \int_{\Omega^e} \nabla B_i \nabla B_k^t d\Omega^e + h_s \int_{\Gamma_2^e} \nabla B_i \nabla B_k d\Gamma_2^e$$
$$+ h_c \int_{\Gamma_3^e} \nabla B_i \nabla B_k d\Gamma_3^e \int_{\Gamma_3^e} \sigma \varepsilon (T^4 - T_{amp}^4) B_i d\Omega \tag{13.19}$$

$$[M]^e = \int_{\Omega^e} \rho c B_i B_k^t d\Omega^e \tag{13.20}$$

$$\{G\}^e = (h_c T_{amp} - E) \int_{\Gamma_3^e} B_i d\Gamma_3^e + h_s T_b \int_{\Gamma_2^e} B_i d\Gamma_2^e + H \int_{\Omega^e} B_i d\Omega^e \tag{13.21}$$

Hence, after assembling the elementary matrices, the global system is

$$\frac{\partial(T_1 + T_2 + T_3)}{\partial T} = \sum_{e=1}^{e}\left\{\frac{\partial(T_1 + T_2 + T_3)}{\partial T}\right\}^{e} = [K]\{T\} + [M]\left\{\frac{\partial T}{\partial t}\right\} - \{G\} = 0 \quad (13.22)$$

where $[K]$ is called the global stiffness matrix, $[M]$ the global mass matrix, and $\{G\}$ is the global load matrix considering boundary conditions.

13.3.2.2 Web-Spline Approximation

Having briefly discussed the necessary background material for web-splines in Chapter 3, temperature distribution analysis of FEM with web-splines is straightforward. Rewriting (13.17) in 3D using web-splines as finite element basis functions, (13.23) is obtained:

$$T_h(i) = \sum_{u}\sum_{v}\sum_{w}\alpha_{u,v,w,i}B_{u,v,w}(x_i, y_i, z_i) \quad (13.23)$$

where B is the web-spline basis function, x,y,z are the coordinates, u,v,w are web-spline parameters, and α is the coefficient of basis functions. Each point in the equation has three coordinates. Summation is done over all the defined control point 3D tensor products for a given xyz location. The basis function for a given location is calculated from the degree of the web-spline using the standard iterative formula [2]. Thus, to obtain the approximate solution of the temperature distribution in the eye, the web-splines are incorporated into the global matrix equation in (13.22), and the linear system of equations are assembled and solved easily with the program written in MATLAB®.

13.3.3 SIMULATION RESULTS

In this section, we investigate the steady state temperature distribution in the 2D and 3D unexposed human eye models, with the use of the web-spline method. For each model, grid convergence analysis has been done. The simulations are performed using linear, quadratic, and cubic b-splines with 0.0625 and 0.0125 grid widths, respectively. To confirm the validity of our results, we compare them with those reported in [35,37], and [38]. We adjust the thermal properties of the eye tissue constants and size of our model to those in [37] and [38] for 2D and 3D simulations, respectively.

13.3.3.1 2D Results

First, to find the optimum grid number, we computed cubic web-spline approximations for different grid widths $h = 0.5, 0.25, 0.125, 0.0625, 0.03125$. This grid convergence test is shown graphically in Figure 13.5. It is deduced from the figure that as the grid number increases, the temperature results on the corneal surface become more stabilized. The optimum number of grids is found to be 193, for which h is 0.0625.

We illustrate in Figure 13.6 the inner (•), outer (○), and extended (▲) b-splines using cubic basis splines in the 2D human eye whose dimensions are given in Figure 13.4.

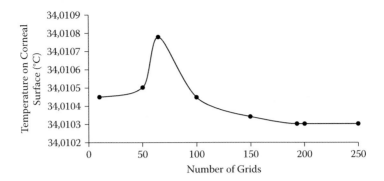

FIGURE 13.5   Grid convergence for the 2D web-spline model.

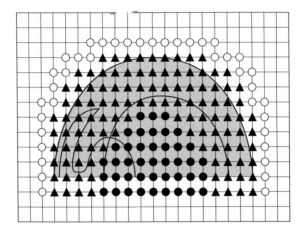

FIGURE 13.6   The standard •, extended inner ▲, and outer o cubic b-splines for the human eye.

The simulations were also performed with linear and quadratic b-splines. With cubic b-splines, 39 outer, 42 standard inner, and 112 extended inner b-splines are used in the simulations.

The thermal model of the 2D human eye is given in Figure 13.7. From this figure it is clearly observed that the lowest temperature, 34.01°C, appears at the corneal surface. The highest temperature occurs as we move away from the cornea toward the sclera.

The latest study regarding the calculation of the temperature distribution at steady state with no exposure to radiation in the 2D human eye has been performed by [35,37] using the method of finite elements. A corneal surface of 33.25°C was obtained in [35] with 496 nodes, and in [37] 33.64°C was approximately found with 8557 triangular elements. Figure 13.8 compares the temperature along the pupillary axis predicted by the two studies with that of the 2D web-spline method. Figure 13.8 reveals that the calculated temperatures along the axis of symmetry are in good agreement with those from the previous 2D finite element studies. In addition, as is evident from

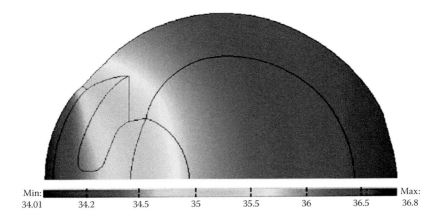

Min: 34.01   34.2   34.5   35   35.5   36   36.5   Max: 36.8

FIGURE 13.7   Thermal pattern of the 2D model without exposure to radiation. (Please see color insert.)

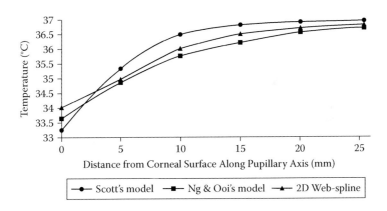

FIGURE 13.8   Comparison between the 2D web-spline model, [35] and [37].

Table 13.2, this low number of grids in the web-spline technique makes the computation time very low such as 0.1 s, 0.2 s, and 0.3 s for linear, quadratic, and cubic b-splines, respectively.

13.3.3.2   3D Results

In this section, we examined the temperature distribution at steady state in the 3D human eye model. The 3D model is constructed by revolving one-half of the 2D model 360° around its horizontal pupillary axis and is depicted in Figure 13.9. First, grid convergence analysis is illustrated in Figure 13.10 for cubic b-splines where the optimum grid width is calculated to be 0.125 (5203 grids) when the gradient of the graph approaches zero. Thus it is assumed that any decreases in the grid width do not change the simulation results.

An overview of the 3D human eye model for two layers with the outer, the extended inner, and the standard inner cubic web-splines for a grid width of 0.125 is shown in

TABLE 13.2

Efficiency Comparison of Web-Splines with Standard FEM Studies

Method	Number of Nodes
[37]	496
[40]	8557
Linear 2D web-spline	137
Quadratic 2D web-spline	164
Cubic 2D web-spline	193

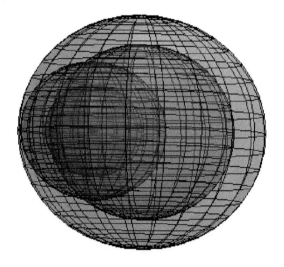

FIGURE 13.9   The 3D human eye model. (Please see color insert.)

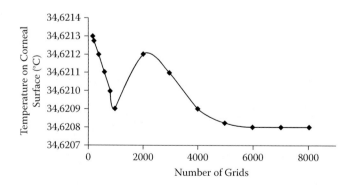

FIGURE 13.10   Grid convergence for the 3D web-spline model. (Please see color insert.)

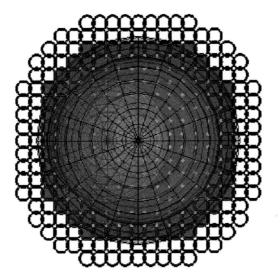

FIGURE 13.11   Grid representation for the 3D human eye model. (Please see color insert.)

Figure 13.11. There are 2843 extended inner b-splines marked with triangles, 1754 outer b-splines marked with white circles, and 606 standard inner b-splines, which appear in the middle layer of the sphere. If a larger grid width had been used, all inner b-splines would be affected by the outer b-splines and become extended inner b-splines.

The numerical value of the temperature in the thermal pattern of the eye model is calculated to be 34.52°C for linear, 34.55°C for quadratic, and 34.62°C for cubic web-splines at the center of the corneal surface. Figure 13.12 plots the local temperature variation along the horizontal pupillary axis for the FEM models developed by [35]'s 2D models, [38]'s 3D models, and the current 3D cubic web-spline model. The temperature distribution of the 3D web-spline model is very similar to those in [35] and [38]. Slight differences in the compared results are mostly attributable to the differences in the modeling of the human eye. In Figure 13.13, the comparison between the different 3D models, namely the one in Ng [38] and the web-spline methods, is shown for the linear, quadratic, and cubic web-splines. In the simulations, it appears that the temperature is minimized at the center of the corneal surface.

The simulation results are compared with the values reported by [37] in which they summarized the results of the corneal surface temperature obtained from the previous studies including the experimental and numerical studies with the mean value of 34.65°C. Upon investigations, it was found that the 3D cubic web-spline model gives only a temperature difference of 0.03°C as compared to the 0.64°C for the 2D cubic web-spline model.

Table 13.3 summarizes the comparisons between the FEM results on the corneal surface inside the human eye model and the web-spline model. When we compare the simulation results with the mean value of 34.65°C on the corneal surface, the current 3D model obtained a discrepancy of only 0.178% while the result of [37] produced a discrepancy of 0.455% and [38] produced a discrepancy of 0.33%. There are some deviations in the results. The reasons for these deviations are the different

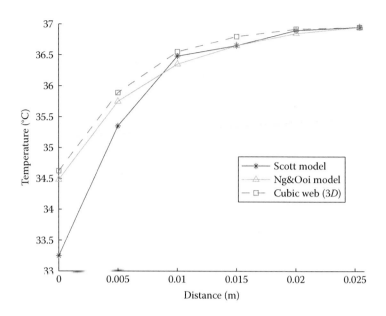

FIGURE 13.12   Comparison of the results for the 3D model using the methods in [35], [38] and the cubic web-spline method. (Please see color insert.)

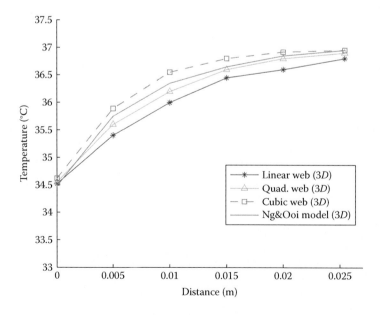

FIGURE 13.13   Comparison of the results for the 3D model using the method in [38] and the linear, quadratic, and cubic web-spline method. (Please see color insert.)

TABLE 13.3

Comparison between the Results of FEM and the Web-Spline Method on the Corneal Surface with the Mean Value of 34.65°C

Author	Method Used	Temperature (°C)	Absolute Difference (°C)	Percentage Difference (°C)
[35]	FEM	33.25	1.4	4.04
[37]	FEM	33.64	1.0	2.91
[38]	FEM	34.48	0.17	0.49
Kunter (3D)	Web-spline (linear)	34.52	0.13	0.38
Kunter (3D)	Web-spline (quadratic)	34.55	0.1	0.29
Kunter (3D)	Web-spline (cubic)	34.62	0.03	0.09

ambient temperature used (20°C versus 25°C) and the different approximations of material properties in the model. The choice of 25°C ambient temperature in the current model is based on a typical laboratory condition in Turkey. In [37], the iris and ciliary body were assumed to have properties similar to aqueous humor whereas the current model obtained different properties for iris and sclera. The number of grids generated in the 3D web-spline model is 2904, 4272, and 5203 for linear, quadratic, and cubic b-splines, respectively, whereas 54,796 elements had been used in [38]. The computation time is 1.2 s, 1.4 s, and 1.5 s for linear, quadratic, and cubic b-splines, respectively.

13.3.4 CONCLUSION

A FEM with web-splines, which models the heat transfer in the normal unexposed 2D and 3D representations of the human eye, has been developed and employed to calculate the steady state temperature distribution based on the properties and parameters reported in the literature. Error analysis indicates that our web-spline-based method is successful in determining the temperature distribution in the eye.

Based on the investigations in this study, the 3D web-spline model was found to yield better accuracy than the 2D web-spline model and is able to give a more precise interpretation of the temperature inside the human eye. The reason the differences become larger in the 2D models is that the actual eye model cannot be sufficient in 2D. Altogether, the 3D heat transfer model is shown to be a more significant representation of the actual human eye than the 2D model.

13.4 WEB-SPLINE COMPUTATION OF TEMPERATURE RISE WITHIN A MODEL OF THE MICROWAVE-IRRADIATED HUMAN EYE

Early theoretical work in the area of the biological effects of electromagnetic radiation is centered on the entire human body irradiation. However, because experimental work indicated that harmful local tissue temperature rises could occur, interest in partial body irradiation was stimulated. Under conditions of partial-body exposure to intense EM waves, significant thermal damage can occur in sensitive tissues. One of the most sensitive organs for EM wave exposure is the human eye.

Exposure of the eye to RF radiation can be sufficient to damage tissues owing to temperature rise. RF energy is generally absorbed in the cornea on the front surface of the eye. A number of models of heat transport in the eye have been proposed, motivated by the development of cataracts after exposure of the eye to infrared and microwave radiation, the most common sources of heat to which the human eye may be exposed.

One of the earliest studies on the thermal effects of microwave radiation in the human eye was done by [29]. They assumed that the eye was spherical and composed of uniform tissue. An analytical solution to the 1D heat transfer problem was developed for steady state conditions and did not account for transient temperature distributions. [28] computed induced temperatures within a model of the microwave-irradiated human eye at 750 MHz and 1.5 GHz. They concluded that at frequencies higher than 1.5 GHz, maximum temperatures could occur within the eye. With the same incident power level, similar temperature values are computed by Guy et al. at 2.45 GHz in the irradiated rabbit's eye. Thus, [28] imply that microwave heating of the rabbit eye and of the human eye can be correlated. Another early investigation that included a finite element heat transport model for the rabbit eye was presented by [32]. The initial temperature distribution of normal rabbit eye and eye exposed to microwave radiation was obtained from experimental measurements carried out on actual rabbits.

As wireless communication and industrial, scientific, and medical applications of radio frequency have rapidly grown, it is important to consider possible health hazards due to this type of non-ionizing radiation. Temperature rises for the human eye exposure to RF energy were investigated in [44,45,46]. Various sources of microwave radiation such as mobile phones [47,48], user antenna in wireless local area networks [49,50] and radar equipment [31,51–53] have been investigated. Results from these numerical investigations enabled exposure limits in the various frequency ranges of microwaves to be defined that would help to reduce the potential hazards of microwave radiation.

This section is the continuation of the previous chapter where only the steady state temperature distribution has been calculated for the unexposed human eye. In this section, we report a calculation of the microwave fields within a model of the human eye. FEM with web-spline computer modeling has been applied to study the corneal surface temperature increase during microwave irradiation. The heat conduction model of the microwave-irradiated eye, which is assumed to be 3D, is also constructed. The mechanism of heat transfer from the eye and the selection of the thermal parameters of the media of the eye are also discussed. The implementation of these parameters in the web-spline solution of the heat conduction is then developed. Furthermore, temperature rises calculated are compared with the values found in the literature pertaining to microwave-induced cataract formation.

13.4.1 THERMAL MODEL OF THE HUMAN EYE

13.4.1.1 Electrical Parameters of the Eye

Due to the lack of experimental data at the microwave frequencies, the evaluation of the complex permittivity values related to the eye tissues is done by using the Debyes dispersion equation. The Debyes equation gives the complex permittivity (ϵ^*) of a dielectric material as a function of the frequency (f), according to ∞

$$\varepsilon^*(f) = \varepsilon'(f) + \frac{\sigma(f)}{j2\pi f \varepsilon_0} = \varepsilon_\infty + \frac{\sigma_s}{j2\pi f \varepsilon_0} + \frac{\varepsilon_s - \varepsilon_\infty}{1 + j\frac{f}{f_r}} \qquad (13.24)$$

where f_r is the relaxation frequency, $\varepsilon_s - \varepsilon_\infty$ is the change in the permittivity due to this relaxation process, and σ_s and ε_∞ are the limits of the conductivity at very low frequencies and of the permittivity at very high frequencies, respectively. Debye parameters for cornea are $f_r = 21.5(GHz)$, $\varepsilon_s = 42.7$, $\varepsilon_\infty = 5.1$, $\sigma_s = 1.21(S/m)$. For the cornea, dielectric and conductivity constants were simplified as polynomial functions [54].

Polynomial function fitting for permittivity and conductivity of the cornea at 1–30 GHz are

$$\varepsilon(f) = -4.9 \times 10^{-5} f^4 + 0.004191 f^3 - 0.112 f^2 + 0.09232 f + 42.62$$
$$\sigma(f) = 5.858 \times 10^{-5} f^4 - 0.005011 f^3 + 0.1342 f^2 - 0.1103 f + 1.308 \qquad (13.25)$$

Dielectric and conductivity variations of cornea tissue are shown in Figure 13.14 with respect to frequency.

In this study, the human eye model is considered as a homogeneous semi-infinite tissue block characterized with known thermal and physical properties [55]. $H(x, t)$ is the heat source due to electromagnetic energy absorbed by tissue. The power deposited in a semi-infinite tissue exposed to incident electromagnetic wave is given as

$$H(x,t) = \frac{2 I_0 \zeta}{\delta} e^{-2x/\delta} U(t) \qquad (13.26)$$

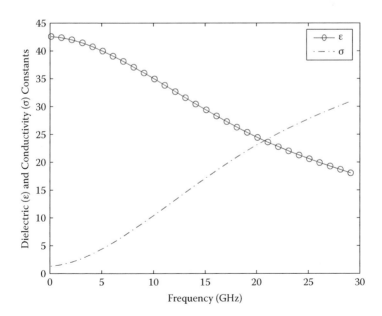

FIGURE 13.14 Dielectric and conductivity variations of cornea tissue. (Please see color insert.)

where I_0 is the power density of incident electromagnetic wave (W/m²), ζ is the power transmission coefficient between air and tissue, δ is the penetration depth, and $U(t)$ is the unit step function. When an incident plane uniform electromagnetic wave is normal to the skin surface, the SAR between the tissue can be determined as $H(x,t)/\rho$, where ρ is the density (kg/m³).

Because biological tissues are a nonmagnetic medium, power transmission coefficient ζ is defined only with permittivities of free space and the tissue [55].

$$\zeta = 1 - \left| \frac{\sqrt{\varepsilon^* \cdot \varepsilon_0} - \sqrt{\varepsilon_0}}{\sqrt{\varepsilon^* \cdot \varepsilon_0} + \sqrt{\varepsilon_0}} \right|^2 \qquad (13.27)$$

The penetration depth δ is given as

$$\delta = \left(\frac{67.52}{f} \right) \left[\sqrt{(\varepsilon')^2 + (\varepsilon'')^2} - \varepsilon' \right]^{-1/2} \qquad (13.28)$$

where f is the frequency in MHz, and ε' and ε'' are the real and imaginary parts of the complex relative permittivity. Table 13.4 depicts the electrical parameters of the cornea at the frequency of interest.

13.4.1.2 Time-Dependent Heat Conduction

The governing differential equation for temperature distribution is the Pennes bio-heat transfer equation:

$$\rho c \frac{\partial T}{\partial t} = \nabla(k\nabla T) + H(x,t) \quad \text{in } \Omega \quad \text{(inside the eye)} \qquad (13.29)$$

where Ω is the domain studied and Γ_1, Γ_2 are its boundaries, as indicated in Figure 13.4. The boundary conditions are specified on the sclera and the cornea, given in (13.30), and (13.31), respectively.

TABLE 13.4
Electrical Parameters of the Cornea at the Certain Frequencies

Frequency f, GHz	Permittivity ε	Conductivity σ, S/m	Energy Transmission Coefficient, ζ	Skin Depth δ, mm
1	42.604	1.326	0.4268	27.445
1.8	42.446	1.515	0.446	23.064
2.45	42.23	1.77	0.4507	19.54
6	39.97	4.47	0.458	7.633
10	36.014	9.199	0.4647	3.547
18	27.194	19.728	0.4834	1.483
30	17.786	30.93	0.517	0.802

$$-k\frac{\partial T}{\partial n}=h_s(T-T_b)\quad\text{on }\Gamma_1\text{(the sclera)}\tag{13.30}$$

$$-k\frac{\partial T}{\partial n}=E+h_c(T-T_{amp})+\sigma\varepsilon(T^4-T_{amp}^4)\text{ on }\Gamma_2\text{(the anterior cornea surface)}$$

$$\tag{13.31}$$

The solution of simplified bioheat equation for the surface temperature ($T(0,t)$) is given in [55] as

$$T(0,t)=\left(\frac{I_0\times\delta\times\zeta}{2k}\right)\times\left[2\sqrt{\frac{t}{\pi\tau}}+e^{t/\tau}erfc(\sqrt{\frac{t}{\tau}})-1\right]\tag{13.32}$$

$$\tau=\frac{\delta^2\rho C}{4k}\tag{13.33}$$

where τ is the time required for thermal energy to diffuse a distance equal to energy penetration depth, and $erfc(x)$ is the complementary error function.

13.4.1.3   Derivation of Finite Element Equations

By multiplying both sides of (13.29) by $\phi^e=\begin{Bmatrix}\phi_1^{(e)}\\\phi_2^{(e)}\end{Bmatrix}$ where $\phi_1^{(e)}$ and $\phi_2^{(e)}$ are the

linear shape functions and integrating over $[x_1^{(e)},x_2^{(e)}]$, we get

$$\int_{x_1^{(e)}}^{x_2^{(e)}}\rho C\begin{Bmatrix}\phi_1^{(e)}\\\phi_2^{(e)}\end{Bmatrix}\frac{\partial T}{\partial t}dx=\int_{x_1^{(e)}}^{x_2^{(e)}}\begin{Bmatrix}\phi_1^{(e)}\\\phi_2^{(e)}\end{Bmatrix}\left[\frac{\partial}{\partial x}\left(k_x\frac{\partial T}{\partial x}\right)+H\right]dx\tag{13.34}$$

By using integration by parts formula, the right side of (13.34) becomes

$$\int_{x_1^{(e)}}^{x_2^{(e)}}\begin{Bmatrix}\phi_1^{(e)}\\\phi_2^{(e)}\end{Bmatrix}\frac{\partial}{\partial x}\left(k_x\frac{\partial T}{\partial x}\right)dx=k_x\frac{\partial T}{\partial x}\begin{Bmatrix}\phi_1^{(e)}\\\phi_2^{(e)}\end{Bmatrix}\Bigg|_{x_1^{(e)}}^{x_2^{(e)}}-\int_{x_1^{(e)}}^{x_2^{(e)}}\begin{Bmatrix}\frac{\partial\phi_1^{(e)}}{\partial x}\\\frac{\partial\phi_2^{(e)}}{\partial x}\end{Bmatrix}\left(k_x\frac{\partial T}{\partial x}\right)dx$$

$$\tag{13.35}$$

$$=\begin{Bmatrix}-k_x\frac{\partial T}{\partial x}\big|_{x=x_1^{(e)}}\\k_x\frac{\partial T}{\partial x}\big|_{x=x_2^{(e)}}\end{Bmatrix}-\int_{x_1^{(e)}}^{x_2^{(e)}}k_x\begin{Bmatrix}\frac{\partial\phi_1^{(e)}}{\partial x}\\\frac{\partial\phi_2^{(e)}}{\partial x}\end{Bmatrix}\frac{\partial T}{\partial x}dx$$

Combining (13.34) and (13.35), and rearranging the terms, we get

$$\int_{x_1^{(e)}}^{x_2^{(e)}} \rho C \left\{ \begin{matrix} \phi_1^{(e)} \\ \phi_2^{(e)} \end{matrix} \right\} \frac{\partial T}{\partial t} dx + \int_{x_1^{(e)}}^{x_2^{(e)}} k_x \left\{ \begin{matrix} \frac{\partial \phi_1^{(e)}}{\partial x} \\ \frac{\partial \phi_2^{(e)}}{\partial x} \end{matrix} \right\} \frac{\partial T}{\partial t} dx = \left\{ \begin{matrix} -k_x \frac{\partial T}{\partial x}\big|_{x=x_1^{(e)}} \\ k_x \frac{\partial T}{\partial x}\big|_{x=x_2^{(e)}} \end{matrix} \right\} + \int_{x_1^{(e)}}^{x_2^{(e)}} \left\{ \begin{matrix} \phi_1^{(e)} \\ \phi_2^{(e)} \end{matrix} \right\}.H \; dx$$

$$(13.36)$$

In the terms on the left side of (13.34) we replace $T(x, t)$ by the finite element inter-

polation $[\phi_1^{(e)}(x)\phi_2^{(e)}(x)] \left\{ \begin{matrix} T_1^{(e)}(t) \\ T_2^{(e)}(t) \end{matrix} \right\}$. Then the term $\int_{x_1^{(e)}}^{x_2^{(e)}} \rho C \left\{ \begin{matrix} \phi_1^{(e)} \\ \phi_2^{(e)} \end{matrix} \right\} \frac{\partial T}{\partial t} dx$ is replaced by

$$\left(\int_{x_1^{(e)}}^{x_2^{(e)}} \rho C \left\{ \begin{matrix} \phi_1^{(e)} \\ \phi_2^{(e)} \end{matrix} \right\} [\phi_1^{(e)}(x)\phi_2^{(e)}(x)] dx \right) \frac{d}{dt} \left\{ \begin{matrix} T_1^{(e)} \\ T_2^{(e)} \end{matrix} \right\}$$

$$(13.37)$$

$$= \left(\int_{x_1^{(e)}}^{x_2^{(e)}} \rho C \left[\begin{matrix} \phi_1^{(e)}\phi_1^{(e)} & \phi_1^{(e)}\phi_2^{(e)} \\ \phi_2^{(e)}\phi_1^{(e)} & \phi_2^{(e)}\phi_2^{(e)} \end{matrix} \right] dx \right) \frac{d}{dt} \left\{ \begin{matrix} T_1^{(e)} \\ T_2^{(e)} \end{matrix} \right\}$$

The term $\int_{x_1^{(e)}}^{x_2^{(e)}} k_x \left\{ \begin{matrix} \frac{\partial \phi_1^{(e)}}{\partial x} \\ \frac{\partial \phi_2^{(e)}}{\partial x} \end{matrix} \right\} \frac{\partial T}{\partial x} dx$ is replaced by

$$\left(\int_{x_1^{(e)}}^{x_2^{(e)}} k_x \left[\begin{matrix} \frac{\partial \phi_1^{(e)}}{\partial x}\frac{\partial \phi_1^{(e)}}{\partial x} & \frac{\partial \phi_1^{(e)}}{\partial x}\frac{\partial \phi_2^{(e)}}{\partial x} \\ \frac{\partial \phi_2^{(e)}}{\partial x}\frac{\partial \phi_1^{(e)}}{\partial x} & \frac{\partial \phi_2^{(e)}}{\partial x}\frac{\partial \phi_2^{(e)}}{\partial x} \end{matrix} \right] dx \right) \left\{ \begin{matrix} T_1^{(e)} \\ T_2^{(e)} \end{matrix} \right\}$$

$$(13.38)$$

As a result, we get

$$\mathbf{M}^{(e)}\dot{\mathbf{T}}^{(e)} + \mathbf{K}^{(e)}\mathbf{T}^{(e)} = \mathbf{F}^{(e)} + \mathbf{Q}^{(e)}$$

$$(13.39)$$

where

$$\mathbf{T}^{(e)} = \left\{ \begin{matrix} T_1^{(e)} \\ T_2^{(e)} \end{matrix} \right\}, \quad \dot{\mathbf{T}}^{(e)} = \frac{d}{dt} \left\{ \begin{matrix} T_1^{(e)} \\ T_2^{(e)} \end{matrix} \right\},$$

$$\mathbf{M}^{(e)} = \int_{x_1^{(e)}}^{x_2^{(e)}} \rho C \left[\begin{matrix} \phi_1^{(e)}\phi_1^{(e)} & \phi_1^{(e)}\phi_2^{(e)} \\ \phi_2^{(e)}\phi_1^{(e)} & \phi_2^{(e)}\phi_2^{(e)} \end{matrix} \right] dx,$$

$$\mathbf{K}^{(e)} = \int_{x_1^{(e)}}^{x_2^{(e)}} k_x \begin{bmatrix} \dfrac{\partial \phi_1^{(e)}}{\partial x} \dfrac{\partial \phi_1^{(e)}}{\partial x} & \dfrac{\partial \phi_1^{(e)}}{\partial x} \dfrac{\partial \phi_2^{(e)}}{\partial x} \\[2mm] \dfrac{\partial \phi_2^{(e)}}{\partial x} \dfrac{\partial \phi_1^{(e)}}{\partial x} & \dfrac{\partial \phi_2^{(e)}}{\partial x} \dfrac{\partial \phi_2^{(e)}}{\partial x} \end{bmatrix} dx$$

$$\mathbf{F}^{(e)} = \int_{x_1^{(e)}}^{x_2^{(e)}} \begin{Bmatrix} \phi_1^{(e)} \\ \phi_2^{(e)} \end{Bmatrix} \cdot H \, dx \qquad (13.40)$$

$$\mathbf{Q}^{(e)} = \begin{Bmatrix} -k_x \dfrac{\partial T}{\partial x}\Big|_{x=x_1^{(e)}} \\[3mm] k_x \dfrac{\partial T}{\partial x}\Big|_{x=x_2^{(e)}} \end{Bmatrix}$$

13.4.1.4 Numerical Time Integration

The time-dependent problem (13.29) is solved numerically by a finite difference scheme. We begin by assuming that the two temperature states $\mathbf{T}_i$ at time t_i and $\mathbf{T}_{i+1}$ at time t_{i+1} are related by

$$\mathbf{T}_{i+1} = \mathbf{T}_i + [(1-\theta)]\dot{\mathbf{T}}_i + \theta\dot{\mathbf{T}}_{i+1}]\Delta t, \quad 0 \le \theta \le 1 \qquad (13.41)$$

where $\Delta t = t_{i+1} - t_i$ denotes the time step. The equation (13.41) follows from the trapezoidal rule, where the parameter θ is chosen by the user. Next we express (13.40) in the global form as

$$\mathbf{KT} + \mathbf{M\dot{T}} = \mathbf{F} \qquad (13.42)$$

By using t_i and t_{i+1}, we have

$$\mathbf{KT}_i + \mathbf{M\dot{T}}_i = \mathbf{F}_i,$$
$$\mathbf{KT}_{i+1} + \mathbf{M\dot{T}}_{i+1} = \mathbf{F}_{i+1} \qquad (13.43)$$

Then, multiplying the first equation in (13.43) by $(1-\theta)$ and the second by θ,

$$(1-\theta)(\mathbf{KT}_i + \mathbf{M\dot{T}}_i) = (1-\theta)\mathbf{F}_i,$$
$$\theta(\mathbf{KT}_{i+1} + \mathbf{M\dot{T}}_{i+1}) = \theta\mathbf{F}_{i+1} \qquad (13.44)$$

which, after adding together, gives

$$\mathbf{M}[(1-\theta)\dot{\mathbf{T}}_i + \theta\dot{\mathbf{T}}_{i+1}] + \mathbf{K}[(1-\theta)\mathbf{T}_i + \theta\mathbf{T}_{i+1}] = (1-\theta)\mathbf{F}_i + \theta\mathbf{F}_{i+1} \qquad (13.45)$$

Now, using (13.41), we delete the time derivative terms and get

$$\frac{\mathbf{M}(\mathbf{T}_{i+1}-\mathbf{T}_i)}{\Delta t}+\mathbf{K}[(1-\theta)\mathbf{T}_i+\theta\mathbf{T}_{i+1}]=(1-\theta)\mathbf{F}_i+\theta\mathbf{F}_{i+1} \tag{13.46}$$

Rewriting this equation, we have

$$\left(\frac{1}{\Delta t}\mathbf{M}+\theta\mathbf{K}\right)\mathbf{T}_{i+1}=\left[\frac{1}{\Delta t}\mathbf{M}-(1-\theta)\mathbf{K}\right]\mathbf{T}_i+(1-\theta)\mathbf{F}_i+\theta\mathbf{F}_{i+1} \tag{13.47}$$

The time integration to solve for **T** is carried out as follows:

- Given a known initial temperature T_0 at time $t = 0$ and a time step Δt;
- Determine T_1 at $t = \Delta t$, which is not known, by using (13.47);
- Use T_1 to determine T_2 at $t = 2\Delta t$; and so on.

13.4.2   3D Transient Analysis

The semidiscrete weak form of (13.29)–(13.31) on an element $\Omega_{(e)}$ with a test function $\phi_j^{(e)}$ is

$$
\begin{aligned}
0 &= \iiint_{\Omega_{(e)}}\left[\rho C\frac{\partial T}{\partial t}-\frac{\partial}{\partial x}\left(k_x\frac{\partial T}{\partial x}\right)-\frac{\partial}{\partial y}\left(k_y\frac{\partial T}{\partial y}\right)-\frac{\partial}{\partial z}\left(k_z\frac{\partial T}{\partial z}\right)+f\right]\phi_j^{(e)}dxdydz\\
&= \iiint_{\Omega_{(e)}}\left[\rho C\phi_j^{(e)}\frac{\partial T}{\partial t}+k_x\frac{\partial\phi_j^{(e)}}{\partial x}\frac{\partial T}{\partial x}+k_y\frac{\partial\phi_j^{(e)}}{\partial y}\frac{\partial T}{\partial y}+k_z\frac{\partial\phi_j^{(e)}}{\partial z}\frac{\partial T}{\partial z}+f\phi_j^{(e)}\right]dxdydz\\
&\quad +\int_{\Gamma_1}\phi_j^{(e)}h_{bl}(T-T_{bl})dS+\int_{\Gamma_2}\phi_j^{(e)}[h_{amb}(T-T_{amb})+\sigma\varepsilon(T^4-T_{amb}^4)+E]ds\\
&\quad -\int_{\Gamma_1^{(e)}\Gamma_{1,2}}\phi_j^{(e)}k\frac{\partial T}{\partial n}dS
\end{aligned}\tag{13.48}
$$

where $k\frac{\partial T}{\partial n}=k_x\frac{\partial T}{\partial x}n_x+k_y\frac{\partial T}{\partial y}n_y+k_z\frac{\partial T}{\partial z}n_z$. We approximate $T(x, y, z, t)$ on the element $\phi_j^{(e)}$ by the semidiscrete approximation

$$T(x,y,z,t)\approx\sum_{i=1}^{n}T_j^{(e)}(t)\phi_i^{(e)}(x,y,z) \tag{13.49}$$

where $\phi_i^{(e)}$ are the interpolation shape functions. Substituting the approximation (13.49) for T, we get the local finite element equations

$$
\left\{ \iiint_{\Omega_{(e)}} \left[\rho C \phi_i^{(e)} \phi_j^{(e)} \frac{\partial T_i}{\partial t} dxdydz + \left(k_x \frac{\partial \phi_i^{(e)}}{\partial x} \frac{\partial \phi_j^{(e)}}{\partial x} + k_y \frac{\partial \phi_i^{(e)}}{\partial y} \frac{\partial \phi_j^{(e)}}{\partial y} \right. \right. \right.
$$

$$
\left. \left. \left. + k_z \frac{\partial \phi_i^{(e)}}{\partial z} \frac{\partial \phi_j^{(e)}}{\partial z} \right) dxdydz + \int_{\Gamma_{1,2}} (h_{bl} + h_{amb}) \phi_i^{(e)} \phi_j^{(e)} dS \right] T_i \right\} + \iiint_{\Omega_{(e)}} f \phi_j^{(e)} dxdydz
$$

$$
- \int_{\Gamma_{1,2}} (h_{bl} T_{bl} + h_{amb} T_{amb} - E) \phi_j^{(e)} dS = 0, \quad \text{for} \quad j = 1, 2, \ldots n \qquad (13.50)
$$

or, in the matrix notation,

$$
\mathbf{M}^{(e)} \dot{\mathbf{T}}^{(e)} + \mathbf{K}^{(e)} \mathbf{T}^{(e)} = \mathbf{F}^{(e)}, \qquad (13.51)
$$

where

$$
M_{ij}^{(e)} = \iiint_{\Omega_{(e)}} \rho C \phi_i^{(e)} \phi_j^{(e)} dxdydz,
$$

$$
K_{ij}^{(e)} = \iiint_{\Omega_{(e)}} \left(k_x \frac{\partial \phi_i^{(e)}}{\partial x} \frac{\partial \phi_j^{(e)}}{\partial x} + k_y \frac{\partial \phi_i^{(e)}}{\partial y} \frac{\partial \phi_j^{(e)}}{\partial y} + k_z \frac{\partial \phi_i^{(e)}}{\partial z} \frac{\partial \phi_j^{(e)}}{\partial z} \right) dxdydz
$$

$$
\qquad (13.52)
$$

$$
+ \int_{\Gamma_{1,2}} (h_{bl} + h_{amb}) \phi_i^{(e)} \phi_j^{(e)} dS,
$$

$$
F_{ij}^{(e)} = \int_{\Gamma_{1,2}} (h_{bl} T_{bl} + h_{amb} T_{amb} - E) \phi_j^{(e)} dS + \iiint_{\Omega_{(e)}} f \phi_j^{(e)} dxdydz, \qquad j = 1, 2, \ldots n.
$$

13.4.3 SIMULATION RESULTS

Considerable work has been done in developing exposure standards for radio frequency (RF) radiation. Exposure standards for microwave energy (in particular, ANSI/IEEE C95.1-1992 and ICNIRP) specify times over which the exposure is to be averaged. In ANSI/IEEE and ICNIRP, these times range from 6 to 30 min, with shorter times at frequencies above 1 GHz. Thus, to calculate our simulation results with the standards and with [55], temperature rise that occurred by incident power density of 5 mW/cm² and 10 mW/cm² in the surface of cornea was calculated respectively at certain frequencies for an exposure time of 6 min.

In this study, the temperature rise in the human eye is computed as follows. First, all tissues in the multilayer model of the eye are assigned a temperature of 37°C. By using (13.29) (with $H(x,t) = 0$), the temperature in the steady state is computed to obtain the initial temperature distribution in the eye in the absence of microwave

TABLE 13.5

Temperature Increment Values on the Cornea Surface for Plan Wave Exposure

Frequency (GHz)	$I_0 = 5$ mW/cm²				$I_0 = 10$ mW/cm²			
	$n = 1$	$n = 2$	$n = 3$	Ozen	$n = 1$	$n = 2$	$n = 3$	Ozen
1	0.023	0.061	0.097	0.093	0.045	0.121	0.194	0.185
1.8	0.023	0.066	0.110	0.108	0.045	0.131	0.220	0.216
2.45	0.026	0.073	0.122	0.121	0.052	0.146	0.243	0.242
6	0.096	0.171	0.204	0.199	0.191	0.341	0.408	0.397
10	0.122	0.220	0.264	0.251	0.244	0.439	0.527	0.502
18	0.111	0.239	0.328	0.296	0.222	0.477	0.656	0.591
30	0.058	0.195	0.369	0.330	0.116	0.390	0.738	0.660

exposure. Secondly, the $H(x,t)$ in the eye exposed to microwave is added to (13.29). This is used as the heat source in (13.29) to compute the temperature rise to the steady state within the eye. Finally, the temperature difference before and after microwave exposure is derived as the temperature rise. The human eye tissue parameters were given in Section 13.3.

Web-spline simulation results with the results of the simplified bioheat equation for the surface temperature (13.32, 13.33) are given in Table 13.5 for linear, quadratic, and cubic web-spline. Results are also given in graphics in Figure 13.15 and Figure 13.16 for 5 mW/cm² and 10 mW/cm² incident power densities, respectively, at the frequency range of 1–30 GHz.

It is shown in the simulated figures that as the degree of the spline functions increases, temperature increase agrees well with [55] solutions.

Variation of temperature rise of cornea surface to exposure time by means of ICNIRP and ANSI/IEEE exposure limits at 30 GHz for 5 mW/cm² and 10 mW/cm² is shown in Figure 13.17.

For comparison, temperature rises of cornea surface versus exposure times are simulated with linear, quadratic, and cubic web-spline model and [55]'s at 6 GHz with 5 mW/cm² incident power density. Findings are depicted in Figure 13.18. It is clearly seen that the cubic web-spline solution of bioheat equations gives more accurate results than linear and quadratic web-splines when compared with [55]'s model.

Temperature variation depending on depth of skin eye tissue using the web-spline technique was simulated for 6 min exposure times. Skin depth simulations are plotted in Figure 13.19 with the power density of 5 mW/cm² at 2.45 GHz, 6 GHz, and 10 GHz frequencies, respectively for cubic web-splines.

13.4.4 CONCLUSION

Temperature rise on the cornea surface for plane wave exposure has been investigated by using the bioheat equation with web-spline model at the frequency range of 1 GHz and 30 GHz. Since radio frequency EM energy can be absorbed in the cornea on the front of surface of the eye, the threshold temperature rise is 3.0°C for cataract

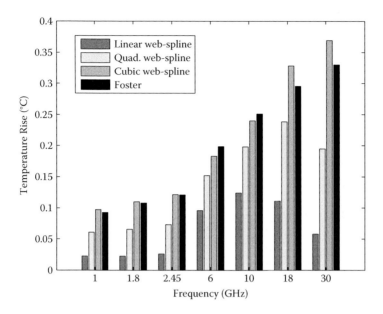

FIGURE 13.15 Temperature rise on the cornea surface at 6 min. duration at 5 mW/cm^2.

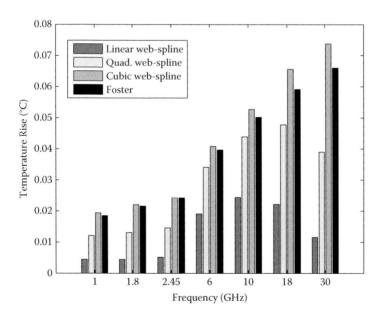

FIGURE 13.16 Temperature rise on the cornea surface at 6 min. duration at 10 mW/cm^2.

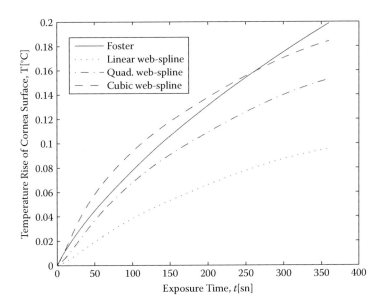

FIGURE 13.17 Temperature rise on the cornea surface at 6 min. duration at 10 mW/cm². (Please see color insert.)

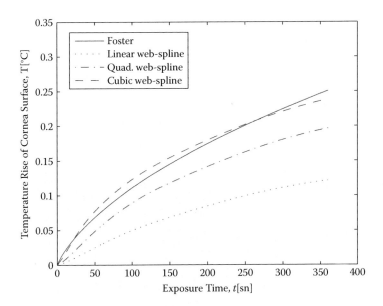

FIGURE 13.18 Temperature rise of cornea surface at 6 min. duration at 6 GHz. (Please see color insert.)

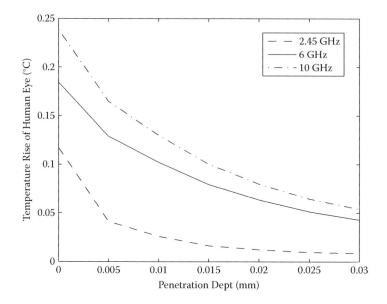

FIGURE 13.19 Cubic web-spline solution of temperature rise on the human eye for $I_0 =$ 5 mW/cm² at 2.45 GHz (– –), 6 GHz (—), 10 GHz (· – · –).

formation. Maximum temperature rise due to power density of 5 mW/cm², which is the maximum permissible exposure limit for controlled environment [ICNIRP 1998], is found to be 0.058°C, 0.195°C, and 0.369°C at 30 GHz for linear, quadratic, and cubic web-splines, respectively. For power density of 10 mW/cm² [ANSI/IEEE 1992], it is found to be 0.116°C, 0.39°C, and 0.66°C at 30 GHz for linear, quadratic, and cubic web-splines, respectively.

REFERENCES

1. de Boor, C.: On Calculating with B-Splines, *Journal of Approximation Theory*, **6**, 50–62 (1972).
2. de Boor, C.: A Practical Guide to Splines, *Applied Mathematics Series,* **27**, Springer-Verlag, New York, 1978.
3. Kipp, A.: Spline Galerkin Approximation, PhD thesis, University of Stuttgart, 1998.
4. Zhou, X.: Physical Spline Finite Element (PSFEM) Solutions to One-Dimensional Electromagnetic Problems, *Progress in Electromagnetics Research*, **40**, 271–294, (2003).
5. Han, J. G., W. X. Ren, Y. Huang: A Spline Wavelet Finite-Element Method in Structural Mechanics, *International Journal for Numerical Methods in Engineering*, **66**, 166–190 (2006).
6. Hollig, K.: Finite Element Methods with B-Splines. *Frontiers in Applied Mathematics*, **26**, Society for Industrial and Applied Mathematics (SIAM), Philadelphia, 2003.
7. Srinivas, V. K., V. K. Rathish, P. C. Das: Weighted Extended B-Spline Method for the Approximation of the Stationary Stokes Problem, *Journal of Computational Applied Mathematics*, **186**, 335–348, 2006.

8. Apaydn, G., S. Seker, N. Ari: Weighted Extended B-Splines for One-Dimensional Electromagnetic Problems, *Applied Mathematics and Computation*, **190**, 1125–1135 (2007).
9. Apaydn, G., S. Seker, N. Ari: Application of Web-Spline Method in Electromagnetics, *International Journal of Electronic and Communication (AEU)*, **62**, 163–173 (2008).
10. Kunter, F. C., G. Apaydin, N. Ari, S. Seker: *Use of Web-Splines for Waveguide of Arbitrary Domain*, Asia Pacific Microwave Conference, Hong Kong and Macau, December 16–20, 2008.
11. Kunter, F. C., G. Apaydin, N. Ari, S. Seker: *Web-Spline Solution of Axisymmetric Cylindrical Problems*, Asia Pacific Microwave Conference, Hong Kong and Macau, December 16–20, 2008.
12. Apaydin, G.: Efficient Finite Element Method for Electromagnetics, *IEEE Antennas and Propagation Magazine*, **51**, 5, 61–71 (2009).
13. Kunter, F. C., S. Seker: *Heat Transfer Model of the Human Eye Using Web-Spline Technique*, 14th Biennal IEEE Conference on Electromagnetic Field Computations (IEEE CEFC2010), May 9–12, Chicago, Illinois, USA, 2010.
14. Kunter F. C., S. Seker: 3D Web-Splines Solution to Human Eye Heat Distribution Using Bioheat Equation, *Engineering Analysis with Boundary Elements*, **35**, 639–646 (2011).
15. Kunter, F. C., S. Seker: Using Bioheat Equation 3D Web-Spline Prediction of Ocular Surface Temperature, *29th Progress in Electromagnetics Research Symposium*, PIERS 2011, Marrakesh, Morocco, March 20–23, 2011.
16. Ho, S. L., S. Yang, J. M. Machado, H. C. Wong: Application of a Meshless Method in Electromagnetics. *IEEE Transactions on Magnetics*, **37**, 5, 3198–3202 (2001).
17. Babushka, I.: The Finite Element Method with Penalty. *Mathematics of Computation*, **27**, 122, 221–228 (1973).
18. Belytschko, T., Y. Krongauz, D. Organ, M. Fleming, P. Krysl: Meshless Methods: An Overview and Recent Developments. *Computation Methods in Applied Mechanics and Engineering*, **139**, 3–47 (1999).
19. Hollig, K., U. Reif, J. Wipper: *Error Estimates for the Web-Method. Mathematical Methods for Curves and Surfaces*: Oslo 2000. Vanderbilt University Press, Nashville, TN, pp. 195–209, 2000.
20. Hollig, K., U. Reif, J. Wipper: Weighted Extended B-Spline Approximation of Dirichlet Problems. *SIAM Journal on Numerical Analysis*, **39**, 2, 442–462 (2001).
21. Hollig, K., U. Reif, J. Wipper: *B-Spline Approximation of Neumann Problems*. Mathematics Institute, University of Stuttgart, 2002.
22. Hollig, K., U. Reif, J. Wipper: Multigrid Methods with Web-Splines, *Numerishe Mathematik*, **91**, 2, 237–256 (2002).
23. Hollig, K.: *Handbook of Computer Aided Geometric Design: Finite Element Approximation with Splines*, Mathematics Institute, Elsevier, Amsterdam, pp. 283–308, 2002.
24. Hollig, K., C. Apprich, A. Streit: Introduction to the Web-Method and Its Application, *Advances in Computational Mathematics*, **23**, 215–237 (2005).
25. Rvachev, V. L.: Analytical Description of Some Geometric Objects, *Dokl AS USSR*, **153**, 4, 765–768 (1963).
26. Rvachev, V. L., A. N. Shevchenko, V. V. Veretelnik: Numerical Integration Software for Projection and Projection-Grid Methods, *Cybernetics and System Analysis*, **30**, 154–158 (1994).
27. Rvachev, V. L., T. I. Sheiko: R-Functions in Boundary Value Problems in Mechanics, *Applied Mechanics Reviews*, **48**, 4, 151–188 (1996).
28. Taflove, A., M. Brodwin: Computation of the Electromagnetic Fields and Induced Temperatures within a Model of the Microwave-Irradiated Human Eye, *IEEE Transactions on Microwave Theory and Technology, MTT-23*, **11**, 888–896 (1975).

29. Al-Badwaihy, K. A., A. B. Youssef: *Biological Effects of Electromagnetic Waves*, Vol. 1, ed. C. C. Johnson and M. L. Shore, HEW Publication, pp. 61–78, 1976.

30. Lagendijk, J. W.: A Mathematical Model to Calculate Temperature Distributions in Human and Rabbit Eyes during Hyperthermic Treatment, *Physics in Medicine and Biology*, **27**, 11, 1301–1311 (1982).

31. Hirata, A., S. Matsuyama, T. Shiozawa: Temperature Rises in the Human Eye Exposed to EM Waves in the Frequency Range 0.6–6 GHz, *IEEE Transactions on Microwave Theory and Technology*, **42**, 4, 386–393 (2000).

32. Emery, A. F., P. Kramar, A. W. Guy, J. C. Lin: Microwave 466 Induced Temperature Rises in Rabbit Eyes in Cataract Research, *International Journal of Heat Transfer*, **97**, 123–128 (1975).

33. Guy, A., J. C. Lin, P. O. Kramar, A. F. Emery: Effect of 2450 MHz Radiation on the Rabbit Eye, *IEEE Transactions on Microwave Theory and Technology*. *MTT-23*, **6**, 492–498 (1975).

34. Amara, E. H.: Numerical Investigations on Thermal Effects of Laser Ocular Media Interaction, *IEEE Transactions on Microwave Theory and Technology*, **38**, 2479–2488 (1995).

35. Scott, J. A.: A Finite Element Model of Heat Transport in the Human Eye, *Physics in Medicine and Biology*, **33**, 2, 227–241 (1988).

36. Scott, J. A.: The Computation of Temperature Rises in the Human Eye Induced by Infrared Radiation, *Physics in Medicine and Biology*, **33**, 2, 243–257 (1988).

37. Ng, E. Y. K., E. H. Ooi: FEM Simulation of the Eye Structure with Bioheat Analysis, *Computer Methods and Programs in Biomedicine*, **82**, 3, 268–276 (2006).

38. Ng, E. Y. K., E. H. Ooi: Ocular Surface Temperature: A 3D FEM Prediction Using Bioheat Equation, *Computers in Biology and Medicine*, **37**, 829–835 (2007).

39. Ooi, E. H., W. T. Ang, E. Y. K. Ng: Bioheat Transfer in the Human Eye: A Boundary Element Approach, *Engineering Analysis with Boundary Elements*, **31**, 494–500 (2007).

40. Ooi, E. H., W. T. Ang, E. Y. K. Ng: A Boundary Element Model of the Human Eye Undergoing Laser Thermokeratoplasty, *Computers in Biology and Medicine*, **38**, 727–737 (2008).

41. Ooi, E. H., W. T. Ang, E. Y. K. Ng: A Boundary Element Model for Investigating the Effects of Eye Tumor on the Temperature Distribution inside the Human Eye, *Computers in Biology and Medicine*, **39**, 667–677 (2009).

42. Ooi, E. H., E. Y. K. Ng: Effects of Natural Convection within the Anterior Chamber on the Ocular Heat Transfer, *International Journal of Numerical Methods in Biomedicine Engineering* (doi: 10.1002/cnm.1411, 2010).

43. Ooi, E. H., E. Y. K. Ng: Ocular Temperature Distribution: A Mathematical Perspective, *Journal of Mechanics in Medicine and Biology*, **9**, 2, 199–227 (2009).

44. Gandhi, O. P., A. Rzai: Absorption of Millimeter Waves by Human Beings and Its Biological Implications, *IEEE Transactions on Microwave Theory and Techniques*, Vol. MTT-34, 228–235 (1986).

45. Sukru, O., S. Comlekci, O. Cerezci, O. Polat: Electrical Properties of Human Eye and Temperature Increase Calculation at the Cornea Surface for RF Exposure, *Biological Effects of EMFs 2nd International Workshop Proceedings*, Vol. 2, Rhodes, Greece, 7–11 October 2002.

46. Sukru, O.: Mikrodalga Frekansli EM Radyasyona Maruz Kalan Biyolojik Dokularda Olusan Isil etkinin Teorik ve Deneysel Incelenmesi, Sakarya Universitesi, Fen Bilimleri Enstitusu, thesis, May 2003.

47. Wang J., O. Fujiwara: FDTD Computation of Temperature Rise in the Human Head for Portable Telephones, *IEEE Transactions on Microwave Theory and Techniques*, **47**, 1528–1534 (1999).

48. Flyckt, V. M. M., B. W. Raaymakers, H. Kroeze, J. J. W. Lagendijk: Calculation of SAR and Temperature Rise in a High-Resolution Vascularized Model of the Human Eye and Orbit when Exposed to a Dipole Antenna at 900, 1500 and 1800 MHz, *Physics in Medicine and Biology*, **52**, 2691–2701 (2007).
49. Bernardi, P., M. Cavagnaro, S. Pisa: *Evaluation of the Power Absorbed in Human Eyes Exposed to Millimeter Waves*, International Symposium on Electromagnetics Compatibility, Rome, Italy, pp. 194–199, 1996.
50. Bernardi, P., M. Cavagnaro, S. Pisa, E. Piuzzi: SAR Distribution and Temperature Increase in an Anatomical Model of the Human Eye Exposed to the Field Radiated by the User Antenna in a Wireless LAN, *IEEE Transactions on Microwave Theory and Techniques*, **46**, 2074–2082, (1998).
51. Hirata A., T. Shiozawa: Heat Transportation Models of the Human Eye for Microwave Exposures, *Proceeding of the International Workshop Ocular Side-Effects by Non-Ionizing Radiation*, Ishikawa, Japan, 2003.
52. Hirata A.: Temperature Increase in Human Eyes Due to Near-Field and Far Field Exposures at 900MHz, 1.5GHz and 1.9GHz, *IEEE Transactions on Electromagnetic Compatibility*, **47**, 68–76 (2005).
53. Hirata, A.: Improved Heat Transfer Modeling of the Eye for Electromagnetic Wave Exposures, *IEEE Transactions on Biomedical Engineering*, **54**, 959–961 (2007).
54. Seker, S., H. Abatay: New Frequency-Dependent Parametric Modeling of Dielectric Materials, *International Journal of Electronics and Communication (AEU)*, **60**, 320–327 (2006).
55. Foster K. R., L. Nozano-Lieto, P. J. Riu: Heating of Tissues by Microwave: A Model Analysis, *Bioelectromagnetics*, **19**, 420–428 (1998).

14 Modeling of Human Eye Exposed to Laser Radiation

Mario Cvetkovic, Dragan Poljak,
and Andres Peratta

CONTENTS

14.1 INTRODUCTION

During the last fifty years, since the first working demonstration of the ruby laser by Teodore Maiman, lasers have become an indispensable tool in a range of industries: entertainment, communications, science, medicine, and others. Due to the fact that light sources had previously been used as a form of treatment [1], particularly in ophthalmology and dermatology, it is logical that these medical disciplines, among the first, happily embraced this new tool. Further development of the novel and versatile laser systems promoted this tool as a "twenty-first-century knife."

Modern lasers implemented in eye surgery procedures cover the electromagnetic spectrum from ultraviolet (UV) to infrared (IR) wavelengths [1–3], including the ArF excimer laser used in laser in situ keratomileusis (LASIK) and photorefractive keratectomy (PRK), ruby laser used in welding of detached retina, Nd:YAG laser used in peripheral iridotomy (treatment of glaucoma) and in posterior capsulotomy (after-cataract treatment), Ho:YAG laser for contactless thermal keratoplasty, and many others. The spread of different types of eye surgeries using the variety of laser wavelengths required an understanding of the basic interaction between the laser light and the eye tissues.

Light incident on a tissue is either transmitted, reflected, scattered, or absorbed inside the tissue [2,3], and among these phenomena, absorption is the most important process due to the fact that absorbed photon energy by a tissue results in re-emitted radiant energy, or in light energy transformed into heat [3], which in turn increases the tissue temperature field.

Consequently, one of the most important issues in surgical application of lasers is assessment of the temperature variation in tissues subjected to the high-intensity laser radiation before an operation takes place. Therefore, to minimize any damage of intraocular tissues due to heating, the mathematical model has proven to be useful to clinicians in this estimation.

14.1.1 Previous Human Eye Models

First attempts to quantify the effects of electromagnetic radiation on the temperature elevation inside an eye were undertaken by Taflove and Brodwin [4] and Emery et al. [5], who calculated the intraocular temperatures due to microwave radiation via the finite difference and the finite element method, respectively. To study cataract formation due to infrared radiation, Scott [6,7] later developed a two-dimensional (2D) finite element model of heat transfer inside the human eye, while Lagendijk [8] used the finite difference method for the calculation of temperatures inside the human and animal eyes undergoing hyperthermia treatment.

Perhaps the earliest effort regarding the analysis of laser–tissue interaction was carried out by Mainster [9], who studied the eye thermal response to infrared laser radiation. In the following two decades, various models were further developed, including the thermal model of the eye exposed to visible and infrared lasers by Amara [10], and a three-dimensional (3D) model of the eye irradiated by argon laser by Sbirlea and L'Huillier [11], to mention just a few.

Recently, a number of human eye models have been developed, ranging from geometrically simple ones [12–14] to detailed 2D [15] and 3D models [16], having taken into account various eye tissues. Furthermore, methods of solving heat transfer problems range from semi-analytical [13] to numerical methods employing finite volume [12,15], finite element [17], or boundary element techniques [16].

14.2   MODEL DESCRIPTION

14.2.1   HUMAN EYE MODELING

Although relatively small in comparison to other organs in the body, measuring some 24 mm along the pupillary axis and 23 mm in diameter, the human eye is a complex system that consists of many tissues. If one aims to model the eye as accurately as possible, various tissues need to be taken into account, which raises the difficulty of the task. This is primarily due to the fact that one is required to have data for all thermal, optical, and electrical properties of comprising tissues, which are usually hard to find in one place.

We have assumed our model of the eye to be a solid structure of given dimensions, consisting of eight homogenous tissues, that is, cornea, aqueous humor, ciliary body, lens, vitreous humor, retina, choroid, and sclera. Having attempted to accurately represent the human eye in terms of dimensional relations between given tissues, we have made some simplifications. Thus neglecting the optic nerve provides a possibility of extending the 2D model to 3D by a simple rotation around the pupillary axis.

Figure 14.1 shows the geometry of our 2D model of the eye, including dimensions of some of the tissues. Figure 14.2 illustrates a 3D model, obtained by rotating the half of a 2D model around the central axis by 360 degrees.

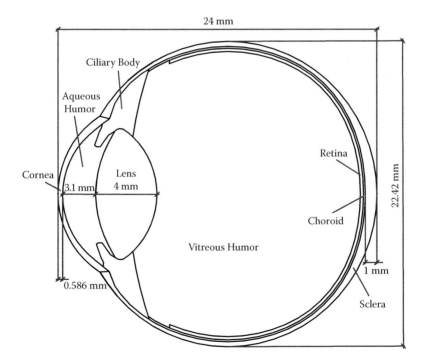

FIGURE 14.1   Two-dimensional model of the human eye.

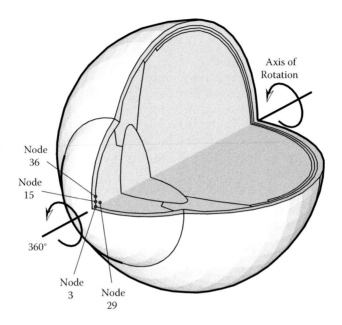

FIGURE 14.2 Three-dimensional model of the human eye.

14.2.2 Modeling Laser–Tissue Interaction

Before proceeding with additional details, it is useful to give an overview of the modeling procedure of a human eye exposed to the laser radiation and to specify the required parameters that one needs to take into account. This is illustrated in Figure 14.3.

The first step would be to calculate the heat generated inside the ocular tissues caused by the internal sources but also due to the external sources such as the laser radiation. Heat generated due to laser radiation depends on the laser parameters such as the wavelength, power density, exposure time, spot size, and the frequency of the applied pulses. Generated heat also depends on the optical properties of the tissue, such as the absorption and scattering coefficients, which are not readily available. This issue will be addressed later on.

Finally, one needs to account for parameters such as the volumetric perfusion rate of blood W_b and the internal volumetric heat generation Q_m (i.e., metabolic rate) since they are always present in the organism and are responsible for the constant temperature of the body.

The heat transfer to surrounding tissues is characterized by tissue thermal properties such as the thermal conductivity k and the specific heat capacity C. The values of these parameters are readily available in the literature (e.g., [18]) and are given in Table 14.1.

14.2.3 Tissue Optical Parameters

The most important among the tissue optical properties is the absorption coefficient, as a result of its strong dependence on the wavelength of the incident laser radiation, as can be seen in Figure 14.4.

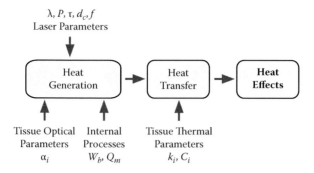

FIGURE 14.3 Parameters required for modeling laser-eye interaction.

TABLE 14.1
Thermal Properties of Various Human Eye Tissues

	Volumetric Perfusion Rate of Blood W_b [kg/m³s]	Internal Heat Generation Q_m [W/m³]	Thermal Conductivity k [J/m s K]	Specific Heat Capacity C [J/kg K]	Density ρ [kg/m³]
Vitreous h.	0	0	0.594	3997	1009
Lens	0	0	0.400	3000	1100
Aqueous h.	0	0	0.578	3997	1003
Cornea	0	0	0.580	4178	1076
Sclera	0	0	0.580	4178	1170
Ciliary body	2700	690	0.498	3340	1040
Choroid	0	0	0.530	3840	1060
Retina	35000	10000	0.565	3680	1039

Medical lasers are based on the principle that different eye tissues are strongly absorbing only at certain wavelengths while weakly absorbing at others [3]. When a beam of light, with wavelength from a visible part of the spectrum, is incident on the eye, on its way to the retina, it passes through the cornea, aqueous, lens, and vitreous humor, which are weakly absorbing on these same wavelengths. On the other hand, the cornea strongly absorbs in the ultraviolet, hence protecting the light-sensitive cells on the retina from the high-energy radiation.

In biological tissues, absorption occurs mainly due to the presence of water molecules, proteins, pigments, and other macromolecules, and is governed by Lambert–Beer's law. In the IR region of the spectrum, strong absorption is primarily attributed to water molecules, while proteins are main absorbers in the UV and visible range of the spectrum [2,3,19,20].

Since absorption coefficient strongly depends on the wavelength of the incident laser radiation, we need to have information about this parameter for the whole range

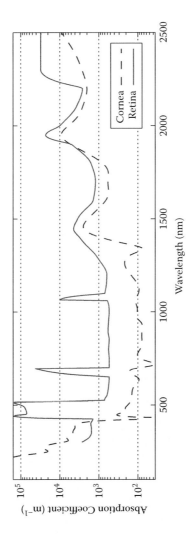

FIGURE 14.4 Wavelength dependence of the absorption coefficient of retina and cornea. (Please see color insert.)

TABLE 14.2
Thicknesses of Eye Tissues Used in Absorption Coefficient Calculation

Tissue Type	Vitreous h.	Lens	Aqueous h.	Cornea	Sclera	Choroid	Retina
Value [mm]	16.97	3.6	3.1	0.586	0.8	0.19	0.3

of wavelengths from UV to IR. Unfortunately, these data are not readily available or they are simply difficult to find for various ocular tissues.

A number of methods are known for measuring the optical properties of tissues, and they are outlined in [21]. Generally, we can classify them as direct techniques, using Lambert–Beer's law, and indirect techniques, where one needs to implement a complex theoretical model of light scattering to obtain the parameter.

One of the easiest methods is based on Lambert–Beer's law and uses the values of transmittances to obtain the absorption coefficient α as

$$\alpha = \frac{1}{d} ln \left| T_{ran} \right| \tag{14.1}$$

where d is the thickness of a specific tissue and T_{ran} is the tissue total transmittance. Values for the tissue thicknesses are listed in Table 14.2.

The values for transmittances were taken from the extensive work of Boettner [22] on spectral transmission of the eye and also from [23].

For the choroid, where the data on the reflectivity of the posterior tissue (sclera) and the anterior tissue (fundus) was available, absorption coefficient has been calculated according to

$$\alpha = \frac{1}{d} ln(\frac{I_0'}{I_0}) \tag{14.2}$$

$$I_0' = I_0[T_{ran}(1 + R_{pi}(1 + R_{ai}))] \tag{14.3}$$

where I_0 and I_0' are the intensities of the incident and the transmitted beams, respectively, R_{pi} is reflectance (%) of the posterior tissue, and R_{ai} is reflectance (%) of the anterior tissue.

Absorption coefficient values from a number of respected papers [10,11,19,24–32] were added to the calculated ones. Graphs of transmittances and calculated absorption coefficients of various human eye ocular tissues, used in our model, can be seen on Figure 14.5 and Figure 14.6, while Table 14.3 summarizes the absorption coefficient values for the selected laser wavelengths, reported in our previous work [33–35].

14.3 HEAT TRANSFER IN THE HUMAN EYE

The temperature distribution inside the human eye can be determined by solving the Pennes' bioheat transfer equation [36]. Even though this equation has been criticized

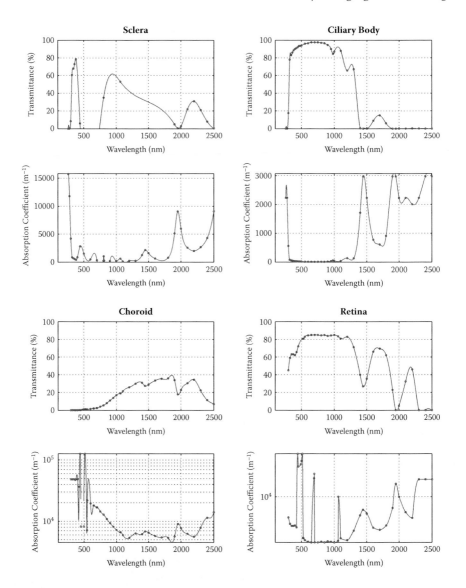

FIGURE 14.5 Transmittances and absorption coefficients of sclera, ciliary body, choroid, and retina. (Please see color insert.)

over the years [37], it is still the foundation for all mathematical analysis of bioheat transfer. The Pennes' equation represents the energy balance between conductive heat transfer, heat generated by the metabolic processes, and the heating or cooling effects due to the flow of arterial blood:

$$\rho C \frac{\partial T}{\partial t} = \nabla(k\nabla T) + W_b C_{pb}(T_a - T) + Q_m + H \qquad (14.4)$$

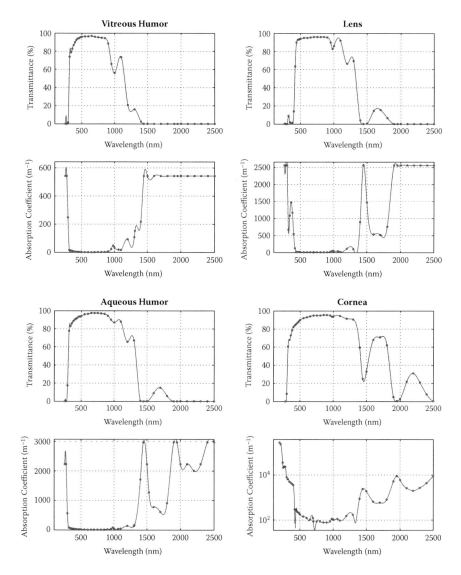

FIGURE 14.6 Transmittances and absorption coefficients of vitreous humor, lens, aqueous humor, and cornea. (Please see color insert.)

where ρ and C are the density and the specific heat capacity of tissue, respectively, W_b is the volumetric perfusion rate, C_{pb} is the specific heat capacity of blood, and Q_m the internal volumetric heat generated by specific tissue.

The bioheat equation also features a new term, H, representing the heat generated inside the tissue due to a certain external source. In our model, H represents the deposited energy due to laser radiation, but could be any other source of electromagnetic radiation [38].

TABLE 14.3

Absorption Coefficient Values of Eye Tissues at Various Laser Wavelengths [1/m]

Tissue Type	2090 nm	1064 nm	694.3 nm	193 nm	1053 nm
Vitreous h.	542.7	20	2	542.7	22.4
Lens	2558.4	43.5	9.5	2558.4	43.2
Aqueous h.	2228.3	35	8.4	2228.3	36.7
Cornea	2923.8	113	124	270000	111.7
Sclera	2923.8	634.8	358.5	28880	560
Ciliary body	2228.3	42.5	8.16	2228.3	42.9
Choroid	6398.2	6615	16848	48475	6671.7
Retina	4370.3	10000	44000	6526.2	594.1

The bioheat equation is supplemented with natural boundary condition equations for the cornea and sclera, respectively:

$$-k\frac{\partial T}{\partial n} = h_c(T - T_{amb}) + \sigma\varepsilon\left(T^4 - T_{amb}^4\right) + E_{vap} \in \Gamma_1 \tag{14.5}$$

$$-k\frac{\partial T}{\partial n} = h_s(T - T_a) \in \Gamma_2 \tag{14.6}$$

where k is the specific tissue thermal conductivity, already given in Table 14.1, h_c and h_s are the heat transfer coefficients of cornea and sclera, respectively, σ is the Stefan–Boltzmann constant, ε is the emissivity of the corneal surface, E_{vap} is the evaporation rate from the corneal surface, T_{amb} is the surrounding air temperature, and T_a is the temperature of the arterial blood. The values of these parameters are given in Table 14.4.

The boundary condition equation (14.5) represents the thermal exchange between the cornea and the surrounding air due to convection, radiation, and evaporation processes, while equation (14.6) represents the thermal exchange between scleral tissue and the ocular globe due to convection only.

To avoid iterative procedures necessary when dealing with nonlinear terms, such as the second term on the righthand side of equation (14.5), representing the heat radiated to the surroundings q_{rad}, we use the following binomial expansion:

$$\left(T^4 - T_{amb}^4\right) = (T - T_{amb})(T + T_{amb})\left(T^2 + T_{amb}^2\right) \tag{14.7}$$

thus linearizing the q_{rad} term to

$$q_{rad} = \sigma\varepsilon T_{app}^3(T - T_{amb}) \tag{14.8}$$

TABLE 14.4

Values for Various Parameters Used in Our Model

Parameter	Label	Value	Unit
Heat transfer coefficient of cornea	h_c	14	W/m²K
Heat transfer coefficient of sclera	h_s	65	W/m²K
Stefan–Boltzmann constant	σ	5.67×10^{-8}	W/m²K⁴
Emissivity of cornea	ε	0.975	—
Evaporation rate of cornea	E_{vap}	40	W/m²
Ambient air temperature	T_{amb}	25	°C
Arterial blood temperature	T_a	36.7	°C

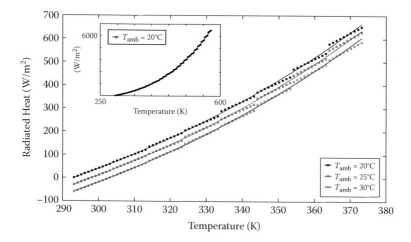

FIGURE 14.7 Approximation of radiation term by segments of 10 K. (Please see color insert.)

where T_{app}^3 is given by

$$T_{app}^3 = (T + T_{amb})\left(T^2 + T_{amb}^2\right) \tag{14.9}$$

We have approximated the value for T_{app} by segments of 10°C, taking into account different values of ambient temperature (20, 25, 30°C). Figure 14.7 shows the plot of actual value of radiation term q_{rad} and the one calculated by using the value of T_{app}, in the range from 20°C to 100°C. Also, the inset on the same figure shows this approximation, in the range from 20°C to 300°C, but only for the value of ambient temperature of 20°C. Some of the approximated values for T_{app} are given in Table 14.5.

A similar linearization approach has been previously utilized by [10], approximating the $(T + T_{amb})$ $(T^2 + T_{amb}^2)$ by T_F^3, where constant value of $T_F = 100°C$ was used, thus underestimating the values for q_{rad}, in particular at higher temperatures that develop when the eye is radiated by a laser.

TABLE 14.5

T_{app} Values for a 10°C Segment*

T_{amb}	<30	<40	<50	<60	<70	<80	<90	<100	<110	<120	<130	<140	<150
20	200	205	215	220	230	235	245	255	260	270	280	290	295
25	200	210	215	225	230	240	250	250	265	275	285	290	300
30	205	210	220	230	235	245	255	260	270	280	285	295	305

* All values are in °C

14.4 HEAT GENERATION (LASER SOURCE MODELING)

When modeling the eye irradiated by a laser, one can use a fact that many laser beams take the form of a Gaussian profile. This is a valid consideration when the beam divergence is very small, as is the case for the laser. We can thus represent the solutions for the electric field and the intensity in the form of a Gaussian function [2]; for example, in cylindrical coordinates (r, z), the intensity distribution at a time t can be written as follows:

$$I(r,z,t) = I_0 e^{-\alpha z} e^{-\frac{2r^2}{w^2}} e^{-\frac{8t^2}{\tau^2}} \qquad (14.10)$$

where I_0 is the incident value of intensity, w is the beam waist, and τ is the pulse duration.

Figure 14.8 illustrates the laser beam propagation in the z-direction, with the typical Gaussian distribution depicted on the left. On each transversal plane along the propagation axis, the beam is of the Gaussian profile.

The last exponential term in the equation (14.10), representing the temporal profile of a power or intensity of a laser pulse used in our model, is depicted in Figure 14.9.

Deposited laser energy $H(r,z,t)$, by the eye tissue at the nth node with cylindrical coordinates (r,z), can be calculated from

$$H(r,z,t) = \alpha I(r,z,t) \qquad (14.11)$$

where α is the wavelength dependent absorption coefficient of the specific tissue and $I(r, z, t)$ is the intensity at the nth node, at time t.

We first calculate the beam intensity at the cornea from

$$I_c = \frac{4P}{d_c^2 \pi} \qquad (14.12)$$

where P is the laser power and d_c is the beam diameter on the cornea.

We then proceed to determine the diameter of the beam formed on a retina. This image will be much smaller than the area of the pupillary opening due to diffraction on this aperture [39]. By taking into account focusing action of the lens, diameter of the image on a retina is related to the wavelength and the size of a pupillary aperture by

$$d_r = 2.44 \frac{\lambda f}{d_p} \qquad (14.13)$$

where λ is the laser wavelength, f is the focal distance of the lens taken to be 17 mm, and d_p is the diameter of a pupillary opening.

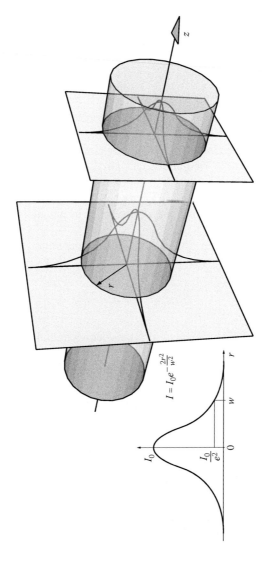

FIGURE 14.8 Gaussian beam propagation along z-axis. (Please see color insert.)

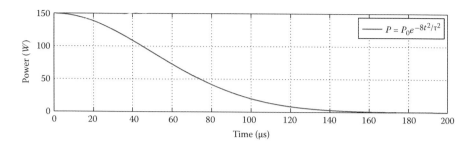

FIGURE 14.9 Laser pulse temporal profile. (Please see color insert.)

Beam intensity on the retina is then calculated from

$$I_r = I_c \frac{d_p^2}{d_r^2} \tag{14.14}$$

From these values of d_r and I_r, we now interpolate the intermediate values for the beam width and intensity at each node along the beam path. This way we have assumed the beam propagation through all the tissues along a pupillary axis, resulting in the absorption of the laser energy depending on the absorption coefficient of those same tissues, given in Table 14.3.

14.5 FINITE ELEMENT SOLUTION

When solving the heat transfer in biological tissues, besides complex mathematical formulation, one often deals with complex geometry. Since the analytic solution of the bioheat equation is limited to a few cases of a simple geometry with a high degree of symmetry, complex domains such as the human eye can be solved using the finite element method (FEM). The basic concept of the method is to discretize a domain of interest into small elements of finite size, and on each of these elements the unknown solution can then be expressed in terms of linear combinations of suitably selected base functions [40]. The solution is obtained after solving a system of linear equations.

The first step is to solve a steady-state variant of the bioheat equation (14.4) accompanied by the boundary conditions, equations (14.5) and (14.6). For the steady-state case, the lefthand side of the equation (14.4) and the last term on the right, representing the source, are taken to be zero, thus reducing the equation to the form

$$\nabla(k\nabla T) + W_b C_{pb}(T_a - T) + Q_m = 0 \tag{14.15}$$

The results obtained with this formula will be subsequently utilized as the initial conditions in the transient analysis, that is, when the eye is subjected to the laser radiation.

Multiplying equations (14.4–14.6) with the set of weight functions W_j and integrating over the entire domain Ω, the following integral formulation is obtained:

$$\int_\Omega \rho C \frac{\partial T}{\partial t} W_j \, d\Omega = \int_\Omega \nabla(k\nabla T)W_j \, d\Omega$$
$$+ \int_\Omega W_b c_b (T_a - T)W_j \, d\Omega + \int_\Omega (Q_m + H)W_j \, d\Omega \tag{14.16}$$

Integrating by parts and using Gauss's generalized theorem:

$$\int_\Omega \nabla(k\nabla T)W_j \, d\Omega = \oint_\Gamma k \frac{\partial T}{\partial n} W_j \, d\Gamma - \int_\Omega k\nabla T \nabla W_j \, d\Omega \tag{14.17}$$

$$\int_\Omega \nabla \vec{A} d\Omega = \oint_\Gamma \vec{A} n d\Gamma \tag{14.18}$$

yields the weak formulation of the Pennes' bioheat equation:

$$\int_\Omega \rho C \frac{\partial T}{\partial t} W_j \, d\Omega = \oint_\Gamma k \frac{\partial T}{\partial n} W_j \, d\Gamma - \int_\Omega k\nabla T \nabla W_j \, d\Omega$$
$$+ \int_\Omega W_b c_b (T_a - T)W_j \, d\Omega + \int_\Omega (Q_m + H)W_j \, d\Omega \tag{14.19}$$

The expressions for boundary conditions are given by

$$-\int_{\Gamma_1} k \frac{\partial T}{\partial n} W_j \, d\Gamma = \int_{\Gamma_1} (h_c + \sigma \varepsilon T_{app}^3)TW_j \, d\Gamma$$
$$- \int_{\Gamma_1} (h_c T_{amb} + \sigma \varepsilon T_{app}^3 T_{app} + E_{vap})W_j \, d\Gamma \tag{14.20}$$

$$-\int_{\Gamma_2} k \frac{\partial T}{\partial n} W_j \, d\Gamma = \int_{\Gamma_2} h_s TW_j \, d\Gamma - \int_{\Gamma_2} h_s T_a W_j \, d\Gamma \tag{14.21}$$

The unknown temperature distribution over a finite element is expressed as a linear combination of the shape functions N_j

$$T^e = \sum_{j=1}^{M} \zeta_j N_j \tag{14.22}$$

where M is the number of local element nodes. For the tetrahedral elements used in our 3D model, $M = 4$.

Equation (14.22) can be written in the matrix form:

$$T^e = \{N\}^T \{\zeta\} = \begin{bmatrix} N_1 & N_2 & N_3 & N_4 \end{bmatrix} \begin{bmatrix} \zeta_1 \\ \zeta_2 \\ \zeta_3 \\ \zeta_4 \end{bmatrix} \quad (14.23)$$

where vector $\{\zeta\}$ represents unknown coefficients of the solution. Temperature gradient expressed in terms of the shape functions can be written as

$$\nabla T = \begin{bmatrix} \dfrac{\partial T}{\partial x} \\[2mm] \dfrac{\partial T}{\partial y} \\[2mm] \dfrac{\partial T}{\partial z} \end{bmatrix} = \begin{bmatrix} \dfrac{\partial N_1}{\partial x} & \dfrac{\partial N_2}{\partial x} & \dfrac{\partial N_3}{\partial x} & \dfrac{\partial N_4}{\partial x} \\[2mm] \dfrac{\partial N_1}{\partial y} & \dfrac{\partial N_2}{\partial y} & \dfrac{\partial N_3}{\partial y} & \dfrac{\partial N_4}{\partial y} \\[2mm] \dfrac{\partial N_1}{\partial z} & \dfrac{\partial N_2}{\partial z} & \dfrac{\partial N_3}{\partial z} & \dfrac{\partial N_4}{\partial z} \end{bmatrix} \begin{bmatrix} \zeta_1 \\ \zeta_2 \\ \zeta_3 \\ \zeta_4 \end{bmatrix} \quad (14.24)$$

Inserting (14.23) and (14.24) into (14.19) and using Galerkin–Bubnov's procedure, where the weighting functions used are the same as the shape functions, $W_j = N_j$, leads to

$$\frac{\rho C}{\Delta t} \int_\Omega T^i W_j\, d\Omega + \int_\Omega (k\nabla T^i \nabla W_j + W_b c_b T^i W_j)\, d\Omega$$

$$+ \int_{\Gamma_1} (h_c + \sigma \varepsilon T_{app}^3) T^i W_j\, d\Gamma_1 + \int_{\Gamma_2} h_s T^i W_j\, d\Gamma_2$$

$$= \int_{\Gamma_1} (h_c T_{amp} + \sigma \varepsilon T_{app}^3 T_{amb} + E_{vap}) W_j\, d\Gamma_1 + \int_{\Gamma_2} h_s T_a W_j\, d\Gamma_2 \quad (14.25)$$

$$+ \int_\Omega (W_b c_b T_a + Q_m + H) W_j\, d\Omega + \frac{\rho C}{\Delta t} \int_\Omega T^{i-1} W_j\, d\Omega$$

We have used the $(T^i - T^{i-1})/\Delta t$ for the time derivative, where T^i is temperature of the nth node at the current time step, while T^{i-1} is the nth node temperature from the previous time step, and Δt represents the time step. Recasting the above equation into matrix form, and solving this system using a code written in MATLAB® [41], we finally compute the values for the temperature T at every node in the domain—that is, we obtain the temperature distribution inside the eye.

14.6   RESULTS

The first part of this section presents the results for the steady-state temperature distribution inside the human eye (i.e., when there is no laser radiation). Comparison between the results obtained by the 2D and 3D model is given, followed by the results for the transient case, when the eye is irradiated by the laser beam.

14.6.1 Steady-State Case

According to the finite element method, domains of 2D and 3D models have been discretized to 21,595 triangular elements (11,079 nodes), and to 148,664 tetrahedral elements (27,625 nodes), respectively. The meshes of both models are illustrated in Figure 14.10.

The steady-state temperature distributions for both models are shown in Figure 14.11. For the 3D model, cross-section cuts along horizontal and vertical axes enable the view of the temperature field inside the eye.

It can be seen from Figure 14.11 that the obtained temperature values for the 2D model are lower in the anterior eye tissues than those for the 3D model. This has been reported previously [42,43] and can be attributed to the absence of heat transfer in the direction perpendicular to the 2D model.

The graph in Figure 14.12 shows temperature distribution along the eye pupillary axis for both models, using the varying values of the ambient temperature. It can be

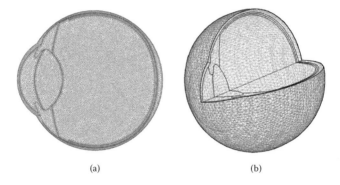

(a)   (b)

FIGURE 14.10 Finite element mesh: (a) 2D model, (b) 3D model. (Please see color insert.)

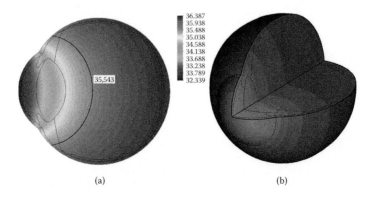

(a)   (b)

FIGURE 14.11 Steady state temperature distribution in the human eye: (a) 2D model, (b) 3D model. (Please see color insert.)

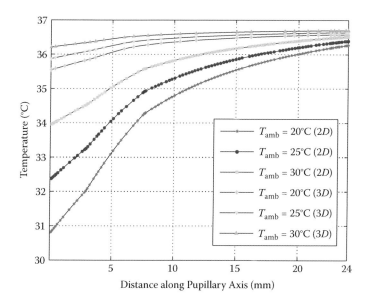

FIGURE 14.12 Steady state temperature along the pupillary axis. Dependence on ambient temperature. (Please see color insert.)

seen that for higher values of this parameter, discrepancy between the two models is lower.

A number of papers reported similar distribution of temperature along the pupillary axis. The biggest discrepancy those papers report is for the corneal surface temperature. This is due to a different value of the ambient temperature [6], heat transfer coefficient of the cornea [6,44,45], or the exclusion of the evaporation term in the boundary condition [10].

The summary of the steady-state values of corneal surface temperatures, obtained by using various techniques, can be found in a work by Ng and Ooi [17]. These values range from 32 to 36.6°C, with a mean value of 34.66°C.

Using the ambient temperature value of 25°C, our 2D and 3D models obtained 32.34°C and 35.54°C, respectively. We can conclude that our steady-state results are in agreement with the results published in a relevant literature, and hence valid.

14.6.2 TRANSIENT CASE

The obtained results from the steady-state analysis will now be utilized as initial conditions for the transient analysis. Due to many laser systems present today, there is an almost unlimited set of laser parameters that can be used. The results for the following lasers are presented: Nd:YAG, Ho:YAG, Ruby, ArF excimer, and Nd:YLF.

Interaction of the last two mentioned lasers is not based on the same mechanism as in the three other laser systems, due to the well-known fact that pulses shorter than 1 μs, if not applied at high frequency, do not cause thermal effects [2]. Interaction mechanisms on which these two lasers are based on are photoablation and plasma-induced ablation, for the ArF excimer and the Nd:YLF laser, respectively.

Photoablation is characterized by the decomposition of a very thin surface layer of tissue, on the order of several micrometers, with the absence of thermal damage to the adjacent tissue [2,46]. When determining the dependence of the depth of ablated tissue on the intensity of the laser, the authors base their assumptions on the Lambert–Beer's law [47], upon which our model is based.

However, we are aware that for any serious analysis, we would need a more detailed model of the cornea, more finely discretized by the finite element method. Furthermore, in addition to the heat transfer, we would need to take into account the mass transfer.

Using our present 3D model, we will therefore show, for illustration purposes only, what happens to the corneal surface when irradiated by ArF laser. Unlike photoablation, the most important parameter in plasma-induced ablation is the value of the electric field induced in the tissues [2]. Therefore, for the Nd:YLF laser we will present values for this parameter in a manner similar to an excimer case, without any inference.

The relation between the value of the electric field and the intensity is given by

$$I = \frac{1}{2}\varepsilon_0 cE^2 \tag{14.26}$$

where ε_0 is the dielectric constant of free space, and c is the speed of light. We will use this relation to obtain the results for the electric field.

14.6.2.1   1064 nm Nd:YAG Laser

Neodymium-YAG is a versatile laser used in procedures such as posterior capsulotomy (after cataract), peripheral iridotomy (treatment of glaucoma), retinal photocoagulation, and many more [1].

Parameters for this laser, used in our model, are one pulse of 1 ms duration, laser power 0.16 W, beam diameter on the cornea 2 mm, and pupil diameter 7.3 mm, similar to [10].

Figure 14.13 shows the temperature distribution in the eye after the end of the pulse application. Results for the 3D model are depicted as horizontal and vertical cross-sections. Also, the inset for the 3D model, with mesh overlaid, details temperature distribution around the posterior parts of the eye, namely vitreous, retina, and choroid, showing the maximum temperature achieved in vitreous humor.

We can note that the 2D model obtains significantly lower temperatures in respect to the 3D model, which can be clearly seen for the case of a node on the retina, where the temperatures are 103.66°C and 120.38°C, for 2D and 3D model, respectively.

Furthermore, it is worth noting that the maximum temperature achieved with the 3D model is in the vitreous humor. As our model aims to focus the laser beam on the retina, it would be more accurate to have maximum temperature achieved on the retina node. However, as clearly seen from Figure 14.13, this is not the case.

This could be achieved by refining the mesh of the retina domain. Currently, this layer is represented with only one element. Since the retinal thickness varies from

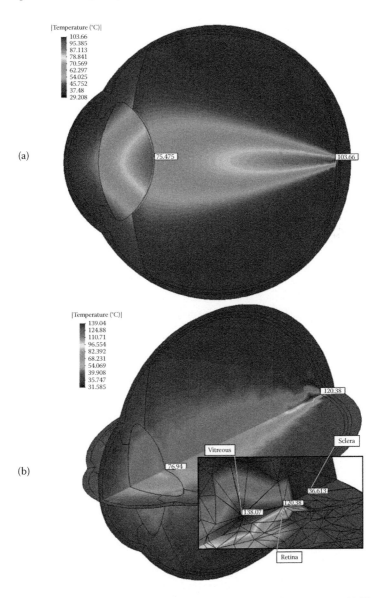

FIGURE 14.13 Comparison between temperature field distribution in the eye: (a) 2D model, (b) 3D model (horizontal and vertical slice). Nd:YAG laser parameters: pulse duration 1 ms, laser power 0.16 W, beam diameter on the cornea 2 mm, and pupil diameter 7.3 mm. (Please see color insert.)

about 0.15 mm anteriorly [48] to around 0.4 mm posteriorly, this would imply the use of a very fine grid, and it is something left for future work.

Finally, one can note the temperature distribution in the lens tissue. The 2D model obtained lower value on a node at the lens-vitreous boundary in respect to the 3D model, 75.47°C versus 76.94°C, but it is interesting to note that the 2D model shows significantly higher temperature gradient throughout the lens tissue. Again, this can be attributed to the absence of a heat transfer in the perpendicular direction.

14.6.2.2 2090 nm Ho:YAG Laser

Holmium:YAG lasers are used in a procedure known as the laser thermokeratoplasty (L-TKP) for the correction of vision [49,50]. Typical treatment consists of delivering several laser pulses in an annular pattern to induce local shrinkage of the corneal collagen.

Parameters used for this laser are seven pulses of 200 μs duration, laser off time between each pulse 2 s, laser power 150 W, beam diameter on the cornea 0.6 mm, and pupil diameter 1.5 mm. Figure 14.14 shows temperature distribution in the 3D eye model during the application of the last laser pulse and 2 s after the laser has been switched off.

Figure 14.15 shows the temperature evolution of selected nodes against calculation step (with respective distance from the cornea center). Location of these nodes is depicted in Figure 14.2. Comparison of 2D and 3D model temperature evolution on selected cornea node (0.35 mm, 0 mm) is shown in Figure 14.16.

Again, the 3D model gives higher maximum temperature at the cornea node in respect to the 2D model (i.e., 230.14°C against 187.44°C). Transient analysis feature of our models obtained significantly higher temperatures after application of seven laser pulses, compared to other authors [13,16]. Those models reported temperatures around 110°C, and in that respect our present model overestimates the temperature.

Temperatures required to initiate shrinkage of corneal tissue are on the order of 100°C, according to [51]. Both our models obtained significantly higher temperatures, so analysis has been carried out to assess the importance of some of the parameters used.

The effects of the pupillary opening, pulse power, and the cornea absorption coefficient are shown in Figures 14.17–14.19, respectively.

The analysis of the parameters showed that the diameter of the pupillary opening has a significant effect on the obtained temperature, as reported in [10,34,35]. In the normal human eye, the pupil diameter varies from 1.5 mm to about 8 mm and is related to the ambient light conditions. It seems that the obtained temperatures, using the pupillary diameter value of 1.0 mm, much better fit the expected values.

Another issue involves the position of the laser beam. Using the current eye model, all seven pulses are applied to the same spot, that is, at the center of the cornea. A more elaborate way would be to take into account annular distribution of the pulses, and thus the lower temperatures would be achieved.

14.6.2.3 694.3 nm Ruby Laser

This was the first laser introduced to ophthalmology in the early 1960s [1], and since then it has been used as a selective heat source to coagulate the retinal tissue in welding detached segments of the retina to the underlying choroid. The temperatures achieved by using this laser should remain below 80°C to prevent unnecessary vaporization and carbonization [2].

Parameters used in our calculation are pulse duration 10 ms, laser power 0.15 W, beam diameter on the cornea 8 mm, and pupil diameter 7.3 mm. A view to a part of

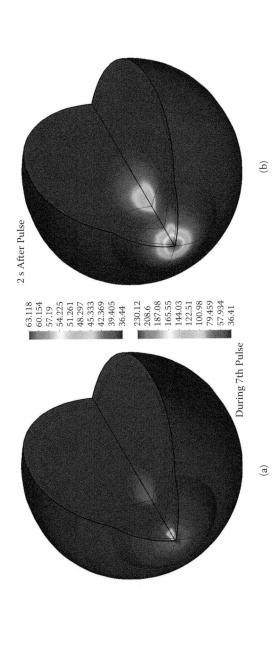

FIGURE 14.14 The temperature field distribution in the human eye; including horizontal and vertical half-slices: (a) at the end of the last pulse, (b) 2 seconds after the last pulse. Ho:YAG laser parameters: 7 pulses of 200 μs duration, laser off time 2 sec, laser power 150 W, beam diameter on the cornea 0.6 mm, and pupil diameter 1.5 mm. (Please see color insert.)

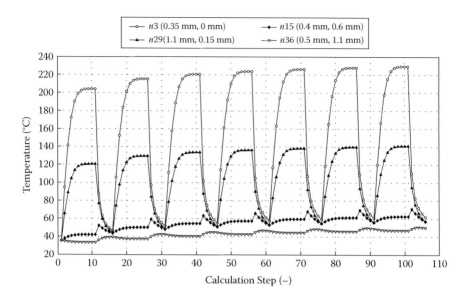

FIGURE 14.15   Ho:YAG laser: Temperature evolution at selected nodes. Numbers in parenthesis represent the distance from the corneal geometric center.

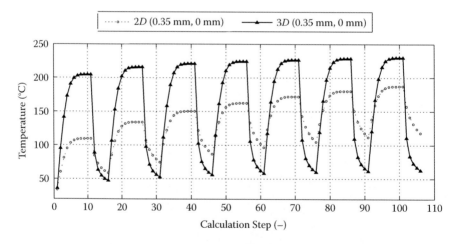

FIGURE 14.16   Ho:YAG laser: Comparison of a temperature evolution on selected cornea node in 2D and 3D model.

temperature distribution around the posterior part of the eye is shown in Figure 14.20, obtained from the 3D model. Maximum temperature of 77°C is again obtained on a node in the vitreous, while the temperature obtained at a node on the vitreo-retinal boundary is 69.16°C. Using the similar laser parameters, Amara [10] obtained a maximum temperature increase of 97°C.

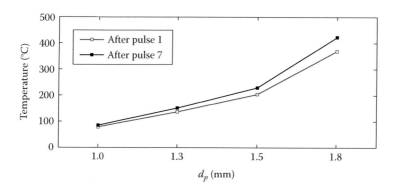

FIGURE 14.17 Ho:YAG laser: The effect of the pupillary opening on the temperature. (Please see color insert.)

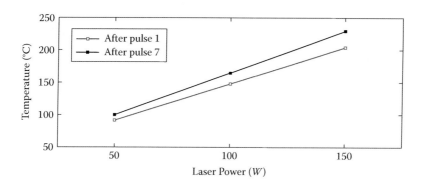

FIGURE 14.18 Ho:YAG laser: The effect of the applied laser power on the temperature. (Please see color insert.)

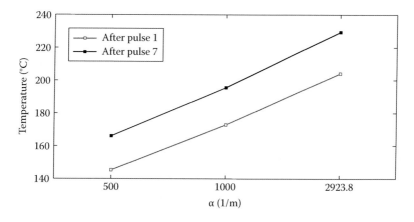

FIGURE 14.19 Ho:YAG laser: The effect of the absorption coefficient of cornea on the temperature. (Please see color insert.)

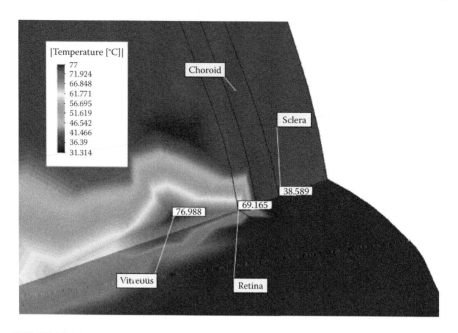

FIGURE 14.20   The temperature field around posterior part of the eye and temperature values for the selected nodes. Ruby laser parameters: pulse duration 10 ms, laser power 0.15 W, beam diameter on the cornea 8 mm, and pupil diameter 7.3 mm. (Please see color insert.)

14.6.2.4   193 nm ArF Excimer Laser

Currently, the two most widely used laser eye surgery methods are the photorefractive keratectomy (PRK) and laser in situ keratomileusis (LASIK), both performed using the ArF excimer laser, due to its ability to provide clean, thin cuts in the cornea by means of ablation [52,53].

Interaction between ArF laser and the eye tissues is based on a different mechanism, so the results presented here can be regarded only as illustrative. ArF laser parameters used are pulse duration 15 ns, laser energy 450 μJ, beam diameter on the cornea 0.2 mm, and pupil diameter 1 mm. Figure 14.21 shows temperature distribution in the anterior of the 3D model, for the vertical and horizontal cross-section, and the inset shows detail at the geometrical center of the cornea.

14.6.2.5   1053 nm Nd:YLF Laser

Neodimium:YLF is a versatile laser due to the fact that it can, alongside the induced thermal effects, produce the effects of plasma-induced ablation and photodisruption. Estimation of the physical parameters of plasma formation are given in [2]: 10 ps pulse duration, power density 8×10^{11} W/cm^2, and the electric field 2.5×10^7 V/cm.

Parameters used for the Nd:YLF laser are pulse duration 30 ps, pulse energy 100 μJ, beam diameter on the cornea 1 mm, and pupil diameter 7.3 mm. Figure 14.22 shows the distribution of the electric field, deposited laser energy, and the temperature around the posterior part of the eye.

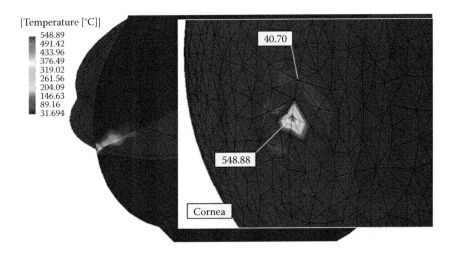

FIGURE 14.21 The temperature around anterior of the eye and detail of the corneal surface. ArF laser parameters: pulse duration 15 ns, laser energy 450 μJ, beam diameter on the cornea 0.2 mm, and pupil diameter 1 mm. (Please see color insert.)

Using our 3D model, we have obtained the value of $1.3 \ 10^{11} \times$ W/cm^2 for the power density and 1.28×10^7 V/cm for the electric field, respectively. Maximum temperature achieved on the retina is around 263°C.

14.7 CONCLUSION

To assess the temperature field inside the human eye during the laser radiation, we have developed a mathematical model based on the space-time dependent Pennes' bioheat transfer equation, having taken into account different types of heat transfer processes.

The detailed geometry of the human eye has been developed to give a realistic representation of the actual eye. Consequently, we have tried to include as many eye tissues as possible, given the available data on various tissue properties.

Laser beam has been considered to be of a Gaussian type and has been modeled by using the Lambert–Beer's law. Deposited laser energy has been included as an additional term in the bioheat equation. Calculation has been carried out for laser wavelengths currently widely used in ophthalmology, covering the electromagnetic spectrum from UV, visible, to IR, while inducing different types of interaction effects.

This work strongly emphasizes the importance of a wavelength-dependent absorption coefficient of various tissues and dedicates a section to this issue.

Transient analysis of Ho:YAG laser radiation showed higher temperatures than the values reported by other respected authors. To elucidate on this matter, parameter analysis has been carried out. Analysis of the pupillary opening parameter showed that lower values could lead to more acceptable results, on the order of temperatures reported by other authors. Also, deposition of the laser pulses in an annular manner would probably additionally lower the temperature.

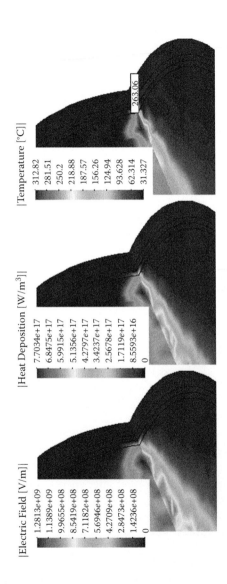

FIGURE 14.22 Distribution of the electric field, deposited laser energy and the temperature. Nd:YLF laser parameters: pulse duration 30 ps, pulse energy 100 μJ, beam diameter on the cornea 1 mm, and pupil diameter 7.3 mm. (Please see color insert.)

Three-dimensional simulations of the Nd:YAG laser radiation showed that we would need to use finer mesh to deliver the laser beam precisely to the node in the retina tissue.

Finer mesh of the cornea could also be useful in studying the effects of the deposited energy of ArF excimer laser, during the process of photoablation.

All in all, modeling the human eye exposed to laser radiation is definitely a challenging task. It requires knowledge of various ocular tissue and laser parameters. When all of these become available, modeling of this interaction can begin, first by determining the heat generated inside the tissue due to laser radiation, followed by the transfer of this heat to the surroundings. The bioheat equation can be analytically solved only for the canonical geometries; therefore one needs to employ numerical methods such as the finite differences, finite elements, or boundary elements to model complex geometries such as a human eye.

REFERENCES

1. K. Thompson, Q. Ren, and J. Parel, "Therapeutic and diagnostic application of lasers in ophthalmology," *Proceedings of the IEEE*, vol. 80, no. 6, pp. 838–860, 1992.
2. M. H. Niemz, *Laser-Tissue Interactions: Fundamentals and Applications,* 3rd, Enlarged Edition. Springer-Verlag, Berlin, 2003.
3. L. Carroll and T. R. Humphreys, "Laser-tissue interactions," *Clinics in Dermatology*, vol. 24, pp. 2–7, 2006.
4. A. Taflove and M. Brodwin, "Computation of the electromagnetic fields and induced temperatures within a model of the microwave-irradiated human eye," *IEEE Transactions on Microwave Theory and Techniques*, vol. 23, pp. 888–896, Jan 1975.
5. A. Emery, P. Kramar, A. Guy, and J. Lin, "Microwave induced temperature rises in rabbit eyes in cataract research," *Journal of Heat Transfer*, vol. 97, pp. 123–128, 1975.
6. J. Scott, "A finite element model of heat transport in the human eye," *Physics in Medicine and Biology*, vol. 33, no. 2, pp. 227–241, 1988.
7. J. Scott, "The computation of temperature rises in the human eye induced by infrared radiation," *Physics in Medicine and Biology*, vol. 33, no. 2, pp. 243–257, 1988.
8. J. Lagendijk, "A mathematical model to calculate temperature distributions in human and rabbit eyes during hyperthermic treatment," *Physics in Medicine and Biology*, vol. 27, no. 11, pp. 1301–1311, 1982.
9. M. A. Mainster, "Ophthalmic applications of infrared lasers—thermal considerations," *Investigative Ophthalmology & Visual Science*, vol. 18, pp. 414–420, Apr 1979.
10. E. Amara, "Numerical investigations on thermal effects of laserocular media interaction," *International Journal of Heat and Mass Transfer*, vol. 38, no. 13, pp. 2479–2488, 1995.
11. G. Sbirlea and J. L'Huillier, "A powerful finite element for analysis of argon laser iridectomy—influence of natural convection on the human eye," *Transactions on Biomedicine and Health*, vol. 4, pp. 67–79, Apr 1997.
12. K. J. Chua, J. C. Ho, S. K. Chou, and M. R. Islam, "On the study of the temperature distribution within a human eye subjected to a laser source," *International Communications in Heat and Mass Transfer*, vol. 32, pp. 1057–1065, 2005.
13. F. Manns, D. Borja, J. M. Parel, W. Smiddy, and W. Culbertson, "Semi-analytical thermal model for subablative laser heating of homogeneous nonperfused biological tissue: application to laser thermokeratoplasty," *Journal of Biomedical Optics*, vol. 8, pp. 288–297, Apr 2003.

14. A. Podol'tsev and G. Zheltov, "Photodestructive effect of IR laser radiation on the cornea," *Optics and Spectroscopy*, vol. 102, no. 1, pp. 142–146, 2007.
15. A. Narasimhan, K. Jha, and L. Gopal, "Transient simulations of heat transfer in human eye undergoing laser surgery," *International Journal of Heat and Mass Transfer*, vol. 53, pp. 482–490, Jan 2010.
16. E. H. Ooi, W. T. Ang, and E. Y. K. Ng, "A boundary element model of the human eye undergoing laser thermokeratoplasty," *Computers in Biology and Medicine*, vol. 38, pp. 727–737, 2008.
17. E. Y. K. Ng and E. H. Ooi, "Ocular surface temperature: A 3D FEM prediction using bioheat equation," *Computers in Biology and Medicine*, vol. 37, pp. 829–835, 2007.
18. S. C. DeMarco, G. Lazzi, W. Liu, J. D. Weiland, and M. S. Humayun, "Computed SAR and thermal elevation in a 0.25-mm 2-D model of the human eye and head in response to an implanted retinal stimulator—Part I: Models and methods," *IEEE Transactions on Antennas and Propagation*, vol. 51, no. 9, pp. 2274–2285, 2003.
19. W. Makous and J. Gould, "Effects of lasers on the human eye," *IBM Journal of Research and Development*, vol. 12, no. 3, pp. 257–271, 1968.
20. J. Krauss, C. Puliafito, and R. Steinert, "Laser interactions with the cornea," *Survey of Ophthalmology*, vol. 31, pp. 37–51, Jan 1986.
21. W. Cheong, S. Prahl, and A. Welch, "A review of the optical properties of biological tissues," *IEEE Journal of Quantum Electronics*, vol. 26, pp. 2166–2185, Jan 1990.
22. E. A. Boettner, "Spectral transmission of the eye," tech. rep., Report of the University of Michigan Ann Arbor Contract AF41(609)-2966, 1967.
23. A. Takata, L. Zaneveld, and W. Richter, "Laser-induced thermal damage of skin," tech. rep., final report. Sep 76–Apr 77, Jan 1977.
24. D. K. Sardar, G.-Y. Swanland, R. M. Yow, R. J. Thomas, and A. T. C. Tsin, "Optical properties of ocular tissues in the near infrared region," *Lasers in Medical Science*, vol. 22, pp. 46–52, Mar 2007.
25. J. Krauss, C. Puliafito, W. Lin, and J. Fujimoto, "Interferometric technique for investigation of laser thermal retinal damage," *Investigative Ophthalmology & Visual Science*, vol. 28, pp. 1290–1297, Jan 1987.
26. A. Lembares, X. H. Hu, and G. W. Kalmus, "Absorption spectra of corneas in the far ultraviolet region," *Investigative Ophthalmology & Visual Science*, vol. 38, pp. 1283–1287, May 1997.
27. L. Kolozsvári, A. Nógrádi, B. Hopp, and Z. Bor, "UV absorbance of the human cornea in the 240- to 400-nm range," *Investigative Ophthalmology & Visual Science*, vol. 43, pp. 2165–2168, Jul 2002.
28. E. Chan, B. Sorg, D. Protsenko, M. O'Neil, and et al., "Effects of compression on soft tissue optical properties," *IEEE Journal of Seleced Topics in Quantum Electronics*, vol. 2, pp. 943–949, Jan 1996.
29. A. Vogel, C. Dlugos, R. Nuffer, and R. Birngruber, "Optical properties of human sclera, and their consequences for transscleral laser applications," *Lasers in Surgery and Medicine*, vol. 11, pp. 331–340, Jan 1991.
30. W. Weinberg, R. Birngruber, and B. Lorenz, "The change in light reflection of the retina during therapeutic laser photocoagulation," *IEEE Journal of Quantum Electronics*, vol. 20, pp. 1481–1489, Jan 1984.
31. C. Cain and A. Welch, "Measured and predicted laser-induced temperature rises in the rabbit fundus," *Investigative Ophthalmology & Visual Science*, vol. 13, pp. 60–70, Jan 1974.
32. W. J. Geeraets, R. C. Williams, G. Chan, W. T. Ham, D. Guerry, and F. H. Schmidt, "The relative absorption of thermal energy in retina and choroid," *Investigative Ophthalmology*, vol. 1, pp. 340–347, Jun 1962.

33. M. Cvetkovic, A. Peratta, and D. Poljak, "Thermal modelling of the human eye exposed to infrared radiation of 1064 nm Nd:YAG and 2090 nm Ho:YAG lasers," *WIT Transactions in Biomedicine and Health*, vol. 14, pp. 221–231, 2009.
34. M. Cvetkovic, D. Poljak, and A. Peratta, "Thermal modelling of the human eye exposed to laser radiation," *2008 International Conference on Software, Telecommunications and Computer Networks*, vol. 10, pp. 16–20, 2008.
35. M. Cvetkovic, D. Cavka, D. Poljak, and A. Peratta, "3D FEM temperature distribution analysis of the human eye exposed to laser radiation," *The Proceedings of the Eighth International Conference on Modelling in Medicine and Biology, BIOMED 2009, Crete*, 2009.
36. H. H. Pennes, "Analysis of tissue and arterial blood temperatures in the resting human forearm. 1948," *Journal of Applied Physiology*, vol. 85, pp. 5–34, Jul 1998.
37. E. Wissler, "Pennes' 1948 paper revisited," *Journal of Applied Physiology*, vol. 85, pp. 35–41, Jan 1998.
38. D. Poljak, A. Peratta, and C. A. Brebbia, "The boundary element electromagnetic–thermal analysis of human exposure to base station antennas radiation," *Engineering Analysis with Boundary Elements*, vol. 28, pp. 763–770, Jan 2004.
39. H. Cember, *Introduction to Health Physics, Third Edition*. McGraw Hill, Inc. New York, 1996.
40. O. C. Zienkiewicz and R. L. Taylor, *The Finite Element Method: The Basis, Fifth Edition*, vol. 1. Butterworth-Heinemann, 2000.
41. The Mathworks, Inc: MATLAB®. http://www.mathworks.com.
42. R. Acharya, E. Ng, and J. Suri, eds., *Image Modeling of the Human Eye*, ch. 11, pp. 229–252. Artech House, Inc., 2008.
43. E. Y. K. Ng, E. H. Ooi, and U. R. Archarya, "A comparative study between the two-dimensional and three-dimensional human eye models," *Mathematical and Computer Modelling*, vol. 48, no. 5–6, pp. 712–720, 2008.
44. E. Y. K. Ng and E. H. Ooi, "FEM simulation of the eye structure with bioheat analysis," *Computer Methods and Programs in Biomedicine*, vol. 82, pp. 268–276, 2006.
45. E. H. Ooi, W. T. Ang, and E. Y. K. Ng, "Bioheat transfer in the human eye: A boundary element approach," *Engineering Analysis with Boundary Elements*, vol. 31, no. 6, pp. 494–500, 2007.
46. M. Kitai, V. Popkov, V. Semchischen, and A. Kharizov, "The physics of UV laser cornea ablation," *IEEE Journal of Quantum Electronics*, vol. 27, pp. 302–307, Jan 1991.
47. R. Srinivasan and V. Mayne-Banton, "Self developing photoetching of poly (ethylene terephthalate) films by far ultraviolet excimer laser radiation," *Applied Physics Letters*, vol. 41, Jan 1982.
48. D. Pavan-Langston, *Manual of Ocular Diagnosis and Therapy, 6th Edition*. Lippincott Williams & Wilkins, 2008.
49. S. Esquenazi, V. Bui, and O. Bibas, "Surgical correction of hyperopia," *Survey of Ophthalmology*, vol. 51, no. 4, pp. 381–418, 2006.
50. H. Stringer and J. Parr, "Shrinkage temperature of eye collagen," *Nature*, vol. 204, pp. 1307–1307, Dec 1964.
51. R. Brinkmann, J. Kampmeier, U. G. A. Vogel, N. Koop, M. Asiyo-Vogel, and R. Birngruber, "Corneal collagen denaturation in laser thermokeratoplasty," *Laser-Tissue Interaction VII, Proceedings of the SPIE*, vol. 2681, pp. 56–63, Jan 1996.
52. J. Parrish and T. Deutsch, "Laser photomedicine," *IEEE Journal of Quantum Electronics*, vol. 20, no. 12, pp. 1386–1396, 1984.
53. M. W. Berns, L. Chao, A. W. Giebel, L. H. Liaw, J. Andrews, and B. VerSteeg, "Human corneal ablation threshold using the 193-nm ArF excimer laser," *Investigative Ophthalmology & Visual Science*, vol. 40, pp. 826–830, Apr 1999.

15 Computational Bioheat Modeling in Human Eye with Local Blood Perfusion Effect

Hui Wang and Qing-Hua Qin

CONTENTS

Symbols

k	Thermal conductivity of tissue (W·m^{-1}·K^{-1})
ρ	Density of tissue (kg·m^{-3})
c	Specific heat of tissue (J·kg^{-1}·K^{-1})
T	Temperature of tissue (K)
t	Time (s)
ω_b	Blood perfusion rate (ml·s^{-1}·ml^{-1})
ρ_b	Density of blood (kg·m^{-3})
C_b	Specific heat of blood (J·kg^{-1}·K^{-1})
T_a	Artery temperature (K)
h_∞	Film coefficient of ambient fluid (W·m^{-2}·K^{-1})
T_∞	Sink temperature of ambient fluid (K)

E_t	Eye tear evaporation (W·m^{-2})
T_c	Body temperature (K)
Q_m	Metabolic heat (W·m^{-3})
Q_i	Spatial heat (W·m^{-3})
σ	Stefan-Boltzmann constant (5.669×10^{-8} W·m^{-2}·K^{-4})
ε_c	Corneal surface emissivity

15.1 INTRODUCTION

The prediction of bioheat transport in a biological system is of importance in many diagnostic and therapeutic applications. However, analytical prediction is usually difficult in practice because some biological tissues, such as those in the human eye, have different physical properties and domains with complex geometries. The application of computational methods in modeling biological systems has thus attracted increasing attention, benefiting from the rapid development of computer science.

Among the numerical methods developed to date, the finite element method (FEM) and boundary element techniques have been widely used to analyze bioheat transfer phenomena in the human eye. For example, finite element (FE) models in cylindrical coordinates and rectangular coordinates for two-dimensional human eye structures were developed by Scott (1988) and Ng and Ooi (2006), respectively. The former is based on the assumption that the human eye is symmetric about the pupillary axis, ignoring the optic nerve region. The latter uses the commercialized software FEMLAB 3.1 as the computing tool. By considering the circulation of aqueous humor, Ooi and Ng (2008) utilized the FE technique to conduct heat transfer analysis for two-dimensional eye problems. A cylindrical eye model based on the FEM was also developed by Brinkmann et al. (1994). In the FEM analysis mentioned above the solution domain is divided into several cells or elements with independent material definition, and in each subdomain the physical fields are approximated by appropriate polynomial interpolations. A weak-form integral functional is developed to produce the final stiffness equations. The finite volume method (FVM) (Chua et al. 2005; Narasimhan, Jha, and Gopal 2010) and the finite difference method (FDM) (Mainster, White, and Tips 1970) have also been employed to study transient temperature changes in the human eye caused by responses to a laser source.

Besides the domain-type methods mentioned above, the boundary element method (BEM) or dual reciprocity BEM (DRBEM) involving boundary integrals only have been applied to numerical thermal analysis in human eye structures (Ooi, Ang, and Ng 2007; Ooi, Ang, and Ng 2008; Ooi, Ang, and Ng 2009; Peratta 2008). Unlike the FEM, FVM, and FDM, in the BEM analysis the time-consuming domain integrals appearing in the FEM are replaced with boundary integrals (one dimension is reduced) via the use of Green's functions. However, the treatment of singular or near-singular boundary integrals is usually quite tedious and inefficient, and an extra boundary integral equation is also required to evaluate the interior fields within the domain. Moreover, for multidomain problems, the BEM establishes the boundary integral equation separately for each subdomain, and complementary equations associated with the continuity conditions on the interface of adjacent subdomains are required. As a result, evaluation of the coefficient matrix of the resulting equations becomes complex. To overcome this problem, a new type of Green's-function-based approach, a hybrid FE model containing non-singular elementary boundary integrals only, was established for heat transfer in the eyeball, and the corresponding iterative algorithm was constructed for the treatment of nonlinear radiation conditions (Wang and Qin 2010). The developed hybrid FE model, referred to as HFS-FEM, displays the advantages of both FEM and BEM.

The studies discussed above have not considered the blood perfusion rate in the eyeball, and thus in their analyses the Pennes bioheat equation could be reduced to the conventional heat conduction equation. In practice, blood perfusion activity exists in local regions of the eyeball (Flyckt, Raaymakers, and Lagendijk 2006), and accurate prediction of the temperature distribution in the eye then depends on how the impact of the blood flow is taken into account. In this study, evaluation of the transient temperature distribution in a two-dimensional eyeball is performed using FE analysis, taking into account the blood perfusion effect in the sclera, the choroid, retina layers, and the optic nerve, based on the classic Pennes bioheat equation. The thermal properties and control parameters in the computation are chosen from the literature, and the predicted thermal variation in the eyeball is verified by comparison with available results from previous studies of human as well as animal eyes.

15.2 MATHEMATICAL MODEL

The human eyeball is a very complex biological system. Figure 15.1 shows a schematic diagram of the physiology of the human eye, from which it can be seen that the eye is an approximately spherical organ. The anterior transparent surface of the eye is the cornea. The lens lies in between the aqueous humor and vitreous humor, which are transparent liquids of different concentrations. The sclera is the outer white coat that provides full protection to the eye. Besides the cornea, iris, aqueous humor, sclera, vitreous humor, and optic nerve, there are two layers of tissues falling in between the sclera and the vitreous humor, namely the retina and the choroid. The retina is permeated with blood vessels and is connected to the brain by the optic nerve. Under the retina the choroid serves to nourish it.

Abstracting from Figure 15.1, a typical two-dimensional mathematical model of the human eye as sketched in Figure 15.2 is taken into consideration for the following computation. In the figure, only cornea, iris, aqueous humor, sclera, vitreous humor, and optic nerve are considered. For simplicity, since the retina and choroid layers are relatively thin, they are modeled together with the sclera and the optic nerve. Moreover, for the sake of convenience, each of the subdomains is assumed to be thermally isotropic and homogeneous.

Exact discrimination between the aqueous and vitreous humors is not possible, nor between the iris and the ciliary body. Because they are water-like, their physical properties are approximately equivalent. Convection of the aqueous humor is not modeled since it is assumed to have a negligible effect on the resulting temperature distribution.

Referring to the rectangular coordinate system (x,y) with the origin at the center of the outer surface of the cornea and the arrangement of the horizontal axis coinciding with the papillary axis, the governing equation representing the bioheat transfer

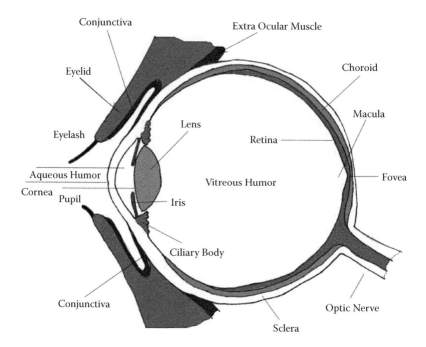

FIGURE 15.1   Schematic diagram of the physiology of the human eye. (From http://www. lookupinfo.org/eye_care/eye_conditions.aspx) (Please see color insert.)

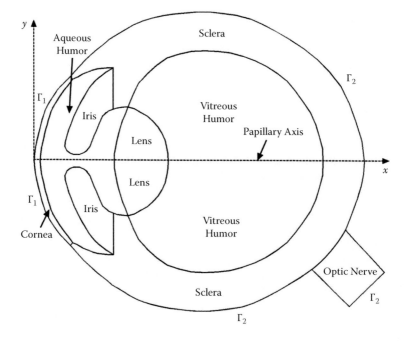

FIGURE 15.2   Simplified mathematical model of the two-dimensional human eye.

in the eyeball domain Ω can be written using the well-known Pennes bioheat equation, which addresses the effect of blood perfusion and metabolic activities in the biological system (Pennes 1948):

$$k\nabla^2 T + \rho_b c_b w_b (T_a - T) + Q_m + Q_i = \rho c \frac{\partial T}{\partial t} \quad \text{in } \Omega \quad (15.1)$$

where $\nabla^2 = \partial^2/\partial x^2 + \partial^2/\partial y^2$ denotes the Laplace operator, t is the time variable, ρ represents the density of the tissue, c stands for the specific heat of the tissue and k is the thermal conductivity of the tissue, w_b is the blood flow rate, that is, the volume of blood flowing through a unit mass of tissue per unit time, ρ_b is the density of blood, c_b is the specified heat of the blood, T represents the unknown tissue temperature, T_b denotes the blood temperature, Q_m stands for the metabolic heat source term, and Q_i represents the external heat generation, which may be caused by an external laser beam, electrical disturbance, radiation of electromagnetic waves, and so on. The relevant thermal properties including thermal conductivity, specific heat and density for the different subdomains are tabulated in Table 15.1, based on data from the literature (Flyckt, Raaymakers, and Lagendijk 2006; Narasimhan, Jha, and Gopal 2010; Ooi, Ang, and Ng 2009; Ng and Ooi 2006).

In addition, the following boundary conditions and initial condition are added to the biological system.

15.2.1 CONVECTION, RADIATION, AND TEAR EVAPORATION ON THE CORNEAL SURFACE Γ_1

Since the cornea is the only region in the eye that is exposed to the environment, the heat loss caused by convection and radiation should be considered. Also, the evaporation of tears on the corneal surface increases its cooling rate. The three forms of cooling mechanism can be combined and the related boundary condition on the surface of cornea is written as

TABLE 15.1
Thermal Properties of Various Parts of the Eyeball

Subdomains	k (W·m⁻¹·K⁻¹)	c (J·kg⁻¹·K⁻¹)	ρ (kg·m⁻³)	ω_b (ml·s⁻¹·ml⁻¹)
Cornea	0.58	4178	1050	0
Aqueous humor	0.58	3997	1000	0
Iris	1.0042	3180	1100	0
Sclera/retina/choroid	1.0042	4178	1000	0.02219
Lens	0.40	3000	1050	0
Vitreous body	0.603	4178	1000	0
Optic nerve	1.0042	3680	1030	0.00371
Blood	0.53	3600	1050	—

Source: Flyckt, Raaymakers, and Lagendijk 2006; Narasimhan, Jha, and Gopal 2010; Ooi, Ang, and Ng 2009; Ng and Ooi 2006.

$$q_1 \equiv -k_1 \frac{\partial T_1}{\partial n} = h_\infty \left(T_1 - T_\infty \right) + \varepsilon_c \sigma \left(T_1^4 - T_\infty^4 \right) + E_t \quad \text{on } \Gamma_1 \qquad (15.2)$$

where n is the unit outward normal to the surface, h_∞ is the heat transfer coefficient between the eye and ambient environment, T_∞ is the sink temperature, σ is the Stefan-Boltzmann constant with value 5.669×10^{-8} W/(m^{2}K^4), ε_c is the corneal emissivity, and E_t is the heat loss term due to tear evaporation.

15.2.2 Convection Condition on the Outer Surface Γ_2 of the Sclera

On the outer surface of the sclera, heat flows run into the eye from the blood acting as heating source from the ophthalmic artery to the sclera. This heating mechanism may be modeled using the following convection boundary condition:

$$q_2 \equiv -k_2 \frac{\partial T_2}{\partial n} = h_b \left(T_2 - T_b \right) \quad \text{on } \Gamma_2 \qquad (15.3)$$

where h_b denotes the blood convection coefficient from the sclera to the body core and T_b is the blood temperature, which is taken as 37°C by assuming that no heat loss occurs when blood flows from the common carotid artery to the ophthalmic artery.

15.2.3 Continuity Conditions on Common Interfaces

Continuous conditions exist on the common interface between two arbitrary adjacent regions R_i and R_j in the eye, which are assumed to be perfectly bonded:

$$\left. \begin{array}{c} T_i = T_j \\ q_i + q_j = 0 \end{array} \right\} \quad \text{on } R_i \cap R_j \qquad (15.4)$$

15.2.4 Initial Condition

In the domain under consideration, the initial temperature is assumed to be

$$T(t = 0) = T_0 \qquad (15.5)$$

with a specific initial temperature T_0 of domain.

15.3 NUMERICAL EXPERIMENTS

FEM is regarded as an appropriate tool for simulating thermal effects in the eye model, which usually consists of several regions. Thermal analysis of biological tissues using FEM can be categorized as a nonstructural solution using capabilities that are offered by the FEM. In the present work, the coordinates of the two-dimensional eye model are taken from the literature (Ooi, Ang, and Ng 2007) and then imported into AutoCAD software to generate a graphic image of the eye. Subsequently the image is imported into FEMLAB 3.2 (COMSOL Inc., Burlington, MA), which is suitable for solving complex partial differential equations (PDE), based on the MATLAB® PDE toolbox. It should be mentioned that the geometrical dimensions of the computing model employed in this chapter are taken from a particular approach in the literature (Ooi, Ang, and Ng 2007) and regenerated. Therefore, the geometrical dimension of the computational model here might be different from that in other publications and the results might show some discrepancy from those in other publications.

To simulate the temperature distribution and investigate the effect of control parameters on the temperature variation in the eye model, the values of control parameters related to the outer boundary conditions are listed in Table 15.2 (Ooi, Ang, and Ng 2007; Ng and Ooi 2006) for consideration.

15.3.1 VALIDATION STUDIES

To verify the FE procedure, 13,256 triangular elements are generated as shown in Figure 15.3, and the number of degrees of freedom to be solved for is 26,659. During the calculation using FEMLAB, to ensure mesh quality and validity of the solution, the mesh is refined until there is less than 0.5% difference in solution

TABLE 15.2
Control Parameters Related to Boundary Conditions

Control Parameters	Value
Blood temperature T_b	37 (°C)
Blood convection coefficient h_b	65 (Wm^{-2}K^{-1})
Ambient temperature T_∞	0~50 (°C)
Ambient convection coefficient h_∞	10~100 (Wm^{-2}K^{-1})
Cornea surface emissivity ε_c	0.975
Evaporation rate of tear	40~320 (Wm^{-2})

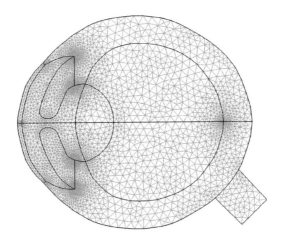

FIGURE 15.3   Triangular FE mesh for two-dimensional human eye model.

between adjacent refinement levels. The ambient temperature is specified as 25°C, the ambient convection coefficient is assumed to be 10 $Wm^{-2}K^{-1}$, the loss of heat flux $E_t = 40$ W/m^2, the initial temperature $T_0 = 0°C$ (Paruch 2007), and the time step is chosen as $\Delta t = 2$ s. A relatively steady state is achieved when the inter-iteration difference between adjacent time instances is less than or equal to a small value (i.e., 10^{-3}). It is necessary to mention that the initial temperature does not affect the final steady state of the temperature distribution, but it can affect the time taken to a steady state heat transfer and can change the manner of heat transfer at the start time.

The heating effect of blood perfusion in the sclera and optic nerve is initially ignored for the purpose of comparison with available experimental and numerical results. At this time, the governing equation (15.1) of the bioheat transfer is reduced to a standard transient Poisson equation. At the time instant $t = 2970$ s a relatively steady state is achieved. The temperature at the center of the outer corneal surface is 34.135°C, which is within the temperature range (from 33.4°C to 34.8°C) presented in Table 3 of Ooi, Ang, and Ng (2007). The calculated value has a percentage relative error 0.87% with 34.435°C obtained using the HFS-FEM (Wang and Qin 2010). In Figure 15.4 the temperature distribution in a human eye for the time at 10, 100, 1000, and 2700 s is presented, and good agreement is observed with results from Paruch (2007). It can be seen from Figure 15.4 that the region with lower temperature associated with the initial temperature becomes smaller as time progresses, and then the heat transfer behavior due to the temperature difference between the ambient fluid outside the cornea and the blood flow outside the sclera dominates. In the absence of blood perfusion, the distribution of temperature along the papillary axis is plotted in Figure 15.5. As expected, at $t = 2970$ s, good agreement is achieved between the current results and those from the HFS-FEM. The temperature on the papillary axis is observed to increase from 34.135°C at the center of the outer corneal surface to 36.618°C at the intersection point of the outer surface of sclera and the horizontal coordinate axis. Simultaneously, the change of heat conduction behavior is clearly illustrated as time progresses. Thus, the computing model presented allows us to obtain a relatively accurate result for the temperature distribution of a human eye and is therefore verified.

15.3.2 EFFECT OF BLOOD PERFUSION RATE

In the analysis of the thermal effects of blood perfusion rate, the value in the literature (Flyckt, Raaymakers, and Lagendijk 2006) is taken into consideration as the control parameter for investigation purposes. This enables us to understand the importance of blood flow in the thermoregulation of the human eye. The effects of blood perfusion on the transient temperature distribution inside the human eye, both at the center of the corneal surface and along the papillary axis, are displayed in Figures 15.6–15.8. It is found from Figure 15.6 that the presence of blood perfusion in parts of the sclera and optic nerve makes the heat transfer more rapidly in the eyeball compared to the case without blood perfusion. Because the blood temperature, which is 37°C here, is the highest in the computing domain, a heating effect rather than a cooling effect takes place, and more heat energy flows from the blood vessels in the sclera region into the eyeball to cause a temperature increase. Figure 15.7 shows the transient temperature variation at the center of the outer corneal surface. We find that a steady

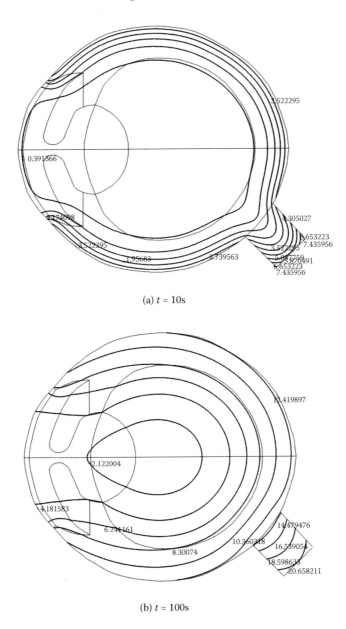

(a) $t = 10s$

(b) $t = 100s$

FIGURE 15.4   Transient temperature distribution in the human eye in the absence of blood perfusion.

(*Continued*)

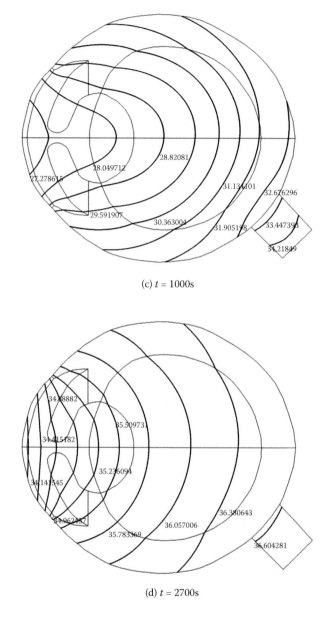

(c) $t = 1000s$

(d) $t = 2700s$

FIGURE 15.4 (*Continued*)   Transient temperature distribution in the human eye in the absence of blood perfusion.

temperature distribution can be obtained at about 1500 s, when the effect of blood perfusion rate is invoked. The steady state temperature at the test point is 34.94°C, which is higher than the corresponding value when the blood perfusion rate is ignored. The results in Figure 15.8 show that the presence of blood perfusion impedes the cooling of the eye with the result that the temperature in the eye is close to that of the

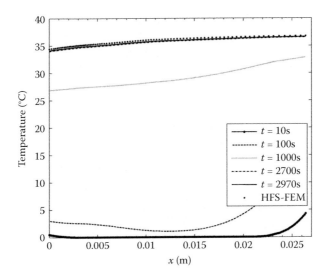

FIGURE 15.5   Temperature variation on the papillary axis in the absence of blood perfusion.

body core. The results obtained from this analysis imply that the blood flow in the eye plays an important role in the overall temperature distribution in the eyeball.

15.3.3   EFFECT OF AMBIENT FLUIDS

The thermal effect of ambient fluid near the outer corneal surface can be analyzed by changing two parameters: ambient temperature and ambient convection coefficient. In the present work, the value of the ambient temperature is restricted to within the range $[0\sim50]°C$ and the ambient convection coefficient is chosen in the range $[10\sim100]$ $Wm^{-2}K^{-1}$ to study the induced temperature response. The evaporation rate is assumed to be 40 Wm^{-2} in the computation. The related numerical results are presented in Figure 15.9 and Figure 15.10. In Figure 15.9, the ambient temperature changes and the convection coefficient of the ambient fluid remains at 10 $Wm^{-2}K^{-1}$. It can be seen from Figure 15.9 that a significant increase in the temperature at the center of the corneal surface can be detected when the ambient temperature increases from 0°C, 25°C to 50°C, each level corresponding to cold, moderate, and extremely hot conditions, respectively. The higher sink temperature allows more heat to flow into the eye and causes a higher corneal surface temperature. In the final steady state, about 3.1°C at the sample point is observed for every increment of 25°C in the ambient temperature. In Figure 15.10, the variation of the convection coefficient is investigated with a sink temperature of $T_\infty =$ 25°C. As expected, we find that the higher value of the convection coefficient of ambient fluid first causes more rapid heating on the cornea surface when $t < 420$ s. It is understandable that in this stage the heat energy flows from the surrounding fluid to the corneal region and the corneal temperature is below 25°C, the sink temperature. Then the higher convection coefficient leads to more heat loss (cooling effect) when $t > 420$ s, and the corresponding steady state temperature is lower, since the corneal surface temperature exceeds the ambient temperature at this stage, and the heat energy flow is reversed.

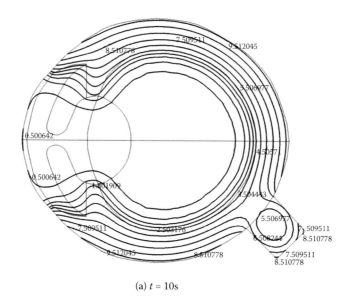

(a) $t = 10$s

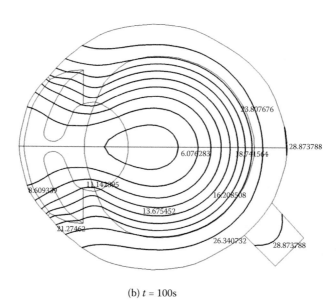

(b) $t = 100$s

FIGURE 15.6   Transient temperature distribution in the human eye with specified blood perfusion.

(Continued)

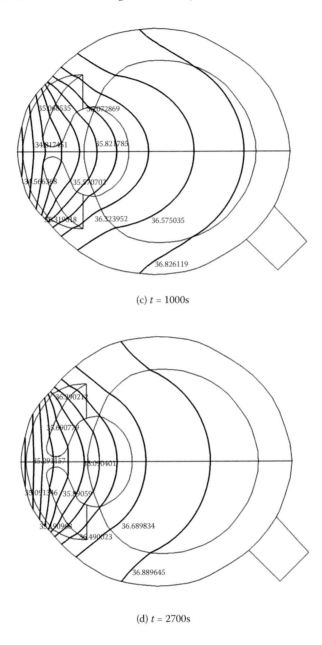

(c) $t = 1000$s

(d) $t = 2700$s

FIGURE 15.6 (Continued)   Transient temperature distribution in the human eye with specified blood perfusion.

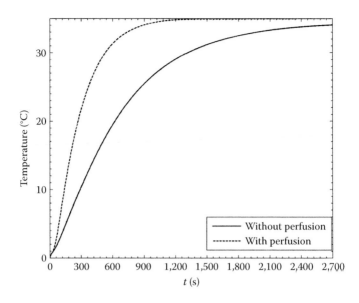

FIGURE 15.7   Transient temperature variation at the center of the corneal surface for two different cases.

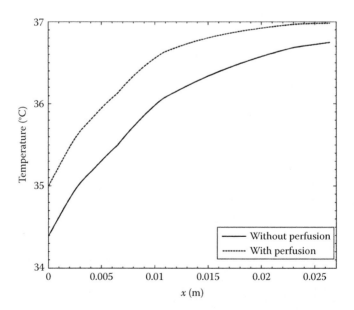

FIGURE 15.8   Steady temperature variation on the papillary axis for two different cases.

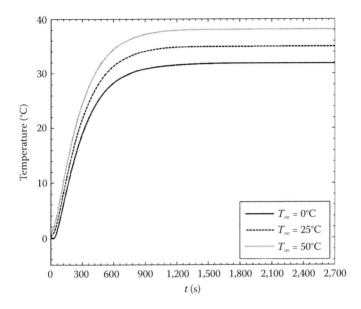

FIGURE 15.9 Temperature variation at the center of the cornea for various ambient temperatures.

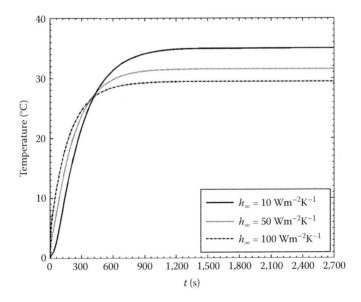

FIGURE 15.10 Temperature variation at the center of the cornea for various ambient fluids.

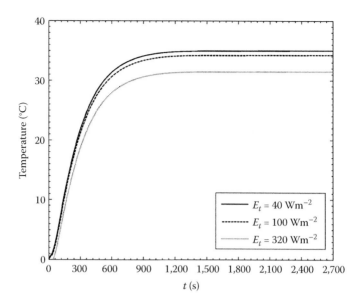

FIGURE 15.11 Temperature variation at the center of the cornea for various tear evaporations.

15.3.4 EFFECT OF TEAR EVAPORATION

There is usually a thin lipid layer covering the corneal surface, the function of which is to prevent evaporation of tears from the corneal surface. When the layer is destroyed, the evaporation rate increases dramatically and can reach as high as 320 Wm^{-2} (Mishima and Maurice 1961), whereas the evaporation rate of normal eyes is in the range of 20–100 Wm^{-2} (Scott 1988). It is therefore important to investigate the effect of evaporation on temperature distribution in the eye model. In the following analysis, the temperature and the convection coefficient of ambient fluid are taken to be 25°C and 10 Wm^{-2}K^{-1}, respectively. The temperature variation at the center of the corneal surface is shown in Figure 15.11, from which it can be seen that the evaporation rate seems to be important in changing the corneal surface temperature. The larger the value of the tear evaporation, the lower is the temperature at the center of the corneal surface. It is understandable that the cooling effect increases as the evaporation rate increases. It is also observed from Figure 15.11 that there is an approximately steady decrease in the value of 0.125°C at the center of the corneal surface for every increment in the value of 10 Wm^{-2} for evaporation rate.

15.4 CONCLUSIONS

In this chapter, a transient FEM model is constructed to perform computer simulation of the thermal states of biological bodies governed by the Pennes bioheat equation. The purpose of this chapter is to investigate the thermal effect in the eyeball caused by blood perfusion rates in the sclera and the optic nerve. It is shown that the eye is very difficult to heat or cool when physiological perfusion is correctly taken into account. Validation of the transient mathematical model including blood perfusion in the eye was performed by comparing the findings with results in the literature. Subsequently, through sensitivity analysis conducted in the presence of blood perfusion in the eyeball, three dominant parameters (ambient temperature, film coefficient of ambient fluid, and tear evaporation rate) were determined, to obtain insight and to weight the importance of each parameter. These parameters significantly affect the surface temperature of the cornea in practice.

ACKNOWLEDGMENT

The work reported in this chapter is partially supported by the Australian Endeavor Awards 2011 and Foundation for University Key Teacher by the Henan Province, China, under the grant no. 2011GGJS-083.

REFERENCES

Brinkmann, R., N. Koop, G. Droege, U. Grotehusmann, A. Huber, and R. Birngruber. 1994. Investigations on laser thermokeratoplasty. *Laser Applications in Ophthalmology, Proceedings of the SPIE*, Budapest, Hungary

Chua, K. J., J. C. Ho, S. K. Chou, and M. R. Islam. 2005. On the study of the temperature distribution within a human eye subjected to a laser source. *International Communications in Heat and Mass Transfer* 32 (8):1057–1065.

Flyckt, V. M. M., B. W. Raaymakers, and J. J. W. Lagendijk. 2006. Modeling the impact of blood flow on the temperature distribution in the human eye and the orbit: Fixed heat transfer coefficients versus the Pennes bioheat model versus discrete blood vessels. *Physics in Medicine and Biology* 51 (19):5007–5021.

Mainster, M. A., T. J. White, and J. H. Tips. 1970. Corneal thermal response to the CO_2 laser. *Applied Optics* 9 (3):665–667.

Mishima, S, and D. M. Maurice. 1961. The effect of normal evaporation on the eye. *Experimental Eye Research* 1 (1):46–52.

Narasimhan, A., K. K. Jha, and L. Gopal. 2010. Transient simulations of heat transfer in human eye undergoing laser surgery. *International Journal of Heat and Mass Transfer* 53 (1–3):482–490.

Ng, E. Y. K., and E. H. Ooi. 2006. FEM simulation of the eye structure with bioheat analysis. *Computer Methods and Programs in Biomedicine* 82 (3):268–276.

Ooi, E. H., W. T. Ang, and E. Y. K. Ng. 2007. Bioheat transfer in the human eye: A boundary element approach. *Engineering Analysis with Boundary Elements* 31 (6):494–500.

Ooi, E. H., W. T. Ang, and E. Y. K. Ng. 2008. A boundary element model of the human eye undergoing laser thermokeratoplasty. *Computers in Biology and Medicine* 38:727–737.

Ooi, E. H., W. T. Ang, and E. Y. K. Ng. 2009. A boundary element model for investigating the effects of eye tumor on the temperature distribution inside the human eye. *Computers in Biology and Medicine* 39 (8):667–677.

Ooi, E. H, and E. Y. K. Ng. 2008. Simulation of aqueous humor hydrodynamics in human eye heat transfer. *Computers in Biology and Medicine* 38 (2):252–262.

Paruch, M. 2007. Numerical simulation of bioheat transfer process in the human eye using finite element method. *Scientific Research of the Institute of Mathematics and Computer Science* 1(6), Częstochowa, Poland.

Pennes, H. H. 1948. Analysis of tissue and arterial blood temperatures in the resting human forearm. *Journal of Applied Physiology* 1 (2):93–102.

Peratta, A. 2008. 3D low frequency electromagnetic modeling of the human eye with boundary elements: Application to conductive keratoplasty. *Engineering Analysis with Boundary Elements* 32 (9):726–735.

Scott, J. A. 1988. A finite element model of heat transport in the human eye. *Physics in Medicine and Biology* 33:227–242.

Wang, H., and Q. H. Qin. 2010. FE approach with Green's function as internal trial function for simulating bioheat transfer in the human eye. *Archives of Mechanics* 62 (6):493–510.

16 Modeling and Simulation of Bioheat Transfer in the Human Eye with Edge-Based Smoothed Finite Element Method (ES-FEM)

Eric Li, GR Liu, Vincent Tan, and ZC He

CONTENTS

16.1   INTRODUCTION

Cancer cells in the eyes can develop into tumors. They are often found in the eyeball, the eyelids, and the orbit. Generally, there are two types of tumors, known as retinoblastoma and melanoma, within the eyes that can badly affect vision. In serious cases, eye tumors can spread to the other parts of the body. Therefore, detection of the eye tumors and early treatment are very important. Various methods have been developed to treat eye tumors. The most popular clinical treatments are surgery, cryosurgery, hyperthermia, and immunotherapy depending on the location, size, and aggressiveness of the tumor. Hyperthermia and cryosurgery are often found to be more powerful and effective. Immunotherapy is still largely experimental. In all these treatments, accurate modeling in the human eye is an effective tool to improve precision. There are many computational models of the human eye currently available. Taflove and Brodwin [1] used the finite difference method (FDM) to simulate heat transfer across the human eye to investigate microwave radiation effects. Ooi [2] analyzed the effects of natural convection on the aqueous humor using the finite element method (FEM). However, very little research on modeling hyperthermia in the human eye is available. The objective of hyperthermia is to raise the tumor temperature above 315 K without damaging the surrounding tissue. The main challenge of hyperthermia is to minimize the damage to healthy tissue. Therefore, it is very important to accurately predict temperature distribution for tumor hyperthermia treatment.

The FDM and FEM have played an important role in the modeling of heat transfer of human eye. However, the FDM is limited to simple geometry. In contrast, the FEM can handle much more complicated geometry, but FEM is limited by the rigid reliance on elements.

To overcome the limitations of the FEM, many meshfree methods have been developed [3–5]. Compared with FEM, numerical treatments in meshfree methods are not confined by the elements/cells. Thus meshfree methods can produce more accurate solutions and display more flexibility in implementation, higher convergence rate, and greater effectiveness. Currently, the node-based smoothed finite element method (NS-FEM) [6–7] is often capable of providing upper bound solution in energy norm using the same mesh as that used in FEM for force-driven elasticity problems [6–7]. In NS-FEM, the shape functions are constructed using point interpolation methods for points on the edges of the smoothing domains. Instead of using compatible strain in the FEM, NS-FEM uses smoothed strains obtained in a boundary integral form. The strain smoothing domains and the integration are all operated over the domains associated with nodes.

However, NS-FEM does not work very well for time-dependent problems due to "overly soft" behavior [6–7] caused by the excessive node-based smoothing operations leading to temporal instability. To overcome this problem, the edge-based smoothed finite element method (ES-FEM) [8–9] for 2D problems with the strain smoothing performed over the edge-based smoothing domain and the face-based smoothed finite element method (FS-FEM) [9–10] for 3D problems with the strain smoothing performed over the face-based smoothing domain have been proposed. Compared with FEM and NS-FEM, ES-FEM (or FS-FEM) often gives close-to-exact stiffness and the solutions are much more accurate and stable both spatially and temporally.

In ES-FEM, strain smoothing domains and the integration are operated over the edge-based (2D) and face-based (3D) smoothing domains, respectively. The smoothing domain of an edge is created by connecting the nodes at two ends of the edge to centroids of two adjacent elements that can be triangular, quadrilateral, and even n-sided polygonal elements. In this work, we formulate the ES-FEM and FS-FEM for accurate solutions to the bioheat transfer in the human eye.

This chapter is organized as follows: Section 16.2 briefly describes the mathematical model of the bioheat transfer problems. Section 16.3 briefs the detailed formulation of ES-FEM and FS-FEM for bioheat transfer problem. Section 16.4 outlines the 2D example of hyperthermia treatment. In Section 16.5, discussions on sensitivity analysis and hyperthermia treatment for the 3D human eye are presented. Finally, the conclusions from the numerical results are made in Section 16.6.

16.2 MATHEMATICAL MODEL FOR HUMAN EYE

The eye anatomy is shown in Figure 16.1. The anterior portion of the eye consists of the cornea, anterior chamber, and iris. The posterior portion includes the lens, vitreous, and sclera. A, B, C, D, and E are points on the corneal surface, anterior of lens, anterior of vitreous, posterior of vitreous, and the sclera. The Pennes bioheat equation [11] is used to analyze heat transfer in the human eye:

$$\rho c \frac{\partial T}{\partial t} = k\nabla^2 T + \omega \rho c_b (T_{bl} - T) + Q_m + Q \tag{16.1}$$

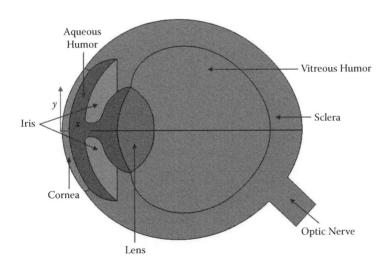

FIGURE 16.1   Anatomy of 2D model of eye [2]. (a) Edge-based smoothing domains in 2D problem for gradient smoothing and integration are created by sequentially connecting the centroids of the adjacent triangles with the end-points of the edge. (b) For 3D problems, the smoothing domain is created using the neighbor tetrahedral elements by connecting vertexes of the triangle (face k) to the centroids of two adjacent elements. (Please see color insert.)

In the Pennes' model, the main assumption is that the net rate heat transfer between blood and tissue is proportional to the product of the volumetric perfusion rate and the difference between the arterial blood temperature and the local tissue temperature. The blood acts as a local distributed, scalar source when positive, or sink when negative. The four terms on the right-hand side of the bioheat equation are blood conduction, blood perfusion, metabolism, and external heat source. Since only a small part in the human eye is responsible for blood perfusion and metabolic heat generation, these two terms can be neglected. Thus, the final governing equation for steady state condition can be written as follows:

$$k\nabla^2 T + Q = 0 \qquad (16.2)$$

where k is the thermal conductivity of tissue of human eye, T is the temperature of tissue of human eye, and Q is the external heat source.

The first boundary condition can be defined as follows:
At the sclera,

$$-k\frac{\partial T}{\partial n} = h_{bl}(T - T_{bl}) \qquad (16.3)$$

Here, n is the outward normal direction on the surface boundary, h_{bl} is the coefficient of ambient convection, and T_{bl} is the blood temperature.

The second boundary condition is at the cornea, where heat is lost to the ambient environment:

$$-k\frac{\partial T}{\partial n} = h_{amb}(T - T_{amb}) + \sigma\varepsilon(T^4 - T_{amb}^4) + E \qquad (16.4)$$

The three terms on the RHS equation denote heat loss due to convection, radiation, and tears evaporation. T_{bl}, σ, ε, and E denote the ambient temperature, the Stefan-Boltzmann constant (5.67×10^{-8} $Wm^{-2}K^{-4}$), emissivity (0.975), and evaporation rate.

The properties of each structure of the eye are listed in Table 16.1 [12].

TABLE 16.1
Properties of the Human Eye

	Thermal Conductivity (Wm⁻¹K⁻¹)	Specific Heat	Density (kgm⁻³)
Cornea	0.58	4178	1050
Aqueous	0.58	3997	996
Iris	1.0042	3180	1100
Lens	0.40	3000	1050
Vitreous body	0.603	4178	1000
Sclera	1.0042	3180	1100

16.3 FORMULATION OF THE ES-FEM AND FS-FEM

16.3.1 DISCRETIZED SYSTEM EQUATIONS

In this section, we first present the formulation of the FEM based on the standard Galerkin weak form [13–14]. The weighted residual equation can be obtained by multiplying Eq. (16.2) with a test function w in the entire domain:

$$\int_{\Omega} (wk\nabla^2 T + wQ)d\Omega = 0 \tag{16.5}$$

Using integration by parts,

$$k\int_{\Omega} \nabla w \cdot \nabla T d\Omega = Q\int_{\Omega} w d\Omega - \int_{\Gamma_2} wh_{bl}(T - T_{bl})\mathrm{d}\Gamma$$
$$- \int_{\Gamma_3} w((h_{amb}(T - T_{amb}) + \sigma\varepsilon(T^4 - T_{amb}^4) + E)\mathrm{d}\Gamma \tag{16.6}$$

The field temperature can be approximated in the following form:

$$T = \sum_{i=1}^{m} \mathbf{N}_i \mathbf{T}_i \tag{16.7}$$

where $\mathbf{N}_i$ is the shape function and $\mathbf{T}_i$ is the unknown nodal temperature. In the Galerkin weak form, the weight function w is replaced by shape function N.

So the standard Galerkin weak form is expressed as

$$k\int_{\Omega} \nabla\mathbf{N} \cdot \nabla\mathbf{T}d\Omega + h_{bl}\int_{\Gamma_2} \mathbf{N} \cdot \mathbf{NT}\mathrm{d}\Gamma + h_{amb}\int_{\Gamma_3} \mathbf{N} \cdot \mathbf{NT}\mathrm{d}\Gamma$$
$$= Q\int_{\Omega} \mathbf{N}d\Omega + \int_{\Gamma_2} \mathbf{N}h_{bl}T_{bl}\,\mathrm{d}\Gamma - \int_{\Gamma_3} \mathbf{N}(-T_{amb} + \sigma\varepsilon(T^4 - T_{amb}^4) + E)\mathrm{d}\Gamma \tag{16.8}$$

The discretized system equation can be finally obtained and written in the following matrix form:

$$[\mathbf{K} + \mathbf{M}]\{\mathbf{T}\} = \{\mathbf{F}\} \tag{16.9}$$

where the stiffness, force, and mass matrices are given by

$$\mathbf{K} = k\int_{\Omega} \nabla\mathbf{N} \cdot \nabla\mathbf{N}d\Omega \tag{16.10}$$

$$\mathbf{F} = Q \int_{\Omega} \mathbf{N} d\Omega + \int_{\Gamma_2} \mathbf{N} h_{bl} T_{bl} \, d\Gamma + \int_{\Gamma_3} \mathbf{N}(T_{amb} + T_{amb}^4 - E) d\Gamma$$

$$- \int_{\Gamma_3} \mathbf{N} \sigma \varepsilon T^4 \, d\Gamma \tag{16.11}$$

$$\mathbf{M} = h_{bl} \int_{\Gamma_2} \mathbf{N} \cdot \mathbf{N} \mathbf{T} d\Gamma + h_{amb} \int_{\Gamma_3} \mathbf{N} \cdot \mathbf{N} \mathbf{T} \, d\Gamma \tag{16.12}$$

It is noted that the presence of the nonlinear term in the force matrix can be dealt with by using an iterative scheme in the solution.

16.3.2 NUMERICAL INTEGRATION WITH EDGE-BASED GRADIENT SMOOTHING OPERATION

This section formulates gradient smoothing domains of ES-FEM for 2D and 3D problems using triangular elements and tetrahedral elements, respectively. The formulation is almost the same for any other 2D and 3D n-side polygonal elements as long as the simple point interpolation method is used to create shape functions [15]. In the process of numerical integrations of ES-FEM for 2D problems, a mesh of three-node triangles is generated first, which can be done easily and automatically using any mesh generator. Afterward, the problem domain Ω is further divided into N smoothing domains associated with edges of the triangles such that $\Omega_1 \cup \Omega_2 \cup \dots$ $\Omega_N = \Omega$ and $\Omega_i \cap \Omega_j = \emptyset$, $i \neq j$, where N is the number of total edges of triangles. As shown in Figure 16.2(a), the smoothing domain Ω_k for edge k is created by connecting sequentially the endpoints of edge k to the centroids of the neighbor triangles. Extending the smoothing domain Ω_k in 3D problems, the domain discretization is the same as that of standard FEM using tetrahedral elements and the smoothing domain is formed associated with the faces of tetrahedrons. As shown in Figure 16.2(b), the smoothing domain Ω_k for face k is created using the neighbor tetrahedral elements by connecting vertexes of the triangle (face k) to the centroids of two adjacent elements.

The boundary of the smoothing domain Ω_k of edge k (or face k) is labeled as Γ_k and the union of all Ω_k forms the global domain Ω exactly. To perform the numerical integration based on the smoothing domains, Eq. (16.10) can be further rewritten as

$$\overline{\mathbf{K}} = \sum_{k=1}^{N} \overline{\mathbf{K}}^{(k)} \tag{16.13}$$

in which

$$\overline{\mathbf{K}}^{(k)} = k \int_{\Omega_k} \overline{\mathbf{B}}^{\mathrm{T}} \overline{\mathbf{B}} d\Omega \tag{16.14}$$

The generalized gradient smoothing technique that works also for discontinuous field functions [16] is now applied over the smoothing domain to obtain the smoothed nodal gradient for the interested node $\mathbf{x}_k$:

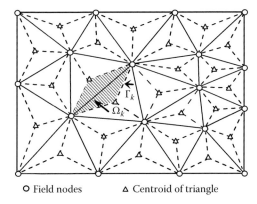

O Field nodes   Δ Centroid of triangle

(a) Edge-based smoothing domains in 2D problem for gradient smoothing and integration are created by sequentially connecting the centroids of the adjacent triangles with the end-points of the edge.

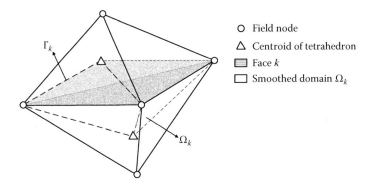

O Field node
Δ Centroid of tetrahedron
▨ Face k
☐ Smoothed domain Ω_k

(b) For 3D problems, the smoothing domain is created using the neighbor tetrahedral elements by connecting vertexes of the triangle (face k) to the centroids of two adjacent elements.

FIGURE 16.2   Illustration of construction of smoothing domain for 2D and 3D problems.

$$\overline{g_i}(\mathbf{x}_k) = \int_{\Omega_k} g_i(\mathbf{x}) W(\mathbf{x} - \mathbf{x}_k) d\Omega \tag{16.15}$$

where g_i is the derivative of the field function (temperature) with respect to x_i, and W is a smoothing function. For simplicity, a piecewise constant function is used:

$$\overline{W}(\mathbf{x} - \mathbf{x}_k) = \begin{cases} 1/V_k & \mathbf{x} \in \Omega_k \\ 0 & \mathbf{x} \notin \Omega_k \end{cases} \tag{16.16}$$

where $V_k = \int_{\Omega_k} d\Omega$ is the area of smoothing domain for edge k in 2D problems. When it comes to 3D problems, the V_k is the volume of smoothing domain for face k.

The temperature gradient for node k and for any point in the smoothing domain is obtained as follows even for discontinuous assumed functions of temperature [30]:

$$\overline{g}_i(\mathbf{x}_k) = \frac{1}{V_k} \int_{\Gamma_k} T n_i \, d\Gamma \qquad (16.17)$$

which is constant in the smoothing domain Ω_k. Using FEM shape functions to construct the field function for temperature, the smoothed gradient for node k can be written in the following matrix form:

$$\overline{\mathbf{g}}(\mathbf{x}_k) = \sum_{I \in D_k} \overline{\mathbf{B}}_I^{\Omega_k} T_I \qquad (16.18)$$

where D_k is the set of all the nodes used in the interpolation for the field function on Ω_k.

$$\overline{\mathbf{g}}^{\mathrm{T}} = \{\overline{g}_1 \quad \overline{g}_2\} \qquad (16.19)$$

$$\left[\overline{\mathbf{B}}_I^{\Omega_k}\right]^T = \left[\overline{b}_{I1} \quad \overline{b}_{I2}\right] \qquad (16.20)$$

$$\overline{b}_{Ip} = \frac{1}{A_k} \int_{\Gamma_k} \mathbf{N}_I(\mathbf{x}) n_p(\mathbf{x}) d\Gamma \qquad (p = 1, 2) \qquad (16.21)$$

For three-dimensional spaces, the corresponding forms are given by

$$\overline{\mathbf{g}}^{\mathrm{T}} = \{\overline{g}_1 \quad \overline{g}_2 \quad \overline{g}_3\} \qquad (16.22)$$

$$\left[\overline{\mathbf{B}}_I^{\Omega_k}\right]^T = \left[\overline{b}_{I1} \quad \overline{b}_{I2} \quad \overline{b}_{I3}\right] \qquad (16.23)$$

$$\overline{b}_{Ip} = \frac{1}{V_k} \int_{\Gamma_k} \mathbf{N}_I(\mathbf{x}) n_p(\mathbf{x}) d\Gamma \qquad (p = 1, 2, 3) \qquad (16.24)$$

where $N_I(X)$ is the shape function for node I.

Using Gauss integration along each segment (or each surface triangle for 3D) of boundary Γ_k of the smoothing domain Ω_k, the above equations can be rewritten in the following summation forms as

$$\bar{b}_{ip} = \frac{1}{A_k} \sum_{q=1}^{N_s} \left[\sum_{r=1}^{N_g} w_r \mathbf{N}_i(\mathbf{x}_{qr}) n_p(\mathbf{x}_q) \right] \tag{16.25}$$

where N_s is the number of segments (or each surface triangle for 3D) of the boundary Γ_k, N_g is the number of Gauss points distributed in each segment (or each surface triangle), and w_r is the corresponding weight for the Gauss point. The smoothed stiffness matrix shown in Eq. (16.13) can be calculated as

$$\overline{\mathbf{K}}^{(k)} = k \int_\Omega \overline{\mathbf{B}}^{\mathrm{T}} \overline{\mathbf{B}} d\Omega = k \overline{\mathbf{B}}^{\mathrm{T}} \overline{\mathbf{B}} A_k \tag{16.26}$$

It can be easily seen from Eq. (16.26) that the resultant linear system is symmetric and banded (due to the compact supports of FEM shape functions), which implies that the system equations can be solved efficiently.

16.4 NUMERICAL RESULTS FOR 2D PROBLEM IN HYPERTHERMIA TREATMENT

16.4.1 BRIEF DESCRIPTION OF HYPERTHERMIA MODEL

Hyperthermia is often used in clinical applications in tumor treatment control by artificially raising the tissue temperature to gain therapeutic benefits. In the hyperthermia treatment, the heat source is localized to the targeted area to elevate the temperature to cause the death of cancerous cells [17]. The heat source can be microwave, radiofrequency, or ultrasound. To simplify the problem, the detail of heat source is ignored. Thus, the knowledge of the temperature distribution and heat transport rates is important in hyperthermia treatments. The goal of this study is to evaluate the potential to apply the ES-FEM and FS-FEM to become a viable method for human eye cancer treatment. The main feature of hyperthermia treatment is to increase the tumor temperature up to 315 K–319 K without major intervention of the surrounding tissue. It is noted that the ambient temperature is kept at 273 K in the hyperthermia treatment simulation. To compare the accuracy of ES-FEM, two sets of mesh as shown in Figure 16.3 are used to analyze the temperature distribution in the hyperthermia treatment. As shown in Figure 16.3, the external heat source is uniformly distributed in a small circle with radius $r = 0.36$ mm, and the power of heat source is $Q_{rm} = 3.5 \times 10^7$ w/m³.

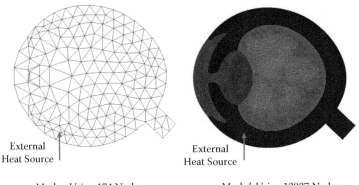

External
Heat Source

External
Heat Source

Mesh *a* Using 174 Nodes   Mesh *b* Using 12827 Nodes

FIGURE 16.3 Four sets of different mesh with heat source distributed in a small circle. Center of heat source: x = 8.5 mm, y = −9.2 mm. (Please see color insert.)

16.4.2 TEMPERATURE DISTRIBUTION

As shown in Figure 16.4, the temperature contours for ES-FEM, FEM using coarse mesh, and reference result using very fine mesh are presented. The model created by ES-FEM clearly provides more accurate results than the FEM model using the same three-node triangular mesh and linear shape functions. This demonstrates our two-dimensional ES-FEM model for bioheat transfer in the human eye. In the hyperthermia treatment, the temperature of healthy tissue must be below the critical threshold. From Figure 16.4, it is also observed that the tissue temperature around the heating source is around 310 K, which has an excellent benefit in hyperthermia treatment. This is one of the most attractive features of internal heating and it is frequently used to thermally kill tumors in deep tissue, although it may cause some mechanical injuries [18]. As shown in Figure 16.4, the maximum temperature always occurs at the heating source in the ES-FEM model, FEM model, and reference model. Thus, it is necessary to analyze the temperature at the heating source.

As illustrated in Figure 16.5, the temperature distribution along the circumference of the heat source in a counterclockwise direction starting from the left horizontal is outlined. The temperature obtained from ES-FEM is closer with the reference solution compared with FEM, which is due to the "softer model" created by the ES-FEM.

The maximum temperature at the heating source is shown in Figure 16.6. Again, the ES-FEM result agrees with the reference solution very well. On the contrary, a large deviation between the FEM and reference result is observed in Figure 16.6. The predicated maximum temperature obtained from the ES-FEM is about 1.49 K away from the reference solution. That of the FEM is, however, about 3.21 K, when the same mesh is used. In the medical treatment, accurate prediction of temperature distribution is extremely important. Therefore, the improvement of ES-FEM on the solution accuracy is significant. Such an improvement is achieved by "a close-to-exact stiffness" property of the ES-FEM [9–10].

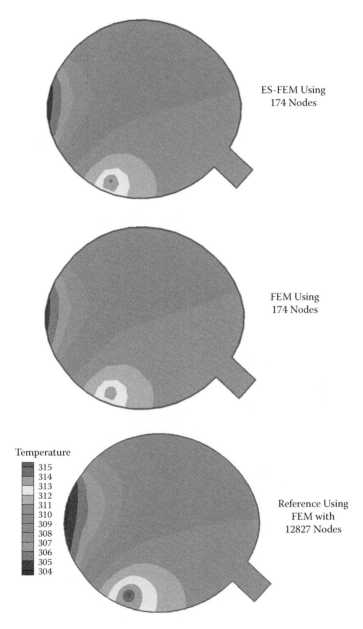

ES-FEM Using
174 Nodes

FEM Using
174 Nodes

Temperature

315
314
313
312
311
310
309
308
307
306
305
304

Reference Using
FEM with
12827 Nodes

FIGURE 16.4 Temperature contour of 2D eye model under hyperthermia treatment. (Please see color insert.)

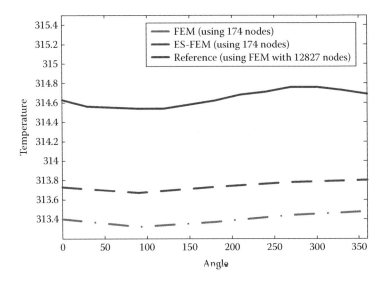

FIGURE 16.5 Temperature distribution at the heating source. (Please see color insert.)

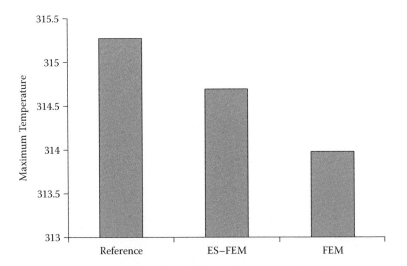

FIGURE 16.6 Comparison for maximum temperature at the heating source. (Please see color insert.)

16.5 NUMERICAL RESULTS FOR 3D ANALYSIS

16.5.1 HYPERTHERMIA MODEL

In this section, the 3D model of the human eye in the hyperthermia treatment is investigated. The 3D model as illustrated in Figure 16.7 is more realistic to predict the temperature distribution accurately in the medical treatment. As shown in

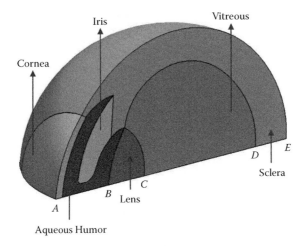

FIGURE 16.7   3D quarter model of human eye. (Please see color insert.)

Figure 16.8, the heating source is uniformly distributed in a small sphere with radius $r = 0.6$ mm. The power of heat source is $Q_{rm} = 4 \times 10^7$ w/m^3.

The computational domain of the 3D human eye is first discretized with 1292 regularly distributed nodes, based on which the four-node tetrahedrons are constructed as shown in Figure 16.8. For the purpose of comparison, the FEM solutions are also calculated using the same tetrahedral mesh. The reference solutions are obtained using FEM with a refined mesh of 17,867 regular nodes.

The computed temperature patterns of the whole domain using FS-FEM are plotted in Figure 16.9, together with linear FEM and reference solutions. Figure 16.9 shows that the temperature contours at the corneal surface obtained from the FS-FEM model are in very good agreement with those of the reference ones compared with the FEM model. The minimum temperature occurs at the corneal surface where there is a large heat transfer between the eye and the cooling ambient. Figure 16.10 presents the temperature contours for section Y-Y obtained from FEM, FS-FEM, and reference model. As shown in Figure 16.10, a large deviation between the FEM model and reference is observed, while the FS-FEM still provides very accurate results compared with FEM using the same coarse mesh. This validates our 3D FS-FEM model for bioheat transfer problems. As shown in Figure 16.10, the location of peak temperature is heating source position. The raised temperature will kill the tumor without damaging the healthy tissue. Thus, the accurate prediction of temperature at the heating source is crucial to determine a successful treatment.

Figure 16.11 presents the peak temperature at the heating source. This figure shows that the FS-FEM results agree well with the reference solutions, and are more accurate than those obtained from linear FEM using the same mesh. The difference of predicated maximum temperature between the FS-FEM and the reference solution is about 1.41 K. That of the FEM is, however, about 3.12 K with the same mesh. This finding demonstrates again that FS-FEM works well even in the 3D model compared with FEM. It is noted that the present FS-FEM formulation is derived from the smoothed

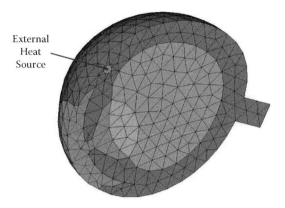

(a) Coarse mesh with 1292 nodes for section Y-Y

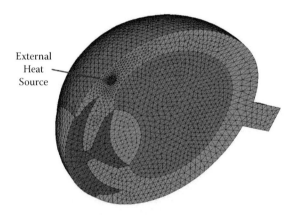

(b) Very fine mesh with 17867 nodes for section Y-Y

FIGURE 16.8   Two sets of different mesh with heat source distributed in a small sphere. (Please see color insert.)

Galerkin weak form, and the FS-FEM model so constructed behaves "softer" compared with the FEM model. The FS-FEM has a "close-to-exact" stiffness feature and hence produces much more accurate results.

16.5.2   Sensitivity Analysis

A similar analysis for the 2D eye model has been done by [2,19–20] to study various factors determining the temperature distribution within the eye. In this section, the 3D FS-FEM model is established to identify the key factors affecting the temperature distribution in the human eye and provide some possibilities to identify the sickness. It is shown in Table 16.2 [2] that all other parameters are under steady state condition when changing the control parameters. The numerical results at five sample points A (the intersection of the anterior corneal surface with the axis of

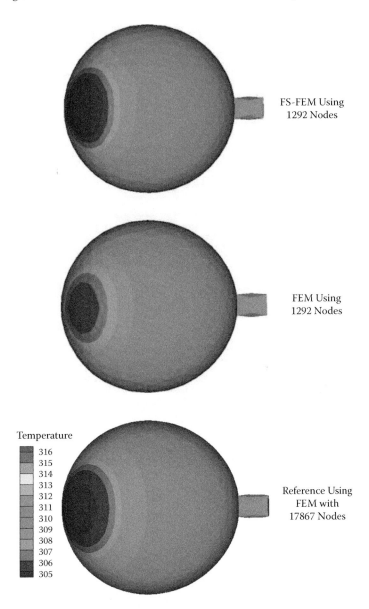

FS-FEM Using
1292 Nodes

FEM Using
1292 Nodes

Temperature

316
315
314
313
312
311
310
309
308
307
306
305

Reference Using
FEM with
17867 Nodes

FIGURE 16.9   Temperature contour of 3D eye model under hyperthermia treatment. (Please see color insert.)

symmetry), B (anterior of lens), C (anterior of vitreous), D (posterior of vitreous), and E (sclera) are calculated to carry out the sensitivity analysis.

In the following investigations, the fine mesh of 17,386 nodes is used for the sensitivity analysis using FS-FEM [20]. To examine the algorithm of FS-FEM, a comparison of numerical results between the FS-FEM and αFEM [20] is made.

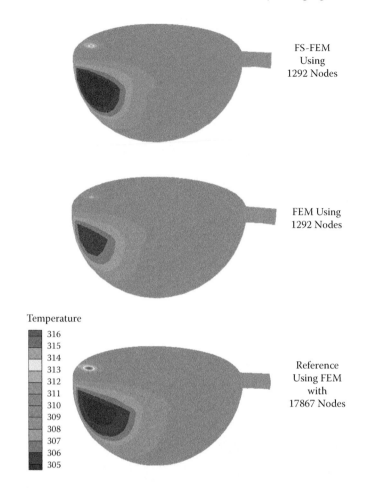

FIGURE 16.10   Temperature contour of 3D eye model for section Y-Y. (Please see color insert.)

16.5.2.1   Effects of Evaporation Rate

A three-layered structure—a thin mucoid layer, a thick aqueous layer, and an extremely thin oily layer—is inside the cornea surface. The oily layer has the function to retard evaporation from the eye. There are five sets of data used in this investigation. All the test data are between the maximum and minimum values recorded in experiments. Results in Table 16.3 have indicated that evaporation rate is an important factor influencing the temperature distribution. From 30 Wm^{-2} to 230 Wm^{-2}, the temperature is dropped by almost 2 K at the corneal surface. The tear loss and tear production balance the moisture level in the eyes. Excessive or insufficient evaporation rate will break the balance. When this balance is broken, dry spots form on the surface of the eyes and cause irritation. Hence the doctor can check for the symptoms and signs of chronic dry eye through the measurement of ocular temperature.

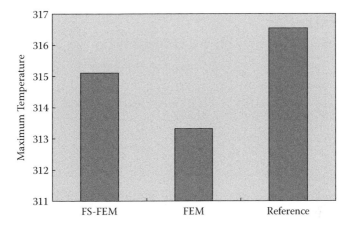

FIGURE 16.11 Comparison for maximum temperature at the heating source. (Please see color insert.)

TABLE 16.2
Parameters under Steady-State Condition

h_{amb}	Ambient convection coefficient	10 Wm^{-2}K^{-1}
h_{bl}	Blood convection coefficient	65 Wm^{-2}K^{-1}
T_{amb}	Ambient temperature	293 K
E	Evaporation rate	40 Wm^{-2}
T_{bl}	Blood temperature	310 K

TABLE 16.3
Effect of Evaporation Rate

	Temperature Distribution (K)				
E (Wm^{-2})	A	B	C	D	E
30	306.83	308.74	309.25	309.87	309.83
80	306.36	308.47	309.17	309.77	309.80
130	305.81	308.25	309.01	309.74	309.78
180	305.33	308.08	308.90	309.71	309.76
230	304.81	307.83	308.77	309.69	309.74

16.5.2.2   Effects of Ambient Convection Coefficient

In this section, the influence of the ambient convection coefficient is investigated. As mentioned in Section 16.2, there is heat exchange between the eye and the ambient. The results in Table 16.4 have shown that the temperature in the human eye decreases with increase of the ambient convection coefficient. The temperature at the corneal surface is the most sensitive to the variation of the ambient convection

TABLE 16.4
Effect of Ambient Convection Coefficient

H (Wm^{-2}K^{-1})	Temperature Distribution (K)				
	A	B	C	D	E
15	306.69	308.34	309.03	309.75	309.84
30	304.33	307.65	308.63	309.66	309.71
50	302.53	306.86	308.23	309.52	309.65
80	300.57	305.92	307.74	309.43	309.52
100	299.67	305.52	307.41	309.36	309.47

TABLE 16.5
Effect of Ambient Temperature

T (K)	Temperature Distribution (K)				
	A	B	C	D	E
273	303.64	307.35	308.55	309.61	309.72
278	304.40	307.69	308.72	309.67	309.75
283	305.21	308.03	308.92	309.70	309.79
303	308.42	309.33	309.65	309.90	309.96
308	309.23	309.67	309.82	309.95	309.99

coefficient. However, the temperature for the inner part of human eye is not overly sensitive to the ambient convection coefficient.

16.5.2.3 Effects of Ambient Temperature

There is heat loss at the corneal surface due to convection and radiation, which is strongly related with the ambient temperature. In addition, the ambient temperature is also one of the factors that affect the amount of tears in the eyes. The best way to relieve the symptoms of dry eye is to keep the eyes moist. In this section, five ambient temperatures listed in Table 16.5 are chosen to investigate the effect of the ambient temperature. It is noticed that there is a significant change at the corneal surface temperature. However, only slight change in the retinal temperature with variation of the ambient temperature is observed.

16.5.2.4 Effect of Blood Temperature

At the unexposed eye, there is a heat exchange between the blood and the retina. Five values—308, 309, 310, 311, and 312 K—are employed to evaluate the effect of blood temperature. It is noted that blood temperatures of 308, 310, and 312 K are undesirable for the human eye. The objective of discussion of these parameters is to provide the possibility of detecting sickness based on the ocular temperature [2]. For example, fever can be detected by the measurement of ocular temperature. Based on the ocular temperature, the doctor can have a better understanding of the patient's condition and provide more effective treatment. From Table 16.6, it is shown that the blood temperature has a great influence on the temperature distribution in the human eye compared with the blood convection coefficient. The temperature is dropped by more than 3 K when the blood temperature varies from 308 K to 312 K. It is no wonder that the blood temperature plays an extremely important role in regulating the human body's temperature.

16.5.2.5   Effect of Blood Convection Coefficient

The movement of the blood flow in the human eye is determined by the blood convection coefficient. In this section, the values 50, 70, 90, 110, and 120 $Wm^{-2}K^{-1}$ are employed to assess the importance of the blood convection coefficient. Table 16.7 shows that the temperature variation at each location is minimally affected. The temperature difference between the maximum and minimum blood convection coefficient is less than 0.5 K.

From the above analysis, it is found that the results obtained from the FS-FEM are very close with the solutions obtained from αEFM [20], which has demonstrated the validity of FS-FEM again. However, the selection of alpha value in the αEFM is still a challenging task, and the implementation of αEFM is more complicated compared with the FS-FEM. Therefore, the ES-FEM and FS-FEM models are excellent candidates to simulate the bioheat heat transfer in the human eye. It is also found that the evaporation, ambient temperature, and blood temperature are the most important factors dominating the temperature distribution in the human eye.

TABLE 16.6
Effect of Blood Temperature

T (K)	Temperature Distribution (K)				
	A	**B**	**C**	**D**	**E**
308	305.11	306.82	307.30	307.85	307.88
309	305.92	307.72	308.25	308.81	308.85
310	306.79	308.68	309.23	309.80	309.82
311	307.61	309.57	310.24	310.81	310.85
312	308.44	310.50	311.19	311.81	311.85

TABLE 16.7
Effect of Blood Convection Coefficient

H ($Wm^{-2}K^{-1}$)	Temperature Distribution (K)				
	A	**B**	**C**	**D**	**E**
50	306.62	308.55	309.15	309.75	309.79
70	306.83	308.72	309.31	309.85	309.88
90	306.91	308.82	309.42	309.92	309.94
110	306.96	308.85	309.45	309.95	309.97
120	306.99	308.88	309.47	309.96	309.98

16.6 CONCLUSION

In this work, ES-FEM and FS-FEM are formulated to determine the temperature distribution of the human eye under hyperthermia treatment. In addition, sensitivity analysis is also conducted to analyze the dominated factors that affect the temperature distribution in the human eye. Apart from that, it is found that temperature in the ocular surface is a good indicator to provide some alternative ways to detect sickness. The following conclusions can be derived:

1. The stiffness of the discretized model in ES-FEM and FS-FEM is reduced compared to the FEM.
2. The ES-FEM using the triangular elements in 2D and FS-FEM using tetrahedral elements in 3D are quite stable and accurate. Compared with FEM, there are no additional parameters in ES-FEM and FS-FEM. Hence this method can be implanted in a straightforward way. However, the FEM does not like such elements and often gives poor solution of accuracy, especially at high temperature gradient region. In the hyperthermia treatment, the temperature changes very quickly at the tumor region. Thus, the results obtained from FEM using triangular elements are poor due to its "overly stiff" behavior.
3. Based on the sensitivity analysis, it has been found that blood temperature, ambient temperature, and evaporation rate are the most important factors affecting the corneal surface temperature.
4. Last but not least, the measurement of ocular surface temperature of the human eye can provide a fast and safe way to detect fever and dry eye, which can help the doctor to improve the diagnosis and treatment.

REFERENCES

1. Taflove A, Brodwin M. Computation of the electromagnetic fields and induced temperatures within a model of the microwave-irradiated human eye. *IEEE Trans. Microw. Theory Tech.* 1975; MTT-23(11): 888–896.
2. Ooi EH, Ng EY. Simulation of aqueous humor hydrodynamics in human eye heat transfer. *Comput. Biol. Med.* 2008; 38 (2): 252–262.
3. Lucy LB. A numerical approach to testing of the fission hypothesis. *Astron. J.* 1977; 8(12): 1013–1024.
4. Monaghan JJ. An introduction to SPH. *Comput. Phys. Commun.* 1998; 48(1): 89–96.
5. Liu GR, Liu MB. *Smoothed Particle Hydrodynamics—A Meshfree Particle Method*, World Scientific: Singapore, 2003.
6. Liu GR, Nguyen TT, Nguyen XH, Lam KY. A node-based smoothed finite element method (NS-FEM) for upper bound solutions to solid mechanics problems. *Comput. Struct.* 2009; 87: 14–26.
7. Liu GR, Zhang GY. Upper bound solution to elasticity problems: A unique property of the linearly conforming point interpolation method (LC-PIM). *Int. J. Numer. Method Engrg* 2008; 74: 1128–1161.
8. Liu GR, Nguyen TT, Lam KY. An edge-based smoothed finite element method (E-SFEM for static and dynamic problems of solid mechanics. *J. Sound Vibr.* 2009; 320: 1100–1130.
9. Li E, Liu GR, Tan V, He ZC. Simulation of hyperthermia treatment using the edge-based smoothed finite-element method. *Numer. Heat Transfer A* 2010; 57(11): 822–847.

10. Nguyen TT, Liu GR, Lam KY, Zhang GY. A face-based smoothed finite element method (FS-FEM) for 3D linear and nonlinear solid mechanics problems using 4-node tetrahedral elements. *Int. J. Numer. Methods Eng.* 2009; 78: 324–353.

11. Pennes HH. Analysis of tissue and arterial blood temperatures in the resting forearm. *J. Appl. Physiology* 1948; 1: 93–122.

12. Ng EYK, Ooi EH. FEM simulation of the eye structure with bioheat analysis. *Comput. Meth. Programs Biomed.* 2006; 82: 268–276.

13. Zienkiewicz OC, Taylor RL. *The Finite Element Method*, 5th ed., Butterworth-Heinemann: Oxford, 2000.

14. Liu GR, Quek SS. *The Finite Element Method: A Practical Course.* Butterworth Heinemann: Oxford, 2002.

15. Dai KY, Liu GR, Nguyen TT. An *n*-sided polygonal smoothed finite element method (nSFEM) for solid mechanics, *Finite Elements Anal. Design* 2007; 43: 847–860.

16. Liu GR. A generalized gradient smoothing technique and the smoothed bilinear form for Galerkin formulation of a wide class of computational methods, *Int. J. Numer. Meth.* 2008; 5: 199–236.

17. Karaa S, Zhang J, Yang FQ. A numerical study of a 3D bioheat transfer problem with different spatial heating, *Appl. Math. Comput.* 2005; 68: 375–388.

18. Shen WS, Zhang J, Yang FQ. *Modeling and Numerical Simulation of Bioheat Transfer and Biomechanics in Soft Tissue.* Technical Report No. 391-04, Department of Computer Science, University of Kentucky, Lexington, KY. 2004.

19. Scott JA. A finite element model of heat transport in the human eye. *Phys. Med. Biol.* 1988; 33(2): 227–241.

20. Li E, Liu GR, Tan V, He ZC. Modeling and simulation of bioheat transfer in the human eye using the 3D alpha finite element method (αFEM). *Int. J. Numer. Meth. Biomed.* 2010; 26:955–976.

17 A Numerical Approach to Bioheat and Mass Transfer in the Human Eye

Andreas Karampatzakis and Theodoros Samaras

CONTENTS

17.1 INTRODUCTION

The study of temperature distribution and heat transfer inside the human eye has been a field of study for many years. Both experimental and computational techniques have appeared in the literature on this subject.

Calculation of the rises in temperature when the eye is heated is an important aspect with possible applications including the dosimetry of nonionizing radiation (Guy et al. 1975, Scott 1988b, Hirata et al. 2000a, 2000b, 2007), the developments of infrared (IR) and radiofrequency (RF) safety guidelines and regulations (Elder 2003) and the investigation and assessment of common clinical procedures on the eye, such as RF (Berjano et al. 2005, 2003, Peratta 2008, Jo and Aksan 2010) and laser (Ooi et al. 2008, Narasimhan et al. 2010) thermokeratoplasty, hyperthermia, and various thermotherapy treatments (Schipper and Lagendijk 1986, Shields et al.

2002, Rem et al. 2001, Harbour et al. 2003). Furthermore, the effects of artificial prosthetics and wear such as contact lenses (Ooi et al. 2007) and artificial intraocular lenses (Karampatzakis and Samaras 2010) can be studied.

Early experiments had an invasive nature and could therefore be performed on animals only, especially pigs or rabbits, since these animals present an ocular structure similar to that of humans. Doss and Albillar (1980) used thermocouples (20 or 50 μm diameter copper-constantan wires) to measure the rise of temperature at several depths in a pig eye undergoing thermokeratoplasty. Bolometers (Mapstone 1968) and infrared imaging (Morgan et al. 1993) have also been used. Nevertheless, these noninvasive techniques cannot provide much information on the temperature distribution with depth, as they can only measure the temperature on the surface. Infrared imaging is still the method of choice when it comes to profiling the temperature on the human eye.

17.2 MODELS OF HEAT TRANSFER IN THE EYE

The impossibility of conducting even semi-invasive experiments on living human eyes, for obvious reasons, made the development of reliable mathematical models essential to acquire depth-related temperature information. Various models of the eye anatomy have been developed. The advances in computational power allow researchers to model the extremely complicated morphology of the eye to an acceptable extent; it is now possible to take into account the surrounding anatomy, the different properties of the tissues, and the effect of fluid dynamics in the anterior chamber, as well as the effect of blood perfusion and metabolic heat generation, in realistic three-dimensional (3D) geometries.

One of the earliest computational models was developed by Guy et al. (1975) to study the cataractogenic effects of temperature rises on a rabbit eye under near-zone 2450 MHz radiation exposure. This was a two-dimensional (2D) model, which employed the finite element method (FEM) to simulate and validate the conditions and results of the experimental (thermocouple) measurements of temperature. A cataractogenic threshold of a 150 mW cm^{-2} incident power density was found for a 100 min exposure, and the pattern of absorption indicated that the lens might be the most susceptible part of the eye to that specific radiation.

Taflove and Brodwin (1975) developed a detailed model of the human eye and calculated the electromagnetic fields inside it for 750 MHz and 1.5 GHz radiation exposure in three dimensions, by studying the eye in two 2D planes. The finite difference in time domain (FDTD) method was employed for solving the time-dependent Maxwell's equations. To simplify the heat transfer equations, the thermal parameters of the eye were considered constant and unchanged with regard to position, temperature, and time, and equal to the corresponding values of water. Justification was given in the grounds of aqueous and vitreous humors consisting of water by 99%. A hot spot of 40.4°C was found deep inside the eye, near the centroid of the bulb, for a radiation of incident power density of 100 mW cm^{-2} at 1.5 GHz.

Lagendijk (1982) conducted experiments to determine the actual thermal properties of the lens and the vitreous body of the rabbit eye, as well as the convection coefficients between the cornea and ambience and between the sclera and the body core. The latter two were found to be $h_c = 20$ W m^{-2} K^{-1} and $h_s = 65$ W m^{-2} K^{-1}, respectively. The value of thermal conductivity of the lens was empirically found to be much lower than that of water. The calculation of these values improved significantly the validity of the computational models, which until then had used the values of water for the tissue parameters. The computational model developed by Lagendijk employed the FEM as well, and was used to calculate the transient and steady state temperature distribution in normal, unexposed human and rabbit eyes, as well as in human and rabbit eyes heated by various techniques. The model, however, neglected different tissues such as the cornea and iris, which are now known to have diverse thermal properties and could have altered the results.

A few years later, Scott (1988a)—led by the increasing incidence of reports of cataracts among workers in the glass industry, who were undergoing prolonged exposures to high levels of infrared radiation—constructed an axisymmetric FEM model by rotating a 2D model around the pupillary axis. The model took into account six different regions inside the eye, namely cornea, aqueous humor, lens, iris, ciliary body, and vitreous humor. All regions were considered homogeneous and isotropic. Boundary conditions were enforced at the cornea and the sclera. The cooling mechanisms assumed at the cornea surface included evaporation, natural convection, and radiation. Heat exchange with the human body was considered by means of the high blood flow in the sclera/choroid/retina regions implemented in the form of the convective boundary for the sclera introduced by Lagendijk (1982). The highest temperatures were found on the axis of symmetry, as expected, since it was the farthest from the cooling mechanisms. A thorough sensitivity analysis showed that the values of thermal conductivity of the lens, as well as the convection coefficient h_s, which depended on the choroidal blood flow, played the most important role in the temperature distribution in the anterior regions of the eye. The ambient and blood temperatures were found to be important as well. In the second part of the study (Scott 1988b), the model was used to predict temperature changes due to exposure to IR radiation. It was calculated that short exposure to a radiation source of 1500°C could lead to a temperature rise of 1–2°C in the lens, while extreme exposure conditions could lead to substantially larger increases.

Flyckt et al. (2006) took a different approach; they created a new model of the eye and orbit consisting of twenty-one different tissue types. The impact of the blood flow was taken into account either by calculating the thermal impact of the individual vessels around the eye or by applying the Pennes bioheat transfer equation (BHTE) (Pennes 1948) to represent the blood perfusion per tissue type. The main finding was that the heat transfer coefficient between the sclera and the body core (h_s), calculated at around 250–300 W m^{-2} K^{-1}, was much higher than the one measured by Lagendijk (1982), which had been widely used in previous studies (Scott 1988a, 1988b, Hirata et al. 2000a, 2000b).

Ng and Ooi (2006) published a new and improved FEM model to predict the temperature profile of the eye in two dimensions. Later, they (Ng and Ooi 2007) extended the model into 3D to allow a more precise representation of the actual human eye. Based on the BHTE and with boundary conditions similar to those of Scott (1988a), the authors calculated the steady state temperature distribution under normal conditions and under electromagnetic wave radiation. A peak temperature of 38.18°C was predicted for the 750 MHz radiation and 41.19°C was computed for the 1500 MHz radiation. It was shown that the most sensitive point to temperature changes was the tip of the cornea; good agreement with the existing 2D models was found.

17.3   MODELS OF MASS TRANSFER IN THE EYE

It is known from experimental and clinical observation that the aqueous humor (AH) is not stagnant in the anterior chamber of the eye; it is constantly circulating, secreted into the posterior chamber by the ciliary body and subsequently drained out of the eye via the trabecular meshwork. The anterior chamber models, which study AH circulation, consider mainly the buoyancy-driven flow.

Canning et al. (2002) have studied the transport of particulate matter in the anterior chamber using both an analytical and a numerical approach and working essentially with a 2D model on the midplane slice. They considered a constant temperature difference ΔT between the corneal endothelium at the front of the chamber and the iris/pupil at the back of it and created an equation to calculate the maximum velocity of the fluid:

$$v_{max} = \Delta T \times 1.98 \times 10^{-4} \text{ m s}^{-1} \text{ K}^{-1} \tag{17.1}$$

In their analysis they concluded that the flow through the pupil aperture could be ignored for most practical situations, except for the case when buoyancy-driven flow became small—for example, when a person is lying asleep and the closed eyelids reduce the aforementioned temperature gradient.

Heys and Barocas (2002) used a finite element analysis of a realistic numerical model of the frontal part of the eye. They modeled as velocity boundary conditions both the inflow of the AH from the ciliary body to the posterior chamber behind the iris and its drainage into the trabecular meshwork. They were interested in the motion of particles inside the anterior chambers as well, but also gave temperature distributions that showed how fluid dynamics changed the symmetrical profile on the interior surface of the cornea, leading to a minimum at a point below the corneal apex.

Wyatt (2004) studied in a geometrically simplified model of the anterior chamber the transport of substances, considering diffusional, convectional, and secretory flow. The author concluded that, although the velocity of secretory flow was small compared to that due to natural convection, it could have substantial effects near the surface of the anterior chamber.

El-Shahed and Elmaboud (2005) and Fitt and Gonzalez (2006) essentially used the model introduced by Canning et al. (2002) for their calculations, whereas Avtar and Srivastava (2006) extended it to account for the fluid permeability of the cornea.

An interesting work was that by Kumar et al. (2006), who treated the drainage of the AH from the trabecular meshwork as flow through a multilayered porous zone of specified pore size and void fraction. Their model was based on the morphology of the anterior chamber of a typical rabbit eye, with a fixed temperature difference between the inner side of the cornea and the lower iris/pupil base of the anterior chamber. The approach of modeling the trabecular meshwork as a porous layer was also taken by Chai et al. (2008), who created a 3D mathematical model of the anterior chamber of a rabbit eye to predict the intraocular pressure reduction achieved by partial thickness scleral drainage channels created with a femtosecond laser.

Ooi and Ng (2008) investigated the importance of the convectional flow inside the anterior chamber of the eye as a whole, since all the previous models of the anterior chamber alone could not show the effects that the flow had on the cornea and other parts of the eyeball. A 2D model was developed, and the flow was modeled by solving numerically with the FEM the incompressible Navier-Stokes equations. The circulation of AH was found to increase the temperature and distort the symmetric temperature profile in the cornea and the anterior chamber that previous heat transfer models of the eye had suggested. The importance of AH flow was further investigated by an artificial heat source placed inside the human eye, suggesting that heat transfer is affected by the flow, especially at the anterior regions of the eye. However, the implied infinitely long cylindrical geometry was not very realistic and could affect the validity of the results, as the authors noted. The same authors used the boundary element method on a 2D model of the anterior chamber to perform a parametric study (Ooi and Ng 2011) of the temperature gradient in it.

Karampatzakis and Samaras (2010) studied the effect of the AH flow on the steady state temperature distribution inside a realistic 3D FEM model. No symmetrical conditions were used, and as an extension to the previously developed models the metabolic heat generation was taken into consideration. Moreover, no constant temperature difference was assumed for the anterior chamber; the temperature of the cornea's back surface was allowed to vary according to the ambient conditions imposed on the boundary of the external cornea surface. The main finding was that, in the standing position, the coolest area of the cornea was inferior to its geometric center, when flow was taken into account, backed up with experimental evidence by Morgan et al. (1993) and Tan et al. (2009). Supine position was also examined in respect to the changes of the velocity profile due to gravity. Furthermore, the effect of an anisotropic thermal conductivity in the cornea, due to its stromal structure as suggested by Berjano et al. (2002), was examined; the results showed that such an anisotropy partially counteracted the effect of the AH flow.

17.4 MODEL DEVELOPMENT

Taking all the above into account, in this chapter we focus on the development of a detailed, anatomically realistic 3D model of the human eye that includes secretory inflow, drainage and circulation of the AH, as well as blood perfusion and metabolic heat generation in the tissues. In this direction we extended the FEM model presented in Karampatzakis and Samaras (2010) (Figure 17.1) to accommodate the in- and outflow of the aqueous humor.

The eye is now modeled by seven different compartments (regions), namely—from the exterior to the interior—the cornea, the anterior chamber, the trabecular meshwork, the iris, the lens, the vitreous humor, and the sclera. In the actual eye, there exist two more layers beneath the sclera, those of the choroid and the retina. As they are relatively thin compared to the sclera, they were all modeled as one for simplicity. The small region of the posterior chamber behind the iris and in front of

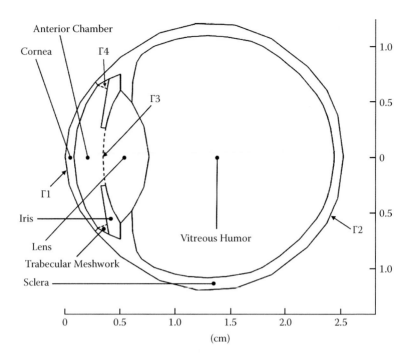

FIGURE 17.1 A mid-plane projection of the model. The different subdomains are outlined, as well as the boundary conditions: Γ1 on the frontal corneal surface, Γ2 on the sclera, Γ3 on the pupil, and Γ4 on the interface between the anterior chamber and the trabecular meshwork (TM).

the lens was also neglected to simplify the calculations, as it would result in a large number of finite elements due to its opening to the anterior chamber. The biological materials in each of the regions are considered homogeneous and isotropic, and their physical properties can be found in Table 17.1. The pupillary axial diameter is 25.2×10^{-3} m and the vertical diameter is 24×10^{-3} m^{-3}.

17.4.1 GOVERNING EQUATIONS

The steady state general heat transfer equation (17.2), including the effects of blood perfusion and mass transfer (where applicable), was solved to calculate the temperature distribution inside the eye:

$$\nabla\left(-k\nabla T\right) = A - B\left(T - T_{bl}\right) - \rho c\left(\bar{v} \cdot \nabla T\right) \tag{17.2}$$

where T is the temperature, ρ is the mass density, c is the specific heat, k is the thermal conductivity, T_{bl} is the blood temperature, A is the metabolic heat generation rate, and B is the term associated with the blood perfusion rate. The vector $\bar{v}$ represents the AH velocity and is associated with heat exchange due to fluid convection.

TABLE 17.1

Thermal Properties of the Biological Materials Present in the Eye

Material	Thermal Conductivity k (W m^{-1} K^{-1})	Density ρ (kg m^{-3})	Specific Heat c (J kg^{-1} K^{-1})	Blood Perfusion Power Equivalent (W m^{-3} K^{-1})	Basal Metabolism (W m^{-3})
Cornea	0.58	1050	4178	—	—
Anterior chamber	0.58	996	3997	—	—
Trabecular meshwork	0.58	996	3997	—	—
Iris	0.52	1050	3600	35000	10000
Lens	0.4	1000	3000	—	—
Vitreous humor	0.603	1100	4178	—	—
Sclera	0.58	1050	3800	8000	22000

Source: For the original references of values see Karampatzakis and Samaras (2010), Numerical model of heat transfer in the human eye with consideration of fluid dynamics of the aqueous humor. *Phys. Med. Biol.* 55, 5653.

The flow of AH inside the anterior chamber is modeled by solving the steady state, three-dimensional, incompressible Navier-Stokes equation:

$$\rho(\vec{v}\cdot\nabla)\vec{v} = \nabla[-p\vec{I} + \eta(\nabla\vec{v} + (\nabla\vec{v})^{T})] + \vec{F} \tag{17.3}$$

where p is the pressure, η is the dynamic viscosity with a value of 0.00074 N s m^{-2} (Ooi and Ng 2008), and $\vec{F}$ is a volume (body) force field, such as gravity.

Fluid convection was included in the equation through the effect of buoyancy due to the presence of a temperature gradient between the back surface of the cornea and the iris/pupil at the bottom of the anterior chamber. To this purpose the Boussinesq approximation (Nield and Bejan 2006) was included in the volume force term of equation (17.3):

$$\vec{F} = \rho\vec{g}\beta(T - T_{mean}) \tag{17.4}$$

where ρ is the reference density of the aqueous humor, g is the gravity acceleration, β is the volume expansion coefficient of aqueous humor set to 3×10^{-4} K^{-1} (Kumar et al. 2006), and T_{mean} is a reference temperature. The latter is calculated during the simulation as the mean temperature on the frontal surface of the anterior chamber (endothelium of the cornea).

In the two regions at the base of the anterior chamber, which comprise the trabecular meshwork, the momentum equation introduced by Amiri and Vafai (1998) to study the incompressible flow through a packed bed is used:

$$\rho(\vec{v}\cdot\nabla)\vec{v} = \nabla\left[-p\vec{I} + \frac{\eta(\nabla\vec{v} + (\nabla\vec{v})^{T})}{\varepsilon}\right] - \frac{\eta}{\kappa}\vec{v} - \frac{\rho\varepsilon C_{f}}{\sqrt{\kappa}}\vec{v}|\vec{v}| \tag{17.5}$$

where ε is the porosity taken equal to 0.5 (Kumar et al. 2007) and κ is the permeability of the porous zone set to 1.25×10^{-16} m^2 (Chai et al. 2008). The dimensionless friction coefficient is calculated as

$$C_f = \frac{1.75}{\sqrt{150\,\varepsilon^3}} \qquad (17.6)$$

The convective term on the left-hand side of equation (17.5) can be neglected, since it is very small (Amiri and Vafai 1998). In laminar flows through porous media, the term proportional to the velocity dominates the pressure drop, so the second right-hand term of (17.5) can also be neglected for computational simplification (Kumar et al. 2006); however, it is included in the following calculations.

Aqueous humor is assumed to enter the anterior chamber from the pupil opening in front of the lens ($\Gamma 3$ on Figure 17.1) at the constant velocity of 2.12×10^{-6} m s^{-1} to achieve a normal secretion rate of 2.5 mm^3 min^{-1} (Canning et al. 2002). As Kumar et al. (2006) showed, this is a reasonable approximation, since the velocity profile and flow pattern in the anterior chamber is buoyancy-driven and the inlet profile has insignificant effects. Of course the diameter of the pupil is variable in reality, depending on the ambient light intensity; however, in this model it is assumed constant.

17.4.2 Boundary Conditions

Heat exchange between the cornea and the ambient environment (at boundary $\Gamma 1$ of Figure 17.1) is modeled by the boundary equation:

$$-k\frac{\partial T}{\partial \hat{n}} = h_c(T - T_{amb}) + \varepsilon\sigma(T^4 - T_{amb}^4) + E \qquad (17.7)$$

where the first, second, and third terms on the right-hand side of the equation denote heat transfer from the eye to the ambience due to convection, radiation, and tear-film evaporation, respectively. Parameter h_c is the heat transfer coefficient between the cornea and the environment, T_{amb} is the ambient temperature, ϵ is the corneal surface emissivity, σ is the Stefan-Boltzmann constant, E is the heat loss due to tear evaporation, and $\hat{n}$ is the unit normal vector pointing away from the cornea.

The second boundary condition (at boundary $\Gamma 2$ of Figure 17.1) is imposed on the sclera. The eye is assumed to be embedded in a homogeneous anatomy that represents the network of blood vessels, and under constant blood temperature, we specify the heat transfer due to convection by

$$-k\frac{\partial T}{\partial \hat{n}} = h_s(T - T_{bl}) \qquad (17.8)$$

where h_s is the heat transfer coefficient between the surrounding body and the eye and T_{bl} is the blood temperature. The control values of the parameters used in equations (17.7) and (17.8) are included in Table 17.2.

Regarding the boundaries for the fluid dynamics calculations, all surfaces are set to a no-slip boundary condition ($\bar{v} = 0$), except from the pupil, which is assigned an

TABLE 17.2
Control Values of the Parameters Used in Boundary Conditions

Parameter	Description	Value
T_{bl}	Blood temperature, °C	37
T_{amb}	Ambient temperature, °C	23
h_s	Body heat transfer coefficient, W m^{-2} K^{-1}	65
h_c	Ambient heat transfer coefficient, W m^{-2} K^{-1}	10
E	Evaporation rate, W m^{-2}	40
σ	Stefan-Boltzmann constant, W m^{-2} K^{-4}	5.67×10^{-8}
ϵ	Emissivity of cornea surface	0.975

inlet velocity boundary ($\vec{v} = -v_o\,\hat{n}$) with $v_o = 2.12 \times 10^{-6}$ m s^{-1} as mentioned above. The interface between the anterior chamber and the trabecular meshwork (boundary Γ4 on Figure 17.1) is assigned a pressure outlet condition with a constant pressure set at 9 mmHg.

17.4.3 NUMERICAL TECHNIQUE

The coupled problem at steady state is solved by the FEM software Comsol Multiphysics 3.5a (COMSOL AB, Stockholm, Sweden). The mesh consists of about 110,000 tetrahedral elements, which are quadratic in the case of the heat transfer problem and linear for the fluid dynamics equations. A direct algorithm (SParse Object Oriented Linear Equations Solver, SPOOLES) is used for solving the equation system with a stopping (convergence) criterion of a relative tolerance of 10^{-6}.

17.5 NUMERICAL RESULTS AND SENSITIVITY ANALYSIS

The temperature distribution in the middle plane of the eye is shown in Figure 17.2. Gravity is applied on the vertical axis (y-axis) to simulate the standing position. AH flow, which forms a velocity field with a counterclockwise direction (Figure 17.3a), contributes in creating an asymmetric temperature profile around the pupillary axis, leading to the coolest area (variation of 1.69°C for the control values) on the corneal surface to be inferior to its geometric center by 2 mm, as shown in Figure 17.3b. The peak velocity of the AH flow vortex is found to be 310.7×10^{-6} ms^{-1}, which comes to good agreement with previous studies, although it is in the lower end of the velocity range found in the literature and close to the values reported by Wyatt (2004).

To determine the most important parameters affecting the temperature distribution, a sensitivity analysis is carried out, in a similar manner to the works of Scott (1988a) and Ng and Ooi (2006).

17.5.1 EFFECT OF AMBIENT TEMPERATURE

The model is tested against a variety of ambient temperatures. The main points of interest are the cornea and the lens, as temperature rises on the latter are connected with cataractogenesis.

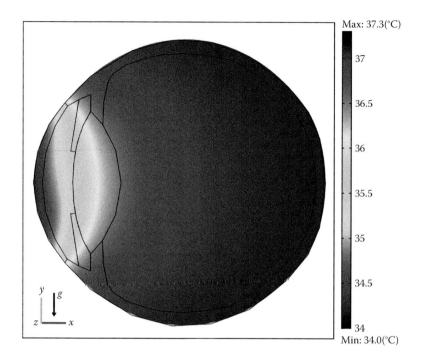

FIGURE 17.2   Temperature distribution on the $z = 0$ plane, including the AH flow, for the standing position. (Please see color insert.)

It is known that the ambient temperature affects more the anterior parts of the eye; therefore, the cornea is expected to show the bigger changes. Table 17.3 and Figure 17.4 show that a significant change of 2.43°C in the mean corneal temperature is recorded across 20°C of ambient temperatures. It should also be noted that as the temperature approaches that of blood (37°C), the range of temperatures in the cornea is diminished.

Table 17.4 and Figure 17.5 show the temperature changes calculated in the lens for the same range of ambient temperatures. As the lens is located deeper inside the eye than the cornea, milder changes are found, as expected, though an increase of 0.81°C is recorded for a 12°C increase of ambient temperature over the control value.

The maximum velocity of the AH is also recorded and shown in Table 17.5 and Figure 17.6. As smaller gradients in temperature lead to lower velocity values, the more the ambient temperature approaches that of blood, the slower the vortex becomes.

17.5.2   EFFECT OF EVAPORATION RATE

The second parameter studied is that of the evaporation rate. The evaporation due to the thin tear film on the cornea is included on the corneal boundary condition. In certain medical conditions, this film is destroyed. We can test this effect by excluding the evaporation term, as shown in Figure 17.7 where the temperatures on the

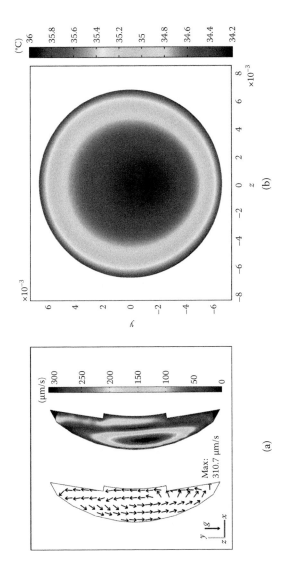

FIGURE 17.3 (a) Direction and magnitude of the velocity field inside the anterior chamber at standing position. (b) Temperature distribution on the corneal surface with consideration of the AH flow. (Please see color insert.)

TABLE 17.3

Minimum, Maximum, Mean, and Range of Temperatures Calculated for the Cornea, for Different Ambient Temperatures

	15°C	20°C	23°C (Control)	25°C	30°C	35°C
Min (°C)	32.92	33.73	34.23	34.47	35.44	36.34
Max (°C)	35.38	35.72	35.92	36.07	36.43	36.81
Mean (°C)	34.15	34.73	35.08	35.27	35.94	36.58
Range (°C)	2.46	1.99	1.69	1.6	0.99	0.47

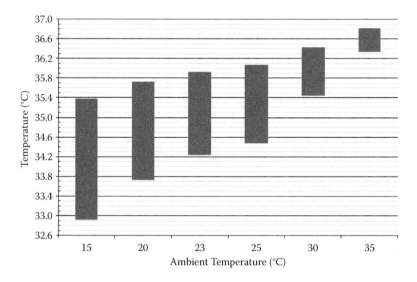

FIGURE 17.4 Temperatures recorded on the cornea for different ambient temperatures.

TABLE 17.4

Minimum, Maximum, Mean, and Range of Temperatures Calculated on the Lens, for a Range of Different Ambient Temperatures

	15°C	20°C	23°C (Control)	25°C	30°C	35°C
Min (°C)	34.58	35.08	35.49	35.6	36.13	36.67
Max (°C)	36.27	36.44	36.55	36.62	36.81	36.99
Mean (°C)	35.43	35.76	36.02	36.11	36.47	36.83
Range (°C)	1.69	1.36	1.06	1.02	0.68	0.32

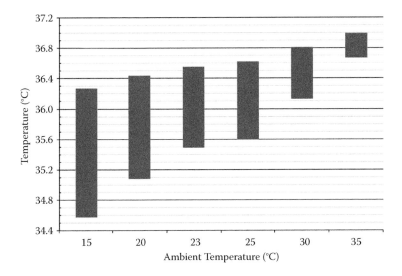

FIGURE 17.5   Range of temperatures recorded in the lens subdomain, for different ambient temperatures.

TABLE 17.5
Maximum Velocities of AH Vortex Recorded for Different Ambient Temperatures

	15 °C	20 °C	23 °C (Control)	25 °C	30 °C	35 °C
v_{max} (µm/s)	431.8	358.8	310.7	276.5	184.7	89.3

vertical midline of the cornea are plotted (all other parameters are identical and match those of the control model). Furthermore, as Ng and Ooi (2006) pointed out, ambient humidity can play a role in affecting the corneal surface temperature, as a more humid environment would reduce the evaporation rate and lead to an increase of the corneal temperature.

As expected, exclusion of evaporation rate increases the overall temperatures, as less heat is being exchanged between the cornea and the ambience. More specifically, a temperature rise of 0.42°C is recorded at the coldest spot of the cornea.

17.5.3 EFFECT OF PERMEABILITY

The permeability value used in equation (17.5) for the porous zone of the trabecular meshwork (TM) is chosen such that the in- and outflow of the AH in the model are balanced. Increasing the permeability by an order of magnitude, to use values

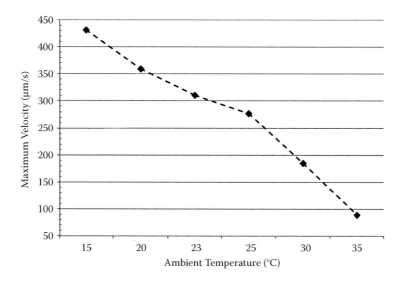

FIGURE 17.6 Maximum recorded vortex velocities for different ambient temperatures. The direction of the flow is always upwards at the back of the anterior chamber and downwards at the cornea.

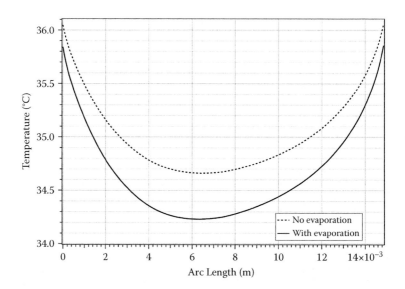

FIGURE 17.7 Temperature across the vertical corneal midline with and without the consideration of tear evaporation. Zero corresponds to the lower limbus.

TABLE 17.6

Effect of Different Permeability Values on the Maximum AH Vortex Velocity and the AH Outflow

Permeability of the Porous Zone (TM) $\kappa(\times 10^{-16}\ m^2)$	Maximum Velocity $V_{max}\ (\times 10^{-6}\ m\ s^{-1})$
1.00	310.9
1.25 (control)	311.0
3.00	311.9
5.00	313.1
10.00	315.4

TABLE 17.7

Calculated Temperatures when Including Mass Transport Mechanisms for the AH

	V_{max} $(\times 10^{-6}\ m\ s^{-1})$	Cornea T_{min} (°C)	Cornea T_{max} (°C)	Lens T_{min} (°C)	Lens T_{max} (°C)
No Flow	N/A	34.19	35.90	35.37	36.55
Flow / No Inflow	320.60	34.28	36.02	35.41	36.59
Flow / Inflow	310.98	34.23	35.92	35.39	36.55
Flow / Inflow (Finer)	314.90	34.23	35.89	35.37	36.54

comparable to those employed by Kumar et al. (2006) or measured by Merchant and Heys (2008), has a minimal effect on the velocity profile, as shown in Table 17.6.

17.5.4 Effect of Aqueous Humor Flow

It is interesting to examine how the inclusion of AH flow affects the temperatures at the points of interest. The model is solved for the stagnant case (No Flow), for the case of convective flow excluding the secretory inflow and drainage (Flow/No Inflow), and for the complete case (Flow/Inflow). The latter is also solved for a finer mesh of about 420,000 tetrahedral elements (Flow/Inflow (Finer)). The results are summarized in Table 17.7.

For the fully solved model, using a finer mesh does not have any effect on the calculated temperatures, while the maximum velocity is increased by only 1.3%. The solution time required, however, is increased by a factor of 6; therefore, using such a fine mesh is not justified with respect to the computational resources required.

For the different models, as Figure 17.8 shows, only the outermost parts of the eye are affected to some extent. The most apparent changes can be seen when plotting the temperature along the vertical midline of the corneal surface (Figure 17.9). The inclusion of in- and outflow seems to partially compensate for the asymmetry that the AH flow introduces.

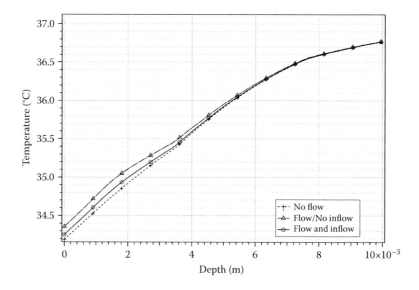

FIGURE 17.8   Temperature distribution across the pupillary axis. Only the outermost (starting from the cornea) 10 mm of the model are shown as any temperature discrepancies are diminished with depth.

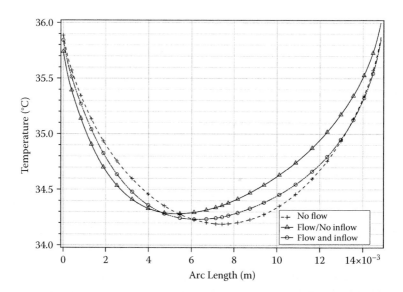

FIGURE 17.9   Temperature distribution along the vertical midline of the cornea. Zero corresponds to the lower limbus.

17.6 DISCUSSION

In this chapter we presented a mathematical model for the calculation of the bioheat transfer in the human eye, taking into account convective mass transport in the anterior chamber. The developed model contains all the necessary anatomical detail for predicting temperature distributions and convective flow velocities of the AH, providing useful information for biomedical and clinical applications. The posterior chamber and the layers behind the sclera were omitted from the model; their inclusion would drastically affect the computational resources necessary to solve the problem without adding to its prediction efficiency (Chai et al. 2008).

It should be noted that in the above model we did not consider particulate mass transport in the eye. To do so, we should have taken into account, apart from convection, the mechanisms of diffusion and gravity settling. However, the presented model is still valid for effects with a short time constant, since, as mentioned by Canning et al. (2002), on time scales on the order of one transit (top to bottom of the anterior chamber) time the effect of diffusion may be ignored; it becomes important for times on the order of hours and above.

The velocity profile inside the eye is difficult to verify directly; therefore pharmacokinetic studies are used to validate the convective flow. Wyatt (2004), in his discussion about the comparison of numerical results to experimental data, found a good agreement between calculations and experiments using superior limbus phenylephrine applications, during which the inferior iris often shows a delayed response compared to the superior iris. Indeed, for a maximum velocity of 330×10^{-6} m s^{-1} (Ooi and Ng 2011) similar to the one reported here, the predicted latency time of activation of 16 min was in excellent agreement with the experimental values.

Temperature distribution on the cornea is, on the contrary, easier to measure, especially with IR imaging. The 3D mathematical models of heat transfer in the eye, especially after the inclusion of the AH flow dynamics (Karampatzakis and Samaras 2010), come to an excellent agreement with experimental results. Therefore, they can be used as good predictors of temperature values resulting under different conditions, when cataractogenesis or other health end-points are researched in epidemiology. The sensitivity analysis shows that environmental and systemic temperatures play a significant role in the final temperature profile inside the eye. Humidity can also become important in conjunction with the tear layer evaporation from the corneal surface. Other studies (Scott 1988b, Hirata et al. 2001, Ng and Ooi 2007) have examined the impact of adding a thermal load to the eye, which is also a very common condition and results in a complicated temperature profile, depending on the spatial distribution of the heat generation rate. Since the temperature gradient between the front and the back of the anterior chamber determines the convective velocity of the AH, it is clear that all the above parameters can lead to completely diverse flows, ranging from fast vortices to stagnation. The biological implications of such situations need to be further studied.

If the temperature distribution is not of main concern, but rather the mechanic effects are of interest, then the developed model can be improved in the future to study glaucoma generation and progression, by fine-tuning the drainage mechanism at the porous media simulating the trabecular meshwork. The model could be then used to predict intraocular pressure and deformation of the cornea for various permeability values. However, this region of the model needs to be redesigned to reflect more anatomical detail, a fact which may result in using only the frontal parts of the model instead of the whole eye, to save on computational resources.

REFERENCES

Amiri, A., and Vafai, K. (1998). Transient analysis of incompressible flow through a packed bed. *Int. J. Heat Mass Tran.* **41**, 4259–79.

Avtar, R., and Srivastava, R. (2006). Modelling the flow of aqueous humor in anterior chamber of the eye. *Appl. Math. Comput.* **181**, 1336–48.

Berjano, E. J., Alió, J. L., and Saiz, J. (2005). Modeling for radio-frequency conductive keratoplasty: implications for the maximum temperature reached in the cornea. *Physiol. Meas.* **26**, 157–72.

Berjano, E. J., Saiz, J., and Ferrero, J. M. (2002). Radio-frequency heating of the cornea: theoretical model and *in vitro* experiments. *IEEE Trans. Biomed. Eng.* **49**, 196–205.

Chai, D., Chaudhary, G., Kurtz, R. M., and Juhasz, T. (2007). Aqueous humor outflow effects of partial thickness channel created by a femtosecond laser in ex vivo human eyes. *Proc SPIE* 6435:64350O-1.

Chai, D., Chaudhary, G., Mikula, E., Sun, H., and Juhasz, T. (2008). 3D finite element model of aqueous outflow to predict the effect of femtosecond laser created partial thickness drainage channels. *Laser. Surg. Med.* **40**, 188–95.

Doss, J. D., and Albillar, J. I. (1980). A technique for the selective heating of corneal stroma. *Contact Intraocul. Lens Med. J.* **6**, 13–17.

Elder, J. (2003). Ocular effects of radiofrequency energy. *Bioelectromagnetics* **24** (Suppl.), S148–61.

El-Shahed, M., and Elmaboud, Y. A. (2005). On the fluid flow in the anterior chamber of a human eye with slip velocity. *Int. Commun. Heat Mass Tran.* **32**, 1104–10.

Fitt, A. D., and Gonzalez, G. (2006). Fluid mechanics of the human eye: aqueous humor flow in the anterior chamber. *Bull. Math. Biol.* **68**, 53–71.

Flyckt, V. M. M., Raaymakers, B. W., and Lagendijk, J. J. W. (2006). Modelling the impact of blood flow on the temperature distribution in the human eye and the orbit: fixed heat transfer coefficients versus the Pennes bioheat model versus discrete blood vessels. *Phys. Med. Biol.* **51**, 5007–21.

Guy, A. W., Lin, J. C., Kramar, P. O., and Emery, A. (1975). Effect of 2450-MHz radiation on the rabbit eye. *IEEE Trans. Microw. Theory Tech.* **23**, 492–8.

Harbour, J. W., Meredith, T. A., Thompson, P. A., and Gordon, M. E. (2003). Transpupillary thermotherapy versus plaque radiotherapy for suspected choroidal melanomas. *Ophthalmology* **110**, 2207–14.

Heys, J. J., and Barocas, V. H. (2002). A Boussinesq model of natural convection in the human eye and the formation of Krukenberg's spindle. *Ann. Biomed. Eng.* **30**, 392–401.

Hirata, A., Matsuyama, S., and Shiozawa, T. (2000a). Temperature rises in the human eye exposed to EM waves in the frequency range 0.6–6 GHz. *IEEE Trans. Electromagn. Compat.* **42**, 386–93.

Hirata, A., Ushio, G., and Shiozawa, T. (2000b). Calculation of temperature rises in the human eye exposed to EM waves in the ISM frequency bands. *IEICE Trans. Commun. E* **83-B**, 541–8.

Hirata, A., Watanabe, S., Fujiwara, O., Kojima, M., Sasaki, K., and Shiozawa, T. (2007). Temperature elevation in the eye of anatomically based human head models for plane-wave exposures. *Phys. Med. Biol.* **52**, 6389–99.

Jo, B., and Aksan, A. (2010). Prediction of the extent of thermal damage in the cornea during conductive keratoplasty. *J. Therm. Biol.* **35**, 167–74.

Karampatzakis, A., and Samaras, T. (2010). Numerical model of heat transfer in the human eye with consideration of fluid dynamics of the aqueous humour. *Phys. Med. Biol.* **55**, 5653.

Kumar, S., Acharya, S., Beuerman, R., and Palkama, A. (2006). Numerical solution of ocular fluid dynamics in a rabbit eye: parametric effects. *Ann. Biomed. Eng.* **34**, 530–44.

Lagendijk, J. J. (1982). A mathematical model to calculate temperature distributions in human and rabbit eyes during hyperthermic treatment. *Phys. Med. Biol.* **27**, 1301–11.

Mapstone, R. (1968). Measurement of corneal temperature. *Exp. Eye Res.* **7**, 237–43.

Merchant, B. M., and Heys, J. J. (2008). Effects of variable permeability on aqueous humor outflow. *Appl. Math. Comput.* **196**, 371–80.

Morgan, B. P., Soh, P. M., and Efron, N. (1993). Potential applications of ocular thermography. *Optometry Vision Sci.* **70**, 568–76.

Narasimhan, A., Jha, K. K., and Gopal, L. (2010). Transient simulations of heat transfer in human eye undergoing laser surgery. *Int. J. Heat Mass Tran.* **53**, 482–90.

Ng, E. Y. K., and Ooi, E. H. (2006). FEM simulation of the eye structure with bioheat analysis. *Comput. Methods Programs Biomed.* **82**, 268–76.

Ng, E. Y. K., and Ooi, E. H. (2007). Ocular surface temperature: a 3D FEM prediction using bioheat equation. *Comput. Biol. Med.* **37**, 829–35.

Nield, D. A., and Bejan, A. (2006). *Convection in Porous Media,* 3rd ed. New York: Springer Science+Business Media.

Ooi, E. H., and Ng, E. Y. K. (2008). Simulation of aqueous humor hydrodynamics in human eye heat transfer. *Comput. Biol. Med.* **38**, 252–62.

Ooi, E. H., and Ng, E. Y. K. (2011). Effects of natural convection within the anterior chamber on the ocular heat transfer. *Int. J. Numer. Meth. Biomed. Engng.* **27**, 408–23.

Ooi, E. H., Ang, W. T., and Ng, E. Y. K. (2008). A boundary element model of the human eye undergoing laser thermokeratoplasty. *Comput. Biol. Med.* **38**, 727–37.

Ooi, E. H., Ng, E. Y., Purslow, C., and Acharya, R. (2007). Variations in the corneal surface temperature with contact lens wear. *Proc. Inst. Mech. Eng. H.* **221(4)**, 337–49.

Pennes, H. H. (1948). Analysis of tissue and arterial blood temperatures in the resting human forearm. *J. Appl. Physiol.* **1**, 93–122.

Peratta, A. (2008). 3D low frequency electromagnetic modelling of the human eye with boundary elements: application to conductive keratoplasty. *Eng. Anal. Bound. Elem.* **32**, 726–35.

Rem, A. I., Oosterhuis, J. A., Journée-de Korver, J. G., van den Berg, T. J., and Keunen, J. E. E. (2001). Temperature dependence of thermal damage to the sclera: exploring the heat tolerance of the sclera for transscleral thermotherapy. *Exp. Eye. Res.* **72**, 153–62.

Schipper, J., and Lagendijk, J. J. W. (1986). The treatment of retinoblastoma by fractionated radiotherapy combined with hyperthermia. *Hyperthermia in Cancer Treatment,* Vol. 3, ed. L. J. Anghileri and J. Robert, Boca Raton, FL: CRC Press, chapter 5, pp. 79–88.

Scott, J. A. (1988a). A finite element model of heat transport in the human eye. *Phys. Med. Biol.* **33**, 227–41.

Scott, J. A. (1988b). The computation of temperature rises in the human eye induced by infrared radiation. *Phys. Med. Biol.* **33**, 243–57.

Shields, C. L., Cater, J., Shields, J. A., Chao, A., Krema, H., Materin, M., and Brady, L. W. (2002). Combined plaque radiotherapy and transpupillary thermotherapy for choroidal melanoma. *Arch. Ophthalmol.* **120**, 933–40.

Taflove, A., and Brodwin, M. (1975). Computation of the electromagnetic fields and induced temperatures within a model of the microwave-irradiated human eye. *IEEE Trans. Microw. Theory Tech.* **23**, 888–96.

Tan, L., Cai, Z. Q., and Lai, N. S. (2009). Accuracy and sensitivity of the dynamic ocular thermography and inter-subjects ocular surface temperature (OST) in Chinese young adults. *Cont. Lens Anterior Eye* **32**, 78–83.

Wyatt, H. J. (2004). Modelling transport in the anterior segment of the eye. *Optometry Vision Sci.* **81**, 271–81.

Index